Advancements in Bio-Medical Image Processing and Authentication in Telemedicine

Rijwan Khan
ABES Institute of Technology, India

Indrajeet Kumar
Graphic Era Hill University, Dehradun, India

A volume in the Advances in Medical Technologies and Clinical Practice (AMTCP) Book Series

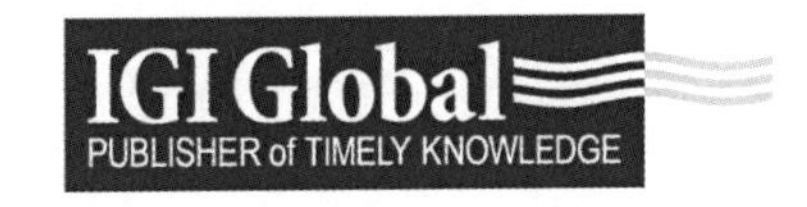

Published in the United States of America by
IGI Global
Medical Information Science Reference (an imprint of IGI Global)
701 E. Chocolate Avenue
Hershey PA, USA 17033
Tel: 717-533-8845
Fax: 717-533-8661
E-mail: cust@igi-global.com
Web site: http://www.igi-global.com

Library of Congress Cataloging-in-Publication Data

Names: Khan, Rijwan, 1981- editor. | Kumar, Indrajeet, 1987- editor.
Title: Advancements in bio-medical image processing and authentication in telemedicine / edited by Rijwan Khan, Indrajeet Kumar.
Description: Hershey, PA : Medical Information Science Reference, [2023] | Includes bibliographical references and index. | Summary: "The main objective of this book is to collect the ideas on Bio Medical Image Processing from the different authors. This book will be combination of bio-medical image processing for medical image processing"-- Provided by publisher.
Identifiers: LCCN 2022051236 (print) | LCCN 2022051237 (ebook) | ISBN 9781668469576 (hardcover) | ISBN 9781668469583 (ebook)
Subjects: MESH: Image Processing, Computer-Assisted--methods | Medical Informatics Computing | Machine Learning | Telemedicine--instrumentation
Classification: LCC RC78.7.D53 (print) | LCC RC78.7.D53 (ebook) | NLM W 26.5 | DDC 616.07/54--dc23/eng/20230125
LC record available at https://lccn.loc.gov/2022051236
LC ebook record available at https://lccn.loc.gov/2022051237

This book is published in the IGI Global book series Advances in Medical Technologies and Clinical Practice (AMTCP) (ISSN: 2327-9354; eISSN: 2327-9370)

British Cataloguing in Publication Data
A Cataloguing in Publication record for this book is available from the British Library.

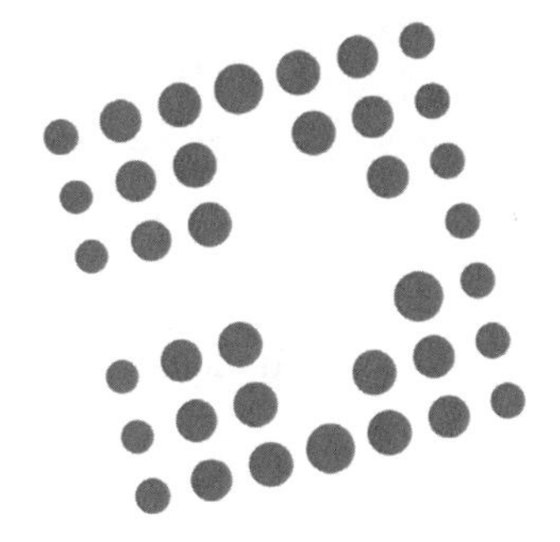

Advances in Medical Technologies and Clinical Practice (AMTCP) Book Series

ISSN:2327-9354
EISSN:2327-9370

Editor-in-Chief: ***Srikanta Patnaik***, SOA University, India, Priti Das, S.C.B. Medical College, India

MISSION

Medical technological innovation continues to provide avenues of research for faster and safer diagnosis and treatments for patients. Practitioners must stay up to date with these latest advancements to provide the best care for nursing and clinical practices.

The **Advances in Medical Technologies and Clinical Practice (AMTCP) Book Series** brings together the most recent research on the latest technology used in areas of nursing informatics, clinical technology, biomedicine, diagnostic technologies, and more. Researchers, students, and practitioners in this field will benefit from this fundamental coverage on the use of technology in clinical practices.

COVERAGE

- Clinical Studies
- Biometrics
- Clinical Nutrition
- Neural Engineering
- Nutrition
- Clinical Data Mining
- Biomedical Applications
- Diagnostic Technologies
- Telemedicine
- Medical Informatics

The Advances in Medical Technologies and Clinical Practice (AMTCP) Book Series (ISSN 2327-9354) is published by IGI Global, 701 E. Chocolate Avenue, Hershey, PA 17033-1240, USA, www.igi-global.com. This series is composed of titles available for purchase individually; each title is edited to be contextually exclusive from any other title within the series. For pricing and ordering information please visit http://www.igi-global.com/book-series/advances-medical-technologies-clinical-practice/73682. Postmaster: Send all address changes to above address.

Titles in this Series

For a list of additional titles in this series, please visit:
http://www.igi-global.com/book-series/advances-medical-technologies-clinical-practice/73682

Recent Advancements in Smart Remote Patient Monitoring, Wearable Devices, and Diagnostics Systems
Furkh Zeshan (COMSATS University Islamabad, Lahore, Pakistan) and Adnan Ahmad (COMSATS University Islamabad, Lahore, Pakistan)
Medical Information Science Reference • © 2023 • 310pp • H/C (ISBN: 9781668464342) • US $345.00

Digital Twins and Healthcare Trends, Techniques, and Challenges
Loveleen Gaur (Amity University, India & Taylor's University, Malaysia & University of the South Pacific, Fiji) and Noor Zaman Jhanjhi (Taylor's University, Malaysia)
Medical Information Science Reference • © 2023 • 293pp • H/C (ISBN: 9781668459256) • US $420.00

Diverse Perspectives and State-of-the-Art Approaches to the Utilization of Data-Driven Clinical Decision Support Systems
Thomas M. Connolly (DS Partnership, UK) Petros Papadopoulos (University of Strathclyde, UK) and Mario Soflano (Glasgow Caledonian University, UK)
Medical Information Science Reference • © 2023 • 380pp • H/C (ISBN: 9781668450925) • US $345.00

Using Multimedia Systems, Tools, and Technologies for Smart Healthcare Services
Amit Kumar Tyagi (National Institute of Fashion Technology, New Delhi, India)
Medical Information Science Reference • © 2023 • 353pp • H/C (ISBN: 9781668457412) • US $380.00

The Internet of Medical Things (IoMT) and Telemedicine Frameworks and Applications
Rajiv Pandey (Amity University, Lucknow, India) Amrit Gupta (MRH, Sanjay Gandhi Postgraduate Institute of Medical Sciences, Lucknow, India) and Agnivesh Pandey (D.A-V. College, Chhatrapati Shahu Ji Maharaj University, Kanpur, India)
Medical Information Science Reference • © 2023 • 340pp • H/C (ISBN: 9781668435335) • US $380.00

For an entire list of titles in this series, please visit:
http://www.igi-global.com/book-series/advances-medical-technologies-clinical-practice/73682

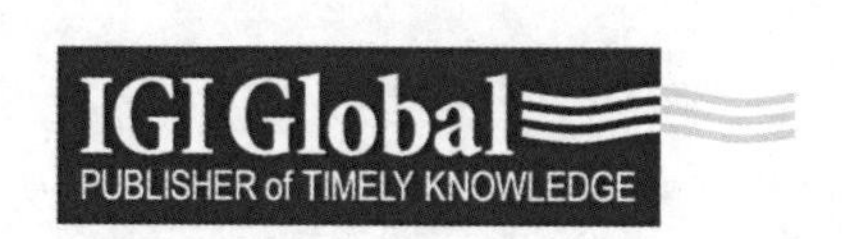

701 East Chocolate Avenue, Hershey, PA 17033, USA
Tel: 717-533-8845 x100 • Fax: 717-533-8661
E-Mail: cust@igi-global.com • www.igi-global.com

Table of Contents

Detailed Table of Contents

Diseases like diabetes, heart disease, kidney disease, thyroid disease, and other diseases are increasing in frequency, and people are suffering globally. Specifically, thyroid and heart diseases affect many people and, without proper treatment, become serious health issues. Different thyroid and heart disease disorders can be detected early with specific symptoms. Here, the authors provide a thorough literature review of the different popular approaches for disease classification using specific symptoms for early identification and treatment using machine learning. This chapter also outlines the different advantages and limitations of specific approaches for disease symptom detection. The experimental results in existing literature has shown significant results on eight disease benchmark datasets using three state-of-the-art algorithms, including the reduced error pruning (REP) tree, random tree, and C4.5 decision tree algorithm.

A trendy technique based on computer science called artificial intelligence (AI) creates software and algorithms to make machines smart and effective at carrying out activities that often call for expert human intellect. Machine learning (ML), deep learning (DL), traditional neural networks, fuzzy logic, and speech recognition are only a few of the subsets of AI that have distinctive skills and functions that might enhance the performance of contemporary medical sciences. Biomedical imaging might undergo a revolution thanks to AI, which could increase the efficiency and precision of picture processing and interpretation. Radiologists could miss tiny abnormalities that can be detected by AI systems that have been taught to spot patterns in those pictures that are challenging for humans to interpret. AI may also be used to generate customized medicine by evaluating a patient's medical pictures and other data to customize treatment regimens, as well as to enhance image processing and visualization.

Recently, disease prediction using diagnostic reports and images are one of the most popular applications of artificial intelligence (AI) and machine learning (ML). Several authors reported significant results in this area by combining cutting-edge hardware with AI and ML-based technologies. In this chapter, the authors present a review of different works carried for the prediction of several chronic diseases by researchers in last five years. Reported AI and ML based methodologies have been used to forecast chronic disease such as heart problems, brain tumors, asthma, diabetes, cholera, arthritis, liver diseases, kidney diseases, malaria, and leukemia. In the literature, the authors also discuss the different user interfaces which have been used to interact with real time AI and ML based disease prediction models. The authors have presented the detailed discussion of each paper including advantages, disadvantages, datasets, performance metrics such as precision, recall, accuracy and F1 score. In the final section, the survey concludes with a description of research gaps that can be addressed by future research attempts.

Colorectal cancer ranks as the second most prevalent cause of death, and proven to be a major cause of morbidity, where one in every six people worldwide dies from cancer. The early diagnostics have always been a torch bearing insight towards better and timely treatment, thus saving the life. In the recent, advanced medical technology has facilitated large amounts of variable data set for analysis, whereas artificial intelligence (AI) technology has the proven role in automatic cancer detection, enabling us to analyze more patients in less time and money hence, commonly used in oncology. The convolutional neural network based models have been quite popular to evaluate cancer imaginary data in current scenario. In this chapter, the authors summarize the computational resources, basic architecture, and applications of advanced AI based methods / soft computing methodologies; i.e. machine learning, deep learning, CNN, RNN, SVM and other machine learning methods for early and faster diagnostics of colorectal cancer with imaginary classification of patient data with challenges.

Skin cancer is amongst the most common forms of cancer and can become life-threatening if not detected early. Due to the rise in the number of cancer cases, there is a growing interest in using computational diagnostics for early cancer detection as the specificity rate of even an expert dermatologist is around 59%. Computer-aided diagnosis can significantly contribute to skin lesion image analysis. Skin cancer prognostication can be achieved with a classification that assigns data objects to particular classes based on extracted features. The steps for image classification are pre-processing where noise is removed and lesion features are highlighted, making it easier to classify the image, detection of the lesion on skin (i.e. segmentation), extracting useful features, and finally applying classification algorithm. This paper provides a review of the recent studies in the bailiwick of skin cancer image classification using machine learning (ML) algorithms.

A visually impaired individual loses vision when a part of the eye or the brain that processes images becomes diseased or damaged. Visually impaired people face many problems during their daily activities such as walking around places, identifying objects, identifying people's feelings or emotions, detecting obstacles, etc. Several solutions work around these problems. The area that needs the attention of researchers is helping the visually impaired people in reading the medical reports, a product's name, and a device's reading. To make them independent, this paper proposed a

diabetic patient population is anticipated to reach 642 million by 2040, implying that one out of every ten people will be diabetic. The data generation and AI based methods—i.e., SVM, kNN, decision tree, Baysian method in medical health –have facilitated the effective prediction and classification of voluminous size of biological data of different types of BMI, skin thickness, glucose, age, tongue and retinal images apart from Omics data, for early diagnostics. The chapter summarizes the basic methods and applications of machine learning and soft computing techniques for diabetes diagnosis and prediction with limitations of integrative approaches.

These days enormous amounts of information is at almost everyone's disposal with a single click of a button, and that too on a hand held device. Data can be present in various forms like still images, and slides of pictures like a video of GIF, over various websites present on the Internet. Because of the excessive use of this data, it also becomes important to secure it as it can be duplicated, transformed, stolen, tampered, or misused pretty easily. Recently, there has been a spike increase in the use of medical images in various E-health applications. In order to counter these potential threats, a number of watermarking techniques are being developed. A watermark is embedded in an image or document in the form of an image or pattern that can be used to authenticate the integrity of the image in question. As time goes by, the complexity of the problems that we are dealing with also keeps on increasing.

Pneumonia is one of the major diseases affecting the large proportion of the population. The detection of pneumonia can be done by an X-ray scan of the patient which is observed by a radiologist to look for abnormalities indicative of pneumonia. This observation is highly subjective and depends on the experience of the radiologist, leading to ambiguity in appropriate diagnosis, and thus producing some false negatives. To overcome these issues, it is imperative that radiologists be provided with a tool that acts as second set of eyes for them and helps them gain confidence in their diagnosis. Keeping in view the aforementioned objectives, many researchers have proposed various computer-assisted classification (CAC) systems based on machine learning and deep learning methods. The present work compared the performance of MobileNetv2, VGG16, and XceptionNet for classifying chest X-ray images into normal and pneumonia classes, reporting the highest accuracy of 96.0% using VGG16.

Pneumonia is a very contagious illness that spreads quickly among newborns. According to UNICEF, pneumonia was to blame for 16% of all baby deaths under the age of five. The main objective of this study is to determine whether a patient has pneumonia using a chest X-ray picture. CNN is used for this for this process, as it's great processing capability makes them the most effective choice for image processing and categorization. By the use of CNN, results will be obtained rapidly, and dependence on medical personnel will be reduced. Additionally, it will produce more precise findings than human vision, which could overlook a little X-Ray feature. More than17,000 chest X-ray pictures of pneumonic and healthy lungs are included in the collection. This model's total accuracy is 88.62%.

The present chapter aims to investigate the occurrence of COVID-19 vaccine administration patterns in Europe for effective vaccination and booster shot scheduling towards COVID-19 pandemic control. Method: Data were obtained from the ECDC on COVID-19 vaccination radar on 5th March 2021 and processed for statistical analysis with IBM's SPSS version 21. Statistically, a significant difference was considered at p less than 0.05. Results: The authors observed statistically significant lower vaccine uptake compared to delivered doses (average at 62.678 ± 3.928%). Uptake for Oxford-AstraZeneca vaccines (50.927 ± 4.626%) compared to Pfizer-Biontech vaccine (86.285 +/- 2.1052%) was observed compared to previous prospective study on the wiliness to receive COVID-19 vaccine in the region (75%). Conclusion: The early COVID-19 acceptance pattern based on vaccine type or manufacturer was observed. The findings will be useful for policymakers to introduce policies on educational campaigns to enhance vaccine and booster uptake for smooth and effective control of the pandemic.

Precise retinal blood vessels segmentation is a vital assignment to diagnose many pathological ailments. Here, an efficient approach has been presented for the segmentation of retinal vessels that includes pre-processing, segmentation, and the post-processing stage. In the pre-processing stage, the retinal images are denoised and restored with the connected vessel lines by utilizing anisotropic diffusion filter. In the next step, retinal images are enhanced by using top hat transform. Further, Gabor filters of various orientations are applied on top hat transformed images to obtain different characteristics of the retinal images. Finally, hysteresis thresholding is applied for the segmentation. The accomplishment of the recommended methodology is inspected with other competitive combined methodologies based on median filter and Gabor filter using different performance indicators. The approach can be used effectively for diagnosis of different ocular disorders, like diabetic retinopathy and glaucoma, which can be followed by different surgical procedures for further treatment.

The conventional methodologies of arrhythmia identification are based on morphological features or certain transformation technique. These conventional techniques are partially successful in arrhythmia identification, because it treats heart as a linear structure. In this chapter, ECG based arrhythmia identification is assessed by employing MIT-BIH arrhythmia dataset. The proposed approach contains two major steps: feature extraction and classification. Initially, a combination of non-linear and linear feature extraction is carried-out using Principal Component Analysis, Kernel Independent Component Analysis and Higher Order Spectrum for achieving optimal feature subsets. The linear experiments on ECG data achieves high performance in noise free data and the non-linear experiments distinguish the ECG data more effectively, extract hidden information and also helps to attain better performance under noisy conditions. After finding the feature information, a binary classifier Support Vector Machine is employed for classifying the normality and abnormality of arrhythmia.

The aim of the present case study is to assess prospectively the HIA of a proposed mobile health intervention to reduce MMR in 10-years. PHIA was carried out on a proposed mHealth intervention to MMR. In addition, an online feasibility pilot study was carried out involving 41 participants from September 1st, 2021, to January 2022. The intervention improved the well-being of pregnant women via education on good nutrition. It reduced MMR, travel costs, frequency of visits to healthcare centers, and increased equality in healthcare accessibility. Due to the reduced frequency of hospital visits, the risk of transportation and road accidents were noticed. About 88% of participants stated the intervention is feasible and worthwhile. While nearly 95% said they are eager and prepared to use the intervention when implemented. The intervention can improve the health of mothers, MMR, and reduce health inequality. Feasibility and willingness to use the new intervention were very high, hence the intervention should be tested on a larger population and in different geographical regions. .

Preface

"The field of bio-medical image processing and authentication in telemedicine has seen significant advancements in recent years, with new technologies and techniques being developed to improve the accuracy and efficiency of medical imaging and telemedicine applications. This edited volume brings together leading experts in the field to provide a comprehensive and up-to-date overview of the latest research and developments in bio-medical image processing and authentication in telemedicine.

The book is organized into four sections, each covering a different aspect of the field. The first section focuses on the latest advancements in bio-medical image processing techniques, including deep learning, machine learning and computer vision. The second section explores the use of biometric and bio-inspired techniques for authentication in telemedicine. The third section presents case studies and real-world applications of bio-medical image processing and authentication in telemedicine. The fourth section discusses the challenges and future directions of the field.

As the editor of this book, I am honored to have brought together such a diverse group of experts from academia and industry to share their knowledge and experience. I believe that this book will serve as a valuable resource for researchers, engineers, and practitioners working in the field of bio-medical image processing and authentication in telemedicine. It provides readers with a deeper understanding of the key issues and trends, as well as practical insights and recommendations for future research and development.

I would like to extend my gratitude to the contributors for their expertise and dedication to this project, as well as to [publisher] for their support in bringing this book to fruition. I hope that this book will be an important resource for anyone interested in the exciting field of bio-medical image processing and authentication in telemedicine."

The below listed titles are research papers or articles that cover a wide range of topics related to the use of machine learning, artificial intelligence, and other technologies in the medical domain. Some of the topics include:

- The use of machine learning algorithms in disease diagnostic models

- The role of Artificial Intelligence in Biomedical Imaging
- The use of AI and ML in colorectal cancer diagnostic
- The use of machine learning techniques for skin lesion image classification
- The use of AI and machine learning in the development of medical assistants for the visually impaired
- The use of blockchain technology in tele healthcare
- The use of machine learning models in diabetes detection
- The use of watermarking in different emerging areas
- The use of deep learning techniques for pneumonia detection using chest x-ray images
- The use of convolution neural network for pneumonia detection through x-ray images
- Investigating COVID-19 vaccination patterns in Europe and the potential for the end of the pandemic
- The use of an enhanced Gabor filter based on heat diffused top hat transform for retinal blood vessel segmentation
- The use of kernel ICA and higher order spectra for arrhythmia recognition and classification
- The prospective health impact assessment of nutritional mHealth interventions on maternal mortality.

All these chapters are focusing on the medical domain and trying to find solutions or advance the existing techniques to improve medical diagnosis and treatment.

ORGANIZATION OF THE BOOK

This book contains 15 chapters. A brief description of each of the chapters is as follows: Chapter 1, titled "An Empirical Review of Machine Learning Algorithms in the Medical Domain", presents a comprehensive overview of the literature on the various well-liked methods for classifying diseases based on specific symptoms to use machine learning for early diagnosis and therapy. Utilizing three cutting-edge algorithms, including the reduced error pruning (REP) tree, random tree, and decision tree method, the experimental results in the literature have demonstrated considerable results and enhance the diagnosis and treatment process.

Chapter 2, titled "Role of Artificial Intelligence in Biomedical Imaging", presents A trendy technique based on computer science called artificial intelligence (AI) creates software and algorithms to make machines smart and effective at carrying out activities that often call for expert human intellect. Machine learning (ML), deep learning (DL), traditional neural networks, fuzzy logic, and speech recognition are only a few of the subsets of AI that have distinctive skills and functions that might enhance the performance of contemporary medical sciences. Biomedical imaging might undergo a revolution thanks to artificial intelligence (AI), which could increase the efficiency and precision of picture processing and interpretation. Radiologists could miss tiny abnormalities that can be detected by AI systems that have been taught to spot patterns in pictures that are challenging for humans to interpret. AI may also be used to generate customized medicine by evaluating a patient's medical pictures and other data to customize treatment regimens, as well as to enhance image processing and visualization.

Chapter 3, titled "Review and Analysis of Disease Diagnostic Models using AI and ML", presents one of the most well-liked uses of artificial intelligence (AI) and machine learning has been the prediction of diseases using medical data and photographs (ML). By fusing state-of-the-art hardware with AI and ML-based technologies, several authors claimed notable breakthroughs in this domain. In this study, we provide a review of various studies conducted over the past five years for the prediction of multiple chronic diseases. Many chronic diseases, including heart issues, brain tumors, asthma, diabetes, cholera, arthritis, liver, renal, malaria, and leukemia, have reportedly been predicted using AI and ML-based approaches. We also talk about the many user interfaces that have been utilized to engage with real-time AI and ML based disease prediction models in the literature.

Chapter 4, titled "Role of AI based methods in colorectal cancer diagnostic-The current updates" presents AI technology has a proven role in automatic cancer detection, enabling us to analyze more patients in less time and money; as a result, it is frequently used in oncology. In recent years, advanced medical technology has made it possible to analyze large amounts of variable data sets. The evaluation of fictitious cancer data using convolutional neural network-based algorithms is quite common today. In this chapter, we provide an overview of the computational capabilities, fundamental architecture, and applications of advanced AI-based methodologies, such as machine learning, deep learning, CNN, RNN, SVM, and other machine learning methods, for the early and rapid diagnosis of colorectal cancer with hypothetical patient data classification problems.

Chapter 5, titled "A Review of Recent Machine Learning Techniques used for Skin Lesion Image Classification" presents analysis of skin lesions can greatly benefit from computer-aided diagnosis. A classification that assigns data objects to specific classes based on extracted properties can be used to predict the likelihood of developing skin cancer. Pre-processing, in which noise is eliminated and lesion features are highlighted to make the classification process easier, detection of the lesion on the skin, or segmentation, extraction of useful features, and application of the classification algorithm are the steps in the classification process. In this study, machine learning (ML) techniques are used to review recent studies in the field of skin cancer picture classification.

Chapter 6, titled "A Medical Assistant for Visually Impaired" presents the tool for people who are visually impaired sometimes struggle with simple tasks like navigating unfamiliar environments, recognizing objects, reading facial expressions, spotting impediments, etc. Many solutions circumvent these issues. Helping those who are blind understand medical records, product names, and device reading is an area that need study attention. This article presented a medical assistant called "M.A.V.I." to aid the blind read medical blood reports, products, regular reports, and LED screens of inaccessible medical devices such a glucose monitor, blood pressure machine, weighing machine, etc. to help them become independent.

Chapter 7, titled "Opportunities and Applications of block chain for empowering tele-healthcare." presents blockchain technology has the potential to empower telehealth care in several ways by providing secure, decentralized, and tamper-proof storage of sensitive health information and enabling new forms of communication and collaboration between patients, healthcare providers, and researchers. while the potential benefits of blockchain for telehealth care are significant, there are also challenges that need to be addressed, such as regulatory compliance, data privacy and security, and scalability. Additionally, blockchain technology is still in its early stages of development, and more research and development is needed to fully realize its potential in telehealth care.

Chapter 8, titled "Applications of Machine Learning Models with Medical Images and Omics Technologies in Diabetes Detection: Machine Learning Models in Diabetes Detection" presents the presence and progression of diabetes-related complications, such as diabetic retinopathy and diabetic nephropathy. ML models can be trained to analyze these images and detect signs of these complications, potentially allowing for earlier diagnosis and intervention. Omics technologies, such as genomics, transcriptomics, and proteomics, can also be used to improve diabetes detection and management. These technologies can provide detailed information about an individual's genetic makeup, gene expression, and protein levels, which can be used to identify biomarkers for diabetes risk or progression. ML models can be trained to analyze this data and identify patterns that are indicative of diabetes or its complications.

Chapter 9, titled "Applications of Watermarking in Different Emerging Areas A Survey" presents watermarking is a technique used to embed hidden information, such as a digital signature or copyright notice, into digital media, such as images, audio, and video. Watermarking can be used for a variety of purposes, including copyright protection, content authentication, and digital rights management. Watermarking can be used to embed patient information or other metadata into medical images, such as X-rays or MRI scans. This can help to ensure that patient privacy is protected and that images are not tampered with. It's important to note that Watermarking as a technique is not foolproof and can be subject to attempts of tampering or removal, but with the advancement of technology, new and robust methods are being developed to make the watermarking more secure.

Chapter 10, titled "Application of Deep Learning Techniques for Pneumonia Detection using Chest X-ray Images" presents the deep learning techniques, specifically Convolutional Neural Networks (CNNs), have been widely applied to the detection of pneumonia using chest X-ray images. These techniques have shown promising results in detecting pneumonia with high accuracy. It's important to note that, while the results of CNNs applied to pneumonia detection have been promising, it is still a complex task and the performance of the model will depend on the quality and diversity of the data used to train and test it.

Chapter 11, titled "Pneumonia Detection through X-Ray Images using Convolution Neural Network" present Pneumonia detection through X-ray images using a convolutional neural network (CNN) is a promising area of research in medical imaging. CNNs are a type of deep learning algorithm that are particularly well-suited for image classification tasks, such as identifying patterns in X-ray images. It is also important to note that the use of a deep learning algorithm like CNNs is not a replacement for radiologists' expertise, it is rather a support tool that can help radiologists to make more accurate and efficient diagnoses.

Chapter 12, titled "Investigating COVID-19 vaccination pattern in Europe, is the end of the pandemic still foreseeable?" presents the vaccination rate in Europe has been increasing, with many countries now reporting that a significant portion of their population has received at least one dose of a COVID-19 vaccine. However, the pace of vaccination has varied widely between countries. For example, some countries in Northern Europe have administered a relatively high number of vaccine doses per 100 people, while other countries in Southern and Eastern Europe have administered fewer doses. It's important to note that the pandemic is a dynamic situation, and the progress of the pandemic and the timeline for ending it will depend on a variety of factors, including the effectiveness of vaccines, changes in the virus itself, and the actions taken by governments and individuals to control its spread.

Chapter 13, titled "An enhanced Gabor filter based on heat diffused top hat transform for retinal blood vessel segmentation: Retinal Blood Vessel Segmentation using GF-HD-THT" presents precise retinal blood vessels segmentation. It is a vital assignment to diagnose of many pathological ailments. Here, an efficient approach has been presented for the segmentation of retinal vessels that includes pre-processing, segmentation, and pot-processing stage. In the pre-processing stage, the retinal images are denoised and restored the connected vessel lines by utilizing anisotropic diffusion filter. In the next step, retinal images are enhanced by using top hat transform. Further, Gabor filter of various orientations are applied on top hat transformed images to obtain different characteristics of the retinal images. Finally, hysteresis thresholding is applied for the segmentation. The accomplishment of the recommended methodology is inspected with other competitive combined methodologies based on median filter and Gabor filter using diffrent performance indicators.

Chapter 14, titled "Arrhythmia recognition and classification using kernel ICA and higher order spectra: SVM method of detection and classification of Arrhythmia" presents the conventional methodologies of arrhythmia identification are based on morphological features or certain transformation technique. These conventional techniques are partially successful in arrhythmia identification, In this chapter, ECG based arrhythmia identification is assessed by employing MIT-BIH arrhythmia dataset. The proposed approach contains two major steps: feature extraction and classification. Initially, a combination of non-linear and linear feature extraction is carried-out using Principal Component Analysis, Kernel Independent Component Analysis and Higher Order Spectrum for achieving optimal feature subsets. The linear experiments on ECG data achieves high performance in noise free data and the non-linear experiments distinguish the ECG data more effectively, extract hidden information and also helps to attain better performance under noisy conditions. After finding the feature information, a binary classifier Support Vector Machine is employed for classifying the normality and abnormality of arrhythmia.

Chapter 15, titled "Prospective Health Impact Assessment on Nutritional mHealth Intervention on Maternal Mortality" presents to evaluate the HIA of a suggested mobile health intervention to lower MMR in 10 years. A PHIA was conducted on a suggested mHealth MMR intervention. In addition, from September 1st, 2021, to January 1st, 2022, a pilot online feasibility study with 41 participants was conducted. Through dietary instruction, the intervention enhanced the wellbeing of expectant mothers. It decreased MMR, travel expenses, the number of times people visited healthcare facilities, and the accessibility of treatment for all. The probability of transportation and traffic accidents was noted when hospital visits decreased. The strategy can lessen health disparities, enhance MMR, and enhance maternal health.

Rijwan Khan
ABES Institute of Technology, India

Indrajeet Kumar
Graphic Era Hill University, India

Chapter 1
An Empirical Review of Machine Learning Algorithms in the Medical Domain

Kumar Abhishek
https://orcid.org/0000-0002-5597-1432
Independent Researcher, USA

Vinay Perni
University of Illinois at Urbana-Champaign, USA

ABSTRACT

Diseases like diabetes, heart disease, kidney disease, thyroid disease, and other diseases are increasing in frequency, and people are suffering globally. Specifically, thyroid and heart diseases affect many people and, without proper treatment, become serious health issues. Different thyroid and heart disease disorders can be detected early with specific symptoms. Here, the authors provide a thorough literature review of the different popular approaches for disease classification using specific symptoms for early identification and treatment using machine learning. This chapter also outlines the different advantages and limitations of specific approaches for disease symptom detection. The experimental results in existing literature has shown significant results on eight disease benchmark datasets using three state-of-the-art algorithms, including the reduced error pruning (REP) tree, random tree, and C4.5 decision tree algorithm.

DOI: 10.4018/978-1-6684-6957-6.ch001

INTRODUCTION

To ensure accurate results, it is critical to handle medical data analysis with precision. Medical data analysis centers around finding unknown patterns that can be used for disease detection and treatment; however, traditional approaches lack accuracy and precision in their prediction.

The following are the main steps traditionally followed when applying machine learning in medicine:

1. Digital Knowledge Base:

The patient case sheet, or profile, is collected from the medical institutes, and the data is digitalized. The patient's profile includes all demographic and clinical data. Demographic data includes the patient's name, age, gender, height, weight, etc. At the same time, clinical data includes diagnoses, symptoms, and medications provided as treatment.

2. Machine Learning (ML) Co-analysis:

Digitalized medical data is pre-processed for better representation as input to the machine learning pipeline. The data undergoes complexity analysis, and different complexities are identified, such as high dimensionality, normalization, feature space selection, outlier, and missing values analysis. The regularized data is prepared and given as input to machine learning algorithms, computer-aided diagnosis is performed, and an effective treatment strategy is identified.

3. Clinical Decision Support:

The results generated by the machine learning analysis are synthesized, medical experts perform a thorough discussion, and finally, clinical decisions are made. The new outcomes are incorporated into the knowledge base.

In supervised learning, a predictive model is built using the training data, and this model is then evaluated on the test data, and, finally, the prediction of unknown instances is made. In unsupervised learning, clustering techniques are applied to the raw data, and a model is built for clustering new cases. One of the most common syndromes worldwide, thyroid disorders and diseases, result from thyroid malfunction (Prerana, 2015), in which the thyroid gland causes lower or higher production of thyroid hormones. The thyroid gland releases triiodothyronine (T3) and thyroxine (T4) into the bloodstream, which are considered principal hormones. The rate of metabolism is regulated by the functions of these thyroid hormones.

In some cases, thyroid hormone secretion is a problem with metabolism control. The most common issues of thyroid disease are hypothyroidism, low or inactive thyroid hormone, and hyperthyroidism, elevated thyroid hormone levels. Early diagnosis is always recommended to prevent the acute effects and improve treatment to maintain the normal thyroid hormone level (Tyagi, 2018).

Autoimmune-mediated thyroid disease is due to immune system dysregulation, genetic predisposition, and environmental factors. Due to variability in disease progression and onset heterogeneity, prognosis and diagnosis are unpredictable. Autoimmunity pre-disposition is highly correlated with genetics and occurs due to a mechanical defect resulting in a loss of self-tolerance. Autoimmune disease prevalence is highly complex, and the diseases are variably represented (Prerana, 2015).

Autoimmune thyroid disease benefits from personalized healthcare for a casual molecular mechanism as an alternative to treating special symptoms. Standard patient care generates multiple clinical data types, including laboratory results and MRI images. Additionally, omics data, like patients' proteomic, transcriptomic, and genomic profiles, have recently become available. Several omics data types can be rapidly used in machine learning models to identify the exact details of autoimmune thyroid disease. Data mining methods have the ability to identify clinically relevant patterns to estimate autoimmune risks, initial and ongoing management, diagnosis, treatment response, and results and observations (Franco, 2013).

Recently, new technology in data mining classification algorithms developed in medical science allows researchers to aid the expert advisory system in diagnosing a greater variety of diseases with increased accuracy. Due to certain errors during the general diagnosis process, medical professionals are using these newly developed systems based on artificial intelligence. These systems assist doctors in reducing the cost and time needed for effective treatment and diagnosis (Stafford, 2020).

Paper Organization

The following section describes the related works of heart and thyroid disease prediction using different data mining algorithms. Further, the recent literature review of disease identification and prediction using machine learning is presented in Section 2. Section 3 illustrates the methodology and dataset description. Section 4 presents the experimental and comparative analyses of the state-of-the-art algorithms. Finally, the research is concluded in Section 5.

RELATED WORKS

Machine Learning Fundamentals

Machine learning is the field of designing algorithms that can self-learn and discover unseen patterns from existing data. The novel patterns can then be used to predict new cases. Machine learning can be subdivided into three main categories: supervised learning, unsupervised learning, and semi-supervised learning. In supervised learning, the main objective is to learn from the data sources with existing class labels. Supervised learning can also be simply understood as classification, as the task of classifying unseen cases using the model built from the labelled training cases. Supervised learning can be performed using classification or regression. Unsupervised learning studies the intrinsic properties of the existing cases without class labels. Unsupervised learning is a recursive process of updating the model as the self-learning process continues and bringing the model to an optimal stage. The above self-learning process of model building is used for clustering unseen cases. Unsupervised learning can be performed using clustering and dimensionality reduction approaches. Semi-supervised learning is a hybrid approach to the prior two learning strategies. In this approach, the data can be both labeled and unlabeled cases for model building.

Recent Literature Review

In (Prasad, 2016), three machine learning algorithms, decision trees, k-nearest neighbor, and logistic regression, were used for thyroid disease prediction and improving accuracy. A machine learning repository thyroid dataset was obtained from UCI archives. Thyroid disease's prediction process and its intuition are described concerning three utilized algorithms with 96.8% accuracy. Furthermore, 1179 thyroid modules were evaluated in (Chaubey, 2021) based on linear and non-linear algorithms using pathological references. For every module, the ultrasonography features were assessed, including shape, aspect ratio, hypoechoic halo, margins, size, calcification pattern, cervicals such as neck and vascularity of the lymph node, echogenicity, and composition. Diagnostic performance was evaluated using the area under the curve (AUC) curve. Kernel support vector machines and random forest algorithms show better AUC values, and the non-linear machine learning algorithm analyzed the thyroid nodule's malignancy risks better.

In (Ouyang, 2019), dimensionality reduction algorithms and multiple classification approaches were used. Machine learning exhibited learning capacity without external modification, and a better observation fit was selected. Similarly, the hypothyroid disease dataset from the UCI data repository was used. The evaluation was performed using the WEKA tool in a Windows 7 environment, with a decision tree or J48 classifier used. Cases were classified as primary, secondary, negative, and compensated thyroid. The accuracy of both approaches was determined using a confusion matrix, with the J48 classifier showing better results (Razia, 2020).

Common thyroid problems, such as hypo- and hyperthyroidism, are classified using a decision tree, radial basis function network, and multilayer perceptron (Banu, 2016). A better classification rate was obtained for the decision tree with the UCI data repository used for validation. However, the factors affecting thyroid identification were not performed (Sonuç, 2021). Moreover, recent machine learning algorithms have diagnosed and predicted thyroid disease. The decision tree approach yielded a better accuracy of 99.4% (Ioniţă, 2016). In another case, classifier performance shows a positive impact by evaluating new features in thyroid data. Naïve Bayes shows 98.92% accuracy when analyzed with a decision tree, data augmentation, K-NN, logistic regression, and SVM. More potential and benefits in the dataset have resulted after analysis which helps doctors obtain more accurate and precise outcomes in lesser time (Raisinghani, 2019).

(Duggal, 2020) proposed different methods of optimization and classification for thyroid illness detection, linked to machine learning classification challenges. These methods include univariate selection, recursive-based elimination method and tree-based optimization. In addition, three classification algorithms are included Naïve Bayes, SVM, and random forest are employed. The experimental evaluation has shown SVMs outperformed other techniques in terms of recognition rate.

(Rao, 2020) introduced a predictive model for thyroid illness via binary classification with decision tree and Naïve Bayes methods. In addition, these strategies also contribute to the reduction of unnecessary redundant data in the patient database. Furthermore, the Thyroid Patient database with the appropriate properties is retrieved, and the existence of thyroid in the patient is determined using the Decision Tree method. These classification approaches simplify the treatment of thyroid patients by decreasing the need for costly additional sophisticated treatments.

The methods used in the suggested model are efficient in terms of cost and output performance. A radiomics model was developed to analyze suspected thyroid patients' immunohistochemical features. Non-redundant and reproducible features were selected using Spearman and test re-test co-efficient. The Kruskal Wallis test was used for feature selection, and a support vector machine developed a feature-based model. Performance was analyzed based on AUC, sensitivity, accuracy, and specificity. An individual non-invasive detection-based galectin, thyroperoxidase, and cytokeratin with respect to CT images were also performed, and benign and malignant thyroid diseases were classified (Abbad Ur Rehman, 2021). Likewise, in (Gu, 2019), thyroid symptom was identified. Two major approaches were used based on the neural network. Overfitting and decision tree were used in Ensemble I, while combinations of boosting and bagging algorithms were utilized in Ensemble II, with Ensemble II showing better results.

In another work (Yadav, 2019), surgical and cytologic pathology diagnoses were recorded and interrelated for every thyroid nodule. The final pathology malignancy was predicted, and follicular cells were identified. The specificity and sensitivity obtained were 90.5% and 92.0%, respectively. Furthermore, in (Elliott Range, 2020), thyroid cancer was determined by generating a prognostic system concerning distant metastasis status, age, primary tumor, and regional lymph nodes. In (Yang, 2019), three neural network classification models, learning vector quantization, probabilistic neural network, and multilayer neural network, were used to diagnose thyroid disease. The UCI data repository was employed for 10- and 3-fold cross-validation techniques. Results were compared with existing studies based on thyroid disease diagnosis. (Temurtas, 2009) explored the thyroid gland's non-functionality, thyroid disease, and autoimmune stage. Various neural network frameworks were utilized for thyroid dysfunctionality identification, and specific parameter evaluation approaches were discussed.

Different machine learning algorithms have been evaluated for early prediction of thyroid disease, and the multilayer perceptron yields 99% accuracy. This approach assists doctors in early diagnosis and provides better treatment. The proposed model fights against thyroid disease and ensures patient welfare (Razia S. &., 2016). Kernel-based classifiers and optimal feature selection are used in thyroid data classification. Multi-kernel support vector machine and grey wolf optimization feature selection process can further enhance the classification process. Thyroid classification results show a 97.4% accuracy rate in the thyroid prediction (Asif, 2020). The thyroid disease dataset was examined using random forest, decision tree, and regression tree algorithms. Using the bagging ensemble approaches, the classifier's results have been enhanced. Prediction accuracy is based on seed and the number fold values. Random forest obtained 99% accuracy, while the decision tree obtained 98% accuracy (Shankar, 2020).

An effective thyroid disease diagnosis was performed using the artificial neural network with three different approaches: artificial neural networks (ANN), multiple regression, and random forest. ANN delivered a higher accuracy than the other two methods at 98.22% (Yadav D. C., 2020).

(Parmar, 2018) used ten different machine learning algorithms to investigate the treatment design strategy for patients suffering from hypothyroidism. Out of all reviewed classifiers, a good accuracy of 84% was achieved with the extra-tree classifier. (Aversano, 2021) reviewed the basic techniques of machine learning for identifying and inhibiting the thyroid, especially using the SVM to predict the approximate probability of a thyroid patient.

(Ramya, 2020) investigated heart disease prediction using many classification algorithms, such as C4.5, ID3, Naive Bayes, and SVM, for early-stage detection and better treatment for affected patients. (Phasinam, 2022) proposed a machine-learning technique for efficiently diagnosing and preventing thyroid disease. The benchmark algorithms, such as KNN, decision trees, and support vector machines, are used for obtaining the model for tracing patients affected by thyroid diseases and ensuring early treatment initiation.

(Tyagi, Interactive thyroid disease prediction system using machine learning technique., 2018) proposed a framework for abnormal thyroid disease detection using features election and ensemble approaches. Moreover, a unique combination of feature selection approaches is employed, such as selecting K best, selecting from the model, and recursive feature elimination, and several benchmark base classifiers, such as random forest, gradient boosting, decision tree, and logistic regression, are used in the framework. The evaluation results have shown that the bagging meta-estimator achieved a significant recognition rate by delivering the highest accuracy in inadequate training and prediction time.

(Akhtar, 2021) provided an investigation technique for thyroid disease prediction using different machine-learning techniques such as a k-nearest neighbor, decision trees, and logistic regression. The percentage of correctly classified instances, i.e., accuracy, is used as one of the evaluation criteria for experimental analysis.

(Chaubey, 2021) proposed a deep neural network architecture with data augmentation techniques for efficient thyroid disease diagnosis in the context of deep learning models. Dimensionality reduction filters, such as feature subset evaluation and correlation-based feature subset selection, are also used for efficient model building. (Zhang, 2022) proposed a multiple-layer neural network architecture for thyroid disease detection for patient-specific case sheet model preparation. The cases of ultrasound imaging and computer tomography (CT) scan inputs were considered through the proposed network for thyroid disease detection and treatment. On the other hand, this study contributes the following main points. First, the framework fused three distinct patient-centric CNN multi-channel topologies that applicability enables doctors to achieve greater diagnostic precision. Additionally, it leads to the potential use of machine learning-driven systems for detection in the clinical field. Second, the approach has dramatically increased the diagnosis accuracy of malignant thyroid nodules. With 11 analyzed models, the author introduced a detailed comparison of experimental data, demonstrating that their neural network of interest, such as Xception, surpassed the majority of CNNs in this scenario. Third, using various medical images, the framework was tested as part of their research. This work contributes to the acceptance of CT scans for thyroid nodule classification, demonstrating that CT pictures' application is as precise and effective as ultrasound imaging.

(Islam, 2022) studied thyroid disease detection and evaluation using 11 machine learning algorithms and investigated the specific context of class imbalance learning using evaluation metrics, such as f-measure, recall, sensitivity, and specificity. The comparison result has revealed that the artificial neural network (ANN) achieved significant results over other state-of-the-art algorithms, including CatBoost and XGBoost. The detailed review demonstrates that ANN delivers better accuracy and F1-score on the benchmark dataset when predicting the thyroid dataset.

(Usman, 2022) applied benchmark machine learning algorithms, such as support vector machine, multi-layer preceptor, and Hammerstein-Weiner techniques, to identify thyroidism status using two independent variables and three evaluation measures. The output of the proposed system demonstrated that SVM, HW, and MLP machine learning models could frame the thyroidism status of each individual as normal or with R-2 values greater than 0.7 in both phases, including training and testing.

(Hu, 2022) investigated the classification of patients with hyper- and hypothyroidism using laboratory tests. They also analyzed using the feature-specific approach for class detection and used different evaluation measures, such as the AUC, specificity, and sensitivity. (Yang F. Z., 2022) proposed various strategies for accelerated drug repurposing using machine learning approaches. They also proposed to apply drug repurposing the COVID-19 medicine therapy. However, the current issues involve the concerns of black-box of unsupervised learning to signaling repurposable medications, which makes it challenging to explain the results' rationale. Additionally, in the context of conventional drug discovery research, it is better to build interpretable unsupervised learning and causal learning.

(Sarker, 2021) reviewed various machine learning approaches for real-world applicability, such as medicine for developing smart and automated applications. In addition, they have covered briefly how several types of ML approaches can be utilized to solve various real-world problems. Furthermore, the relevance of ML techniques to various real-world problems, they also explored several popular application domains. Next, the author summarised and addressed the challenges encountered, as well as the prospective research prospects and future objectives for the field. Therefore, this study stated that issues present promising research prospects, which must be handled with efficient approaches for multiple application domains. The only drawback of this work is that it does not include large datasets for better insights.

METHODOLOGY AND DATASET DESCRIPTION

In this experimental setup, the datasets are validated using different validation measures, such as accuracy, AUC, and error rate. The experimental methodology used for validation is 10-fold cross-validation for ten runs. Most studies utilize 10-fold cross-validation to train and evaluate multiple classifiers. In other words, no additional testing or validation is performed. In addition, cross-validation is used to assess a machine learning model's capability to detect upcoming data. Thus, it can be used to identify issues such as overfitting and biasness, specifically selection bias, and to provide insight into the model that will generalize to a different database.

Dataset Description

Disease prediction is performed using the dataset obtained from the UCI repository. It contains several instances, a minimum of 155 instances for the hepatitis dataset and a maximum of 3,772 instances for the hypothyroid dataset.

Table 1. Description of the datasets

S.No	Dataset	Instances
1	breast-cancer	286
2	heart-statlog	270
3	hungarian-14-heart-disease	294
4	cleveland-14-heart-disease	303
5	pima_diabetes	768
6	wisconsin-breast-cancer	699
7	hepatitis	155
8	hypothyroid	3772

RESULTS AND DISCUSSION

The experimental results are presented in this section using three benchmark algorithms and eight disease datasets. The results are generated on the accuracy, Area under curve (AUC), and Root mean square (RMS) error. The three benchmark algorithms used for simulation are REP tree, random tree, and C4.5 decision tree algorithm.

Table 2. Accuracy results on the diseases datasets

S.No	Dataset	REP Tree	Random Tree	C4.5
1	breast-cancer	69.35	67.37	74.28
2	wisconsin-breast-cancer	94.77	94.19	95.01
3	pima_diabetes	74.46	70.25	74.49
4	cleveland-14-heart-disease	77.02	75.28	76.94
5	hungarian-14-heart-disease	78.56	75.68	80.22
6	heart-statlog	76.15	74.15	78.15
7	hepatitis	78.62	78.29	79.22
8	hypothyroid	99.50	97.60	99.54

Table 2 summarizes the accuracy of different disease datasets on benchmark machine learning algorithms. The C4.5 algorithm performed well on almost all the datasets. Figure 1 presents the pictorial representation of accuracy results and clearly shows that the C4.5 algorithm performed well.

Figure 1. Representation of Accuracy results on three machine learning algorithms REP tree, random tree and C4.5

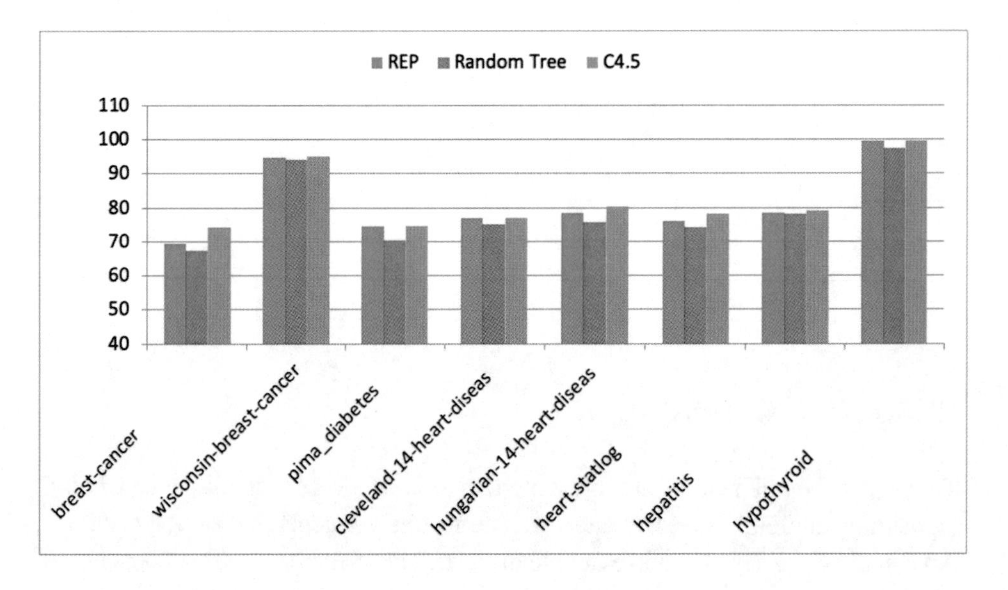

Table 3. AUC results on the diseases datasets

S.No	Dataset	REP Tree	Random Tree	C4.5
1	breast-cancer	0.580	0.605	0.606
2	hungarian-breast-cancer	0.959	0.935	0.957
3	pima_diabetes	0.761	0.674	0.751
4	hungarian-14-heart-disease	0.810	0.753	0.769
5	hungarian-14-heart-disease	0.826	0.753	0.775
6	heart-statlog	0.783	0.738	0.786
7	hepatitis	0.620	0.723	0.668
8	hypothyroid	0.996	0.930	0.996

Table 3 summarizes the AUC of the different disease datasets on the benchmark machine learning algorithms. The REP tree and C4.5 algorithm both performed well on almost all datasets. Figure 2 presents the pictorial representation of AUC results and clearly shows that REP tree and C4.5 algorithms performed well.

Figure 2. Representation of AUC results on three machine learning algorithms REP tree, random tree, and C4.5

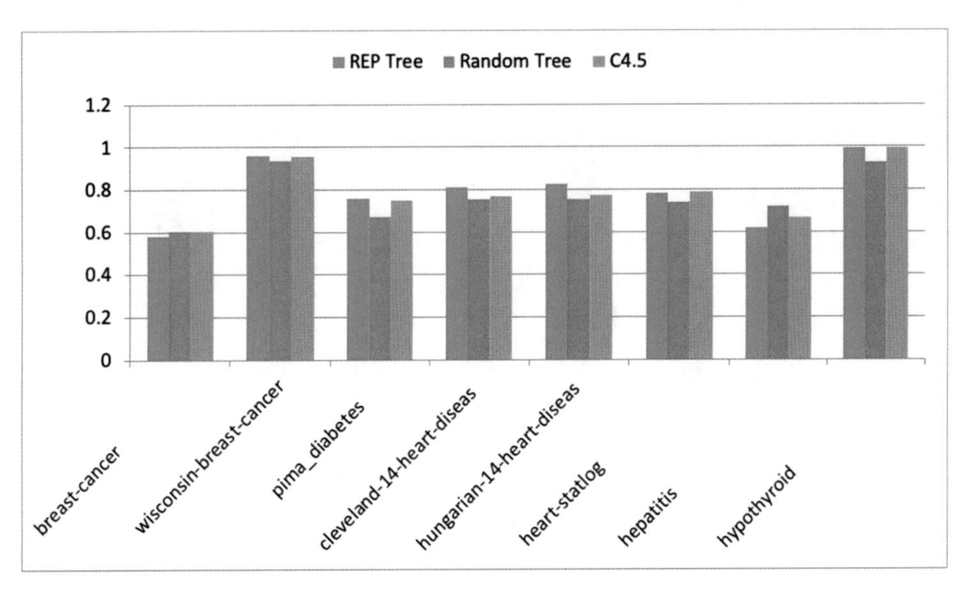

Table 4. RMS error results on the diseases datasets

S.No	Dataset	REP Tree	Random Tree	C4.5
1	breast-cancer	0.466	0.545	0.444
2	wisconsin-breast-cancer	0.209	0.234	0.205
3	pima_diabetes	0.430	0.544	0.439
4	cleveland-14-heart-disease	0.261	0.310	0.281
5	hungarian-14-heart-disease	0.251	0.301	0.252
6	heart-statlog	0.425	0.500	0.429
7	hepatitis	0.402	0.428	0.404
8	hypothyroid	0.045	0.102	0.039

Table 4 summarizes the RMS error of different disease datasets on the benchmark machine learning algorithms. The random tree algorithm performed the worst on almost all the datasets. Figure 3 presents the pictorial representation of RMS error results, and clearly shows the poor performance of the random tree algorithm.

Figure 3. Representation of RMS Error results on three machine learning algorithms REP tree, random tree, and C4.5

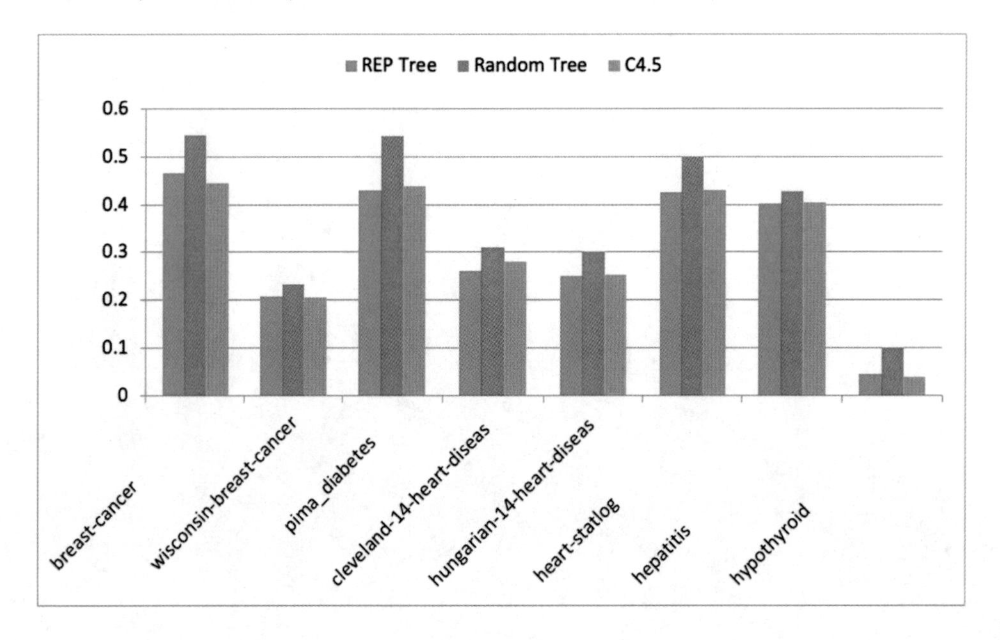

CONCLUSION

In this paper, a literature review of recent medical/disease detection and analysis studies is performed. The survey mainly concentrates on heart and thyroid diseases, which are the principal causes of high mortality. The benchmark algorithms are used for experimental simulation on some of the UCI medical datasets. The experimental results are summarized and discussed for valid reasonability. In future work, the study needs to be conducted on special cases such as uncertain or stream datasets where the ratio of classes dynamically changes.

REFERENCES

Abbad Ur Rehman, H. L., Lin, C.-Y., Mushtaq, Z., & Su, S.-F. (2021). Performance analysis of machine learning algorithms for thyroid disease. *Arabian Journal for Science and Engineering*, *46*(10), 9437–9449. doi:10.100713369-020-05206-x

Akhtar, T. G., Gilani, S. O., Mushtaq, Z., Arif, S., Jamil, M., Ayaz, Y., Butt, S. I., & Waris, A. (2021). Effective Voting Ensemble of Homogenous Ensembling with Multiple Attribute-Selection Approaches for Improved Identification of Thyroid Disorder. *Electronics (Basel)*, *10*(23), 10. doi:10.3390/electronics10233026

Asif, M. A. (2020). Computer aided diagnosis of thyroid disease using machine learning algorithms. *In 2020 11th International Conference on Electrical and Computer Engineering* (pp. 222-225). IEEE.

Aversano, L. B., Bernardi, M. L., Cimitile, M., Iammarino, M., Macchia, P. E., Nettore, I. C., & Verdone, C. (2021). Thyroid disease treatment prediction with machine learning approaches. *Procedia Computer Science*, *192*, 1031–1040. doi:10.1016/j.procs.2021.08.106

Banu, G. R. (2016). A Role of decision Tree classification data Mining Technique in Diagnosing Thyroid disease. *International Journal on Computer Science and Engineering*, 64–70.

Chaubey, G. B., Bisen, D., Arjaria, S., & Yadav, V. (2021). Thyroid disease prediction using machine learning approaches. *National Academy Science Letters*, *44*(3), 233–238. doi:10.100740009-020-00979-z

Duggal, P. (2020). Prediction of thyroid disorders using advanced machine learning techniques. *In 2020 10th International Conference on Cloud Computing, Data Science & Engineering (Confluence)* (pp. 670-675). IEEE.

Elliott Range, D. D., Dov, D., Kovalsky, S. Z., Henao, R., Carin, L., & Cohen, J. (2020). Application of a machine learning algorithm to predict malignancy in thyroid cytopathology. *Cancer Cytopathology*, *128*(4), 287–295. doi:10.1002/cncy.22238 PMID:32012493

Franco, J. S.-A. (2013). Thyroid disease and autoimmune diseases. In *Autoimmunity: From Bench to Bedside*. El Rosario University Press.

Gu, J. Z., Zhu, J., Qiu, Q., Wang, Y., Bai, T., & Yin, Y. (2019). Prediction of immunohistochemistry of suspected thyroid nodules by use of machine learning–based radiomics. *AJR. American Journal of Roentgenology*, *213*(6), 1348–1357. doi:10.2214/AJR.19.21626 PMID:31461321

Hu, M. A. (2022). Development and preliminary validation of a machine learning system for thyroid dysfunction diagnosis based on routine laboratory tests. *Communication & Medicine*, 1–8. PMID:35603277

Ioniţă, I. (2016). Prediction of thyroid disease using data mining techniques. *Broad Research in Artificial Intelligence and Neuroscience*, 115–124.

Islam, S. S., Haque, M. S., Miah, M. S. U., Sarwar, T. B., & Nugraha, R. (2022). Application of machine learning algorithms to predict the thyroid disease risk: An experimental comparative study. *PeerJ. Computer Science*, *8*, 898. doi:10.7717/peerj-cs.898 PMID:35494828

Jha, R. B., Bhattacharjee, V., & Mustafi, A. (2022). Increasing the Prediction Accuracy for Thyroid Disease: A Step Towards Better Health for Society. *Wireless Personal Communications*, *122*(2), 1921–1938. doi:10.100711277-021-08974-3

Ouyang, F. S., Guo, B., Ouyang, L., Liu, Z., Lin, S., Meng, W., Huang, X., Chen, H., Qiu-gen, H., & Yang, S. (2019). Comparison between linear and nonlinear machine-learning algorithms for the classification of thyroid nodules. *European Journal of Radiology*, *113*, 251–25. doi:10.1016/j.ejrad.2019.02.029 PMID:30927956

Parmar, A. K. (2018). A review on random forest: An ensemble classifier. *In International Conference on Intelligent Data Communication Technologies and Internet of Things* (pp. 758-763). Springer.

Phasinam, K. M., Mondal, T., Novaliendry, D., Yang, C.-H., Dutta, C., & Shabaz, M. (2022). Analyzing the Performance of Machine Learning Techniques in Disease Prediction. *Journal of Food Quality*, *2022*, 1–9. doi:10.1155/2022/7529472

Prasad, V. R., Rao, T. S., & Babu, M. S. P. (2016). Thyroid disease diagnosis via hybrid architecture composing rough data sets theory and machine learning algorithms. *Soft Computing*, *20*(3), 1179–1189. doi:10.100700500-014-1581-5

Prerana, P. S. (2015). Predictive data mining for diagnosis of thyroid disease using neural network. *International Journal of Research in Management, Science & Technology*, 75-80.

Raisinghani, S. S. (2019). In International Conference on Advances in Computing and Data Sciences. *Thyroid prediction using machine learning techniques*, 140-150.

Ramya, M. (2020). Prediction And Providing Medication For Thyroid Disease Using Machine Learning Technique (SVM). *Turkish Journal of Computer and Mathematics Education (TURCOMAT)*, 1099-1107.

Rao, A. R. (2020). A machine learning approach to predict thyroid disease at early stages of diagnosis. *In 2020 IEEE International Conference for Innovation in Technology (INOCON)* (pp. 1-4). IEEE. 10.1109/INOCON50539.2020.9298252

Razia, S., & Narasinga Rao, M. R. (2016). Machine learning techniques for thyroid disease diagnosis-a review. *Indian Journal of Science and Technology*, *9*(28), 1–9. doi:10.17485/ijst/2016/v9i28/93705

Razia, S. S. (2020). Machine learning techniques for thyroid disease diagnosis: a systematic review. *Modern Approaches in Machine Learning and Cognitive Science: A Walkthrough*, 203-212.

Sarker, I. H. (2021). Machine learning: Algorithms, real-world applications, and research directions. *SN Computer Science*, 1-21.

Shankar, K. L., Lakshmanaprabu, S. K., Gupta, D., Maseleno, A., & de Albuquerque, V. H. C. (2020). Optimal feature-based multi-kernel SVM approach for thyroid disease classification. *The Journal of Supercomputing*, *76*(2), 1128–1143. doi:10.100711227-018-2469-4

Sonuç, E. (2021). Thyroid Disease Classification Using Machine Learning Algorithms. In Journal of Physics: Conference Series IOP Publishing., 012140.

Stafford, I. S., Kellermann, M., Mossotto, E., Beattie, R. M., MacArthur, B. D., & Ennis, S. (2020). A systematic review of the applications of artificial intelligence and machine learning in autoimmune diseases. *NPJ Digital Medicine*, *3*(1), 1–11. doi:10.103841746-020-0229-3 PMID:32195365

Temurtas, F. (2009). A comparative study on thyroid disease diagnosis using neural networks. *Expert Systems with Applications*, *36*(1), 944–949. doi:10.1016/j.eswa.2007.10.010

Tyagi, A. M. (2018). Interactive thyroid disease prediction system using machine learning technique. *In 2018 Fifth international conference on parallel, distributed and grid computing (PDGC)* (pp. 689-693). IEEE.

Usman, A. G., Ghali, U. M., Degm, M. A. A., Muhammad, S. M., Hincal, E., Kurya, A. U., Işik, S., Hoti, Q., & Abba, S. I. (2022). Simulation of liver function enzymes as determinants of thyroidism: A novel ensemble machine learning approach. *Bulletin of the National Research Center*, *46*(1), 1–10. doi:10.118642269-022-00756-6

Yadav, D. C. (2020). Prediction of thyroid disease using decision tree ensemble method. *Human-Intelligent Systems Integration*, 89-95.

Yadav, D. C., & Pal, S. (2019). To generate an ensemble model for women thyroid prediction using data mining techniques. *Asian Pacific Journal of Cancer Prevention*, *20*(4), 1275–1281. doi:10.31557/APJCP.2019.20.4.1275 PMID:31031212

Yang, C. Q., Gardiner, L., Wang, H., Hueman, M. T., & Chen, D. (2019). Creating prognostic systems for well-differentiated thyroid cancer using machine learning. *Frontiers in Endocrinology*, *10*, 288. doi:10.3389/fendo.2019.00288 PMID:31139148

Yang, F. Z. (2022). Machine learning applications in drug repurposing. *Interdisciplinary Sciences, Computational Life Sciences*, 1–7. PMID:35066811

Zhang, X. L., Lee, V. C. S., Rong, J., Liu, F., & Kong, H. (2022). Multi-channel convolutional neural network architectures for thyroid cancer detection. *PLoS One*, *17*(1), 0262128. doi:10.1371/journal.pone.0262128 PMID:35061759

Chapter 2
Role of Artificial Intelligence in Biomedical Imaging

Avinash Kumar Sharma
ABES Institute of Technology, India

Pranav Kumar Tripathi
ABES Institute of Technology, India

Sushant Sharma
https://orcid.org/0000-0001-8033-3072
ABES Institute of Technology, India

ABSTRACT

A trendy technique based on computer science called artificial intelligence (AI) creates software and algorithms to make machines smart and effective at carrying out activities that often call for expert human intellect. Machine learning (ML), deep learning (DL), traditional neural networks, fuzzy logic, and speech recognition are only a few of the subsets of AI that have distinctive skills and functions that might enhance the performance of contemporary medical sciences. Biomedical imaging might undergo a revolution thanks to AI, which could increase the efficiency and precision of picture processing and interpretation. Radiologists could miss tiny abnormalities that can be detected by AI systems that have been taught to spot patterns in those pictures that are challenging for humans to interpret. AI may also be used to generate customized medicine by evaluating a patient's medical pictures and other data to customize treatment regimens, as well as to enhance image processing and visualization.

DOI: 10.4018/978-1-6684-6957-6.ch002

INTRODUCTION

Biomedical imaging might undergo a revolution thanks to artificial intelligence (AI), which could increase the efficiency and precision of picture processing and interpretation. We will examine the present status of AI in biomedical imaging in this review, along with its uses and drawbacks, and talk about the field's future prospects.

The creation of computer-aided diagnostic (CAD) systems is one of the primary uses of AI in biomedical imaging. These systems evaluate medical photos using machine learning algorithms and offer a diagnosis or suggestion for more testing. Radiology, dermatology, and ophthalmology are just a few of the medical fields where CAD systems have been proven to be useful. In one research, a CAD system outperformed human radiologists in the detection of lung cancer with a sensitivity and specificity of 92% and 96%, respectively.

AI may be used to enhance the processing and visualization of images. For instance, using AI algorithms to improve the quality or contrast of medical photographs might help clinicians more easily spot minute anomalies. AI may also be used to simulate the interior anatomy of the body in three dimensions, which is useful for planning procedures like surgeries and other treatments.

The improvement of tailored medicine is a potential area for AI in biomedical imaging. AI algorithms can assist doctors in creating treatment regimens for each patient by examining their medical imaging and other data, boosting the likelihood of a positive outcome.

Although AI has the potential to revolutionize biomedical imaging, it is crucial to understand its constraints. The requirement for vast quantities of labeled data for training is one of the major obstacles in the development of AI algorithms. In the realm of medicine, where patient privacy is a priority, this might be challenging to get. Additionally, if the data utilized to train AI systems is not inclusive of the entire population, they may be prejudiced. Finally, regulatory and legal restrictions frequently prevent AI from being adopted in medical practice.

Despite these difficulties, AI in biomedical imaging has a promising future. We may anticipate seeing additional uses of AI in the diagnosis and treatment of medical disorders as the area develops. To guarantee that AI is utilized ethically and successfully to enhance patient care, researchers and physicians must continue to collaborate.

BIOMEDICAL IMAGING

In order to diagnose and treat medical diseases, clinicians use biomedical imaging, a vital technology that enables them to see the inside structures and activities of the body. Biomedical imaging has several different modalities, each with unique properties and uses. A common technique that uses radiation to produce pictures of bones and tissues is the X-ray. While magnetic resonance imaging (MRI) utilizes a magnetic field and radio waves to provide precise pictures of the body's soft tissues, computed tomography (CT) employs x-rays to produce detailed images of the interior organs of the body. Both positron emission tomography (PET) and ultrasound employ sound waves and radiation to produce pictures of the body's organs and tissues, respectively.

Recent developments in biomedical imaging have sparked the creation of fresh methods and tools that are enhancing treatment planning and diagnostic precision. Artificial intelligence (AI) is being used, for instance, to evaluate and decipher biological pictures, assisting in the identification of minor anomalies and minimizing the requirement for invasive treatments. The use of various modalities to produce a more complete image of the body's structures and functioning is known as multi-modality imaging, and it is also growing in popularity. A growing trend is image-guided intervention, which makes use of imaging to direct treatments like biopsies and surgery.

The diagnosis and treatment of several medical disorders depend heavily on biomedical imaging. Imaging is used, for instance, to diagnose and stage cancer as well as track the effectiveness of treatment. Imaging is utilized in cardiovascular disease to identify and treat disorders including coronary artery disease and heart failure. Imaging is utilized in neurology to identify and treat disorders including stroke and brain tumors.

Biomedical imaging, in general, is a crucial part of contemporary medicine since it gives medical professionals a non-invasive means to see the body's structures and functioning in order to diagnose and treat a variety of medical diseases. The application of biomedical imaging in medicine is projected to grow even more as the discipline develops new technologies.

AI SUPPORTED CARDIAC MONITORING

Nearly 18 million people died worldwide from cardiovascular diseases (CVD), the leading cause of death, in 2019. Due to their worrisome role as a source of morbidity, CVDs are a major concern, particularly in low- and middle-income nations. Changes in stress levels and way of life become important risk factors for human CVDs in addition to genetics. Heart failure, heart attacks, myocardial infarctions, cardiac arrhythmia, pericarditis, and cardiomyopathy are just a few examples of the several forms of CVDs that can damage the heart's ability to pump blood. The electrocardiogram (ECG), stress test, Holter monitoring device, cardiac computed tomography (CT) scan, and blood biomarker profiling are a few of the instruments that may be used to monitor changes in heart function. Among these, an ECG, a stress test, and biomarker profiling offer a quick and reasonably priced tool for assessing heart function. One of the primary causes of myocardial infarctions is stress. One of the crucial jobs is monitoring physiological stress, which a biosensor may do on an individual basis based on lifestyle, circumstances, and events. By quantifying cortisol, a physiological stress indicator, electrochemical biosensing devices enable stress monitoring(Nakhleh et al., 2016; Karuppaiah et al., 2022).

The current advancements in quick diagnosis techniques for precisely identifying various clinical diseases linked to CVDs are summarized in this review part. Atrial fibrillation (AF), a disorder characterized by an erratic heartbeat, is associated with an increased risk of blood clot development, which may result in cardiovascular problems and potentially a stroke. Since AF is asymptomatic and goes unnoticed until the first thromboembolic episode, a diagnostic problem develops in this case. A thromboembolic event is one in which a blood clot forms in a blood vessel and travels through the circulation to block another blood artery. Long-term continuous monitoring of AF has been done through clinical studies including the Embrace trial (a 30-day screening in patients with cryptogenic stroke) and the Crystal AF trial (a 36-day study of continuous cardiac monitoring to assess AF following cryptogenic stroke). However, as was already indicated, there are bottlenecks in the trials for all suspected cases of AF due to technological issues, inconvenient usage, and inadequate compensation. The technique should be dependable, economical, practical, and equipped with simple instruments for prolonged non-invasive AF detection.

Long-term continuous monitoring of AF has been done through clinical studies including the Embrace trial (a 30-day screening in patients with cryptogenic stroke) and the Crystal AF trial (a 36-day study of continuous cardiac monitoring to assess AF following cryptogenic stroke). However, as was already indicated, there are bottlenecks in the trials for all suspected cases of AF due to technological issues, inconvenient usage, and inadequate compensation. The technique should be dependable, affordable, practical, and equipped with simple equipment for extended non-invasive AF monitoring. One of the modern techniques for real-time monitoring of cardiovascular function is the electrocardiogram (ECG). ECG is helpful in predicting different cardiac disorders since it can show the heart's morphology and functionality. Typically, a 12-lead ECG recorder is used to detect irregular cardiac rhythm. Manually examining an ECG recording takes time, and analyzing a significant amount of data might lead to mistakes. Inconvenient for the user and noisy during ECG measurements, the typical ECG measuring instrument is indeed. Single-channel ECG recorders have improved recently to become sensitive tools for precisely identifying variations in the heartbeat. However, the single-channel ECG recorder generates a massive amount of data, necessitating the use of an automated computer to interpret the data and assess the specificity of the measurement. Accurate diagnosis of arrhythmic heartbeats and accurate abnormality prediction has been achieved by researchers using ML-based algorithms. The distinctive characteristics that may be retrieved from the ECG data can be used to identify cardiac-related diseases such myocardial infarctions, sinus tachycardia, and sleep apnea (Tseng et al., 2020). AI/ML has demonstrated potential in the monitoring of cardiac electrophysiology and cardiac imaging because of developments in cloud computing and the capacity to analyze massive amounts of data. AI (DL/ML)-based systems have been investigated for a number of applications, such as classifying noise in ECG data, identifying arrhythmias, predicting atrial fibrillation, and analyzing whole genome sequences. Figure 1 gives a summary of the function of AI/ML in electrophysiological measurement. In order to improve illness diagnosis, forecast outcomes, and identify novel diseases, AI/ML is trained on data collected from IoMT devices such as smart watches, mobile phone technology, and medical imaging.

Figure 1. AI/function ML's in cardiology. In order to improve the health outcome, classic or contemporary ML algorithms are used to evaluate the biological data obtained by cardiac electrophysiological measurement.

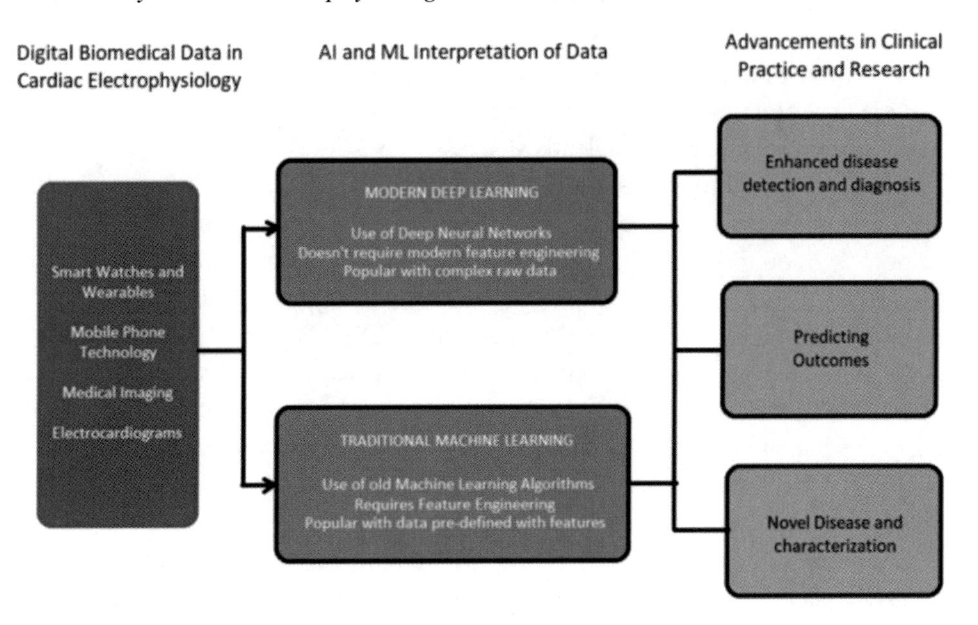

AI IN SURGERY

Biomedical image processing and artificial intelligence (AI) have the potential to transform surgery by increasing the precision and accuracy of diagnostic and therapeutic procedures.The analysis of medical pictures is one of the primary uses of AI in surgery. AI systems, for instance, can be used to automatically find and categorise anomalies in medical imaging, like cancers or lesions. This can facilitate the quicker and more accurate identification of problem regions by surgeons, which may result in better patient outcomes. AI can also be used to track and monitor the development of an illness over time, which can assist medical professionals in making better treatment choices.

The creation of computer-assisted surgical systems is another application of AI in surgery. Real-time imagery and AI algorithms are used by these devices to direct surgeons during difficult operations. For instance, a computer-assisted system might make a precise map of a patient's anatomy using preoperative imaging that the surgeon can use as a guide while performing surgery. Real-time imaging may also be used by the system to monitor the placement of surgical tools and give the surgeon feedback to help them avoid injuring healthy tissue.

Many approaches, including image registration, image segmentation, image enhancement and visualization, computer-aided diagnosis (CAD), and analysis, are being developed in the field of biomedical image processing. These methods can aid medical professionals in diagnosing tumors, planning surgical procedures, and monitoring the course of a patient's sickness.

AI can be used to assess patient data to forecast the possibility of difficulties during surgery and assist clinicians in choosing the most appropriate course of action. By monitoring the patient's progress and spotting potential problems early on, artificial intelligence (AI) can be utilized to assist in post-operative recuperation.

Radiology is one area in particular where AI is being used. Deep learning algorithms are being used in computer-aided diagnosis systems that analyze medical images to spot potential problems like tumors or other anomalies. These systems have the potential to significantly increase the speed and accuracy of diagnosis, which can improve patient outcomes. They have been demonstrated to have a high level of accuracy in detecting specific types of cancers.

Another field is surgical navigation, where AI algorithms are being developed to use medical imaging to create detailed maps of a patient's anatomy. These maps will then be used to guide surgeons during procedures by providing real-time information about the position of surgical instruments and the location of important body structures. These devices have the potential to lower the risk of complications and enhance patient outcomes by enabling surgeons to navigate with more accuracy.

Another application of AI is in image-guided radiation therapy, where it can track the position of tumors and modify the radiation's delivery to reduce harm to healthy tissue. This can lessen the possibility of side effects and increase the efficiency of radiation therapy.

Image registration and image segmentation are two important techniques being researched for biomedical image processing. These methods are used to align images of the same patient that were collected at various times or with various imaging modalities. In order to schedule surgical procedures and track the course of the disease over time, this can help to develop a more thorough and accurate picture of the patient's health. On the other hand, image segmentation is a method for dividing a medical image into its many parts or structures. This can be used to spot tumors, monitor changes over time, or arrange for surgery.

In summary, AI and biomedical image processing have the potential to transform surgery by increasing the precision and accuracy of therapeutic and diagnostic procedures. Researchers and doctors are becoming more aware of the potential of AI in healthcare as a result of the increasing volume of medical imaging data being produced. Although there is still much research to be done, the advancements that have been made so far are encouraging, and we may anticipate seeing more AI and biomedical image processing applications in surgery in the future.

ROLE OF AI IN DIABETES MELLITUS AND CANCER MANAGEMENT

Blood glucose levels must be routinely monitored because diabetes is one of the growing healthcare issues. One of the most important tests for persons with hypoglycemia and hyperglycemia is blood glucose measurement. Around 425 million people worldwide suffer from diabetes, and 12% of global spending is devoted to its control. By 2030, it is anticipated that the cost of diabetes would rise to USD 490 billion. Diabetes retinopathy (DR), which can result in partial or total blindness, can be brought on by chronic diabetes(Grzybowski et al., 2020). A third of diabetics have diabetic macular oedema, which are tiny bulges that protrude from the walls of vessels and leak blood into the retina, causing serious health issues . According to epidemiological studies (i.e., the study of the prevalence and potential causes of the disease), one in three diabetics have DR. Both accurate and regular glucose monitoring are required to stop diabetes-related acute and chronic clinical obstacles. It is crucial to create a technology for patients at a reasonable price without pricking their fingers repeatedly to check the glucose level because the traditional glucose-monitoring approach necessitates puncturing the skin and extracting blood. Systems for POC glucose testing in patients are now on the market and are electrochemically based. The use of glucometers for POC diabetes treatment is growing yearly, despite certain issues with the accuracy and precision of these devices. A continuous glucose-monitoring system (CGM) gives the patient and the carer access to real-time information on glucose levels, as opposed to point-of-use glucose meters, which only offer a snapshot of glucose trends. One of the major obstacles to precise and timely glucose level prediction is the complexity of blood dynamics. Artificial neural networks, natural language processing, and AI/ML-based methods are extremely important for managing diabetes because they can detect diabetes risk and forecast diabetes trends, which makes diabetes care simple(Hasanzad et al., 2022).

To increase clinical accuracy, glucose-monitoring devices now combine AI- and ML-based techniques. For instance, Khanam et al. created a system that uses AI to precisely measure human glucose levels. The algorithm is trained using five input characteristics, including age, pregnancy, BMI, glucose, and insulin levels(Khanam et al., 2021). The data set was assessed using ML techniques including RF, NN, DT, and K-nearest neighbor (KNN) with hidden layers. All models produced an accurate reading of glucose that was >70% dependable. Hamdi et al. used a hybrid system with compartmental models to evaluate the glucose level. The ANN algorithm was used to monitor the glucose levels using the CGM technique. The system comprises a wireless transmitter coupled to a subcutaneous sensor inserted just beneath the skin, which displays the glucose levels. Every 15 minutes, the gadget measures the glucose levels. Data from 12 patients were gathered for the training and validation phases in order to assess the system's performance in clinical analysis. Three layers make up this algorithm: the input layer, the hidden layer, and the output layer.

Figure 2. Artificial neural network representation that uses patient data to determine the best course of action.

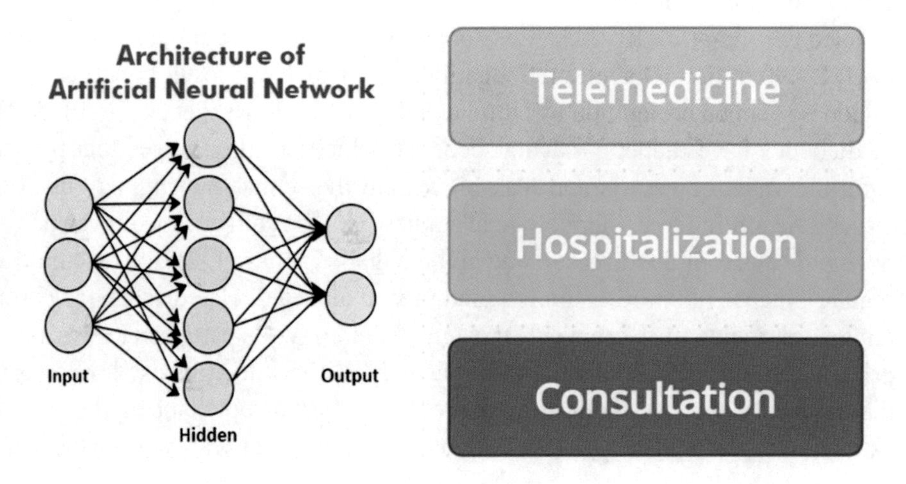

Marcus et al. created a customized SML strategy for predicting blood glucose levels. The non-linear data sets may be analyzed using SML methods to find patterns and correlations. In order to improve the clinical accuracy of the glucose sensors, non-linearity must be addressed. 11 participants' data were gathered to train the system. The CGM devices measured the glucose concentrations in interstitial fluid (ISF). However, it is stated that there is a 5 to 25 minute delay between glucose increases in both compartments. Automated insulin injections (artificial pancreas) are not advised for CGMs due to this delay. Notably, the CGM frequently fails to promptly detect hypoglycemia episodes. This team's algorithm foresees increases in blood sugar levels 30 minutes in advance, allowing for the integration of artificial pancreas devices with CGM(Aljamaan et al., 2021).

It is possible that non-invasive glucose sensing will eventually take the place of the traditional finger-prick method of continuous glucose monitoring. ML-based optical sensors for measuring blood sugar levels have been shown utilizing light sources with various wavelengths. Five distinct ML techniques have been used for glucose analysis and prediction, and more than 21 different light sources with various wavelengths have been employed. By categorizing the data sets into 21 groups, the system's prediction accuracy was increased. The capacity of the system to distinguish between higher, lower, and normal glucose levels was strong. For POC measurement, paper-based analytical devices (PADs) connected to smartphones have been described for colorimetric detection of salivary glucose levels(Mercan et al., 2021). The ability of three distinct chromogenic agent combinations to produce color when glucose interacts on a PAD work surface was investigated. Four different iPhones were used to capture the photographs under seven different lighting situations. The best machine classifiers for each detection circumstance were selected after a variety of ML classifiers were assessed, and thus improved the detection accuracy. After that, the data sets were processed utilizing a cloud-based technology that allows for remote operation of the classifier.

Cancer is a clinical illness marked by uncontrolled cell proliferation and spread throughout the body. Computerized tomography (CT), magnetic resonance imaging (MRI), positron emission tomography (PET), and ultrasound are imaging procedures used to detect cancer(Sakthivel et al., 2021; Sadasivam et al., 2020). To find protein cancer indicators that have been authorized by the FDA early, biomarker-based detection techniques have also been created. Early detection, screening in a large population, classification and stage grading, molecular characterization, patient outcome prediction, treatment response prediction, personalized treatment, automated radiotherapy workflow, and novel anti-cancer drug discovery and clinical trials are just a few of the potential applications of AI-based technologies in cancer research. Additionally, prediction models for evaluating lymph node metastases, treatment response, and prognosis may be developed using AI and ML algorithms.

An ANN model developed by researchers could predict the preoperative stage of stomach cancer with an accuracy of 82% using clinical data, pathological data, and genetic polymorphisms(Jin et al., 2020). Many scientists have created computer models to forecast the course of cancer using AI-based algorithms. Although gene expression has proven to be an effective strategy, it has the disadvantage of having small sample numbers. The AI-coupled ML system has shown to be effective at subtype categorization, diagnosis, and detection. For pattern identification in breast cancer, ML algorithms have been regarded as a favored alternative method. In order to extract the clinical characteristics from the packed datasets, decision-prediction techniques like K-nearest neighbor (KNN), support vector machine (SVM), and decision tree (DT) are used. A 3,3¢-diaminobenzidine (DAB)-based immunohistochemistry technique to identify multiple tumors was developed(Fan et al., 2021). The group correctly identified HER2 overexpressed breast cancer with excellent sensitivity (95%) and selectivity (100%) using the suggested model. The sensitivity limitation of the manual immunohistochemistry approach is solved by the AI-assisted immunohistochemical method.

Figure 3. How AI is trained and it predicts tumors in brain.

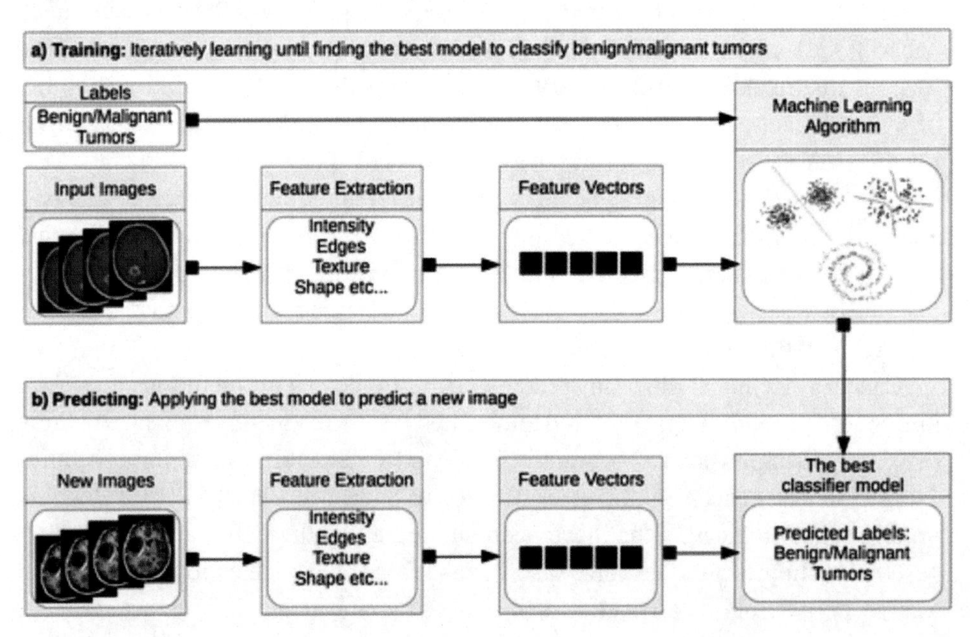

A technique known as deep learning can be used to teach AI to forecast brain cancers using biomedical imaging. This procedure entails teaching a neural network—a type of computer algorithm—to detect patterns in medical photographs. Typically, a collection of medical photographs of brains with and without tumors is used in the procedure. The algorithm is trained using these photos so that it can distinguish the characteristics of tumors in the photographs. Since the algorithm is supervised by the labeled data, this process is known as supervised learning. After the algorithm has been trained, new, unlabeled photos may be analyzed to determine whether or not a tumor is present. Because of the neural network design used in the process, the algorithm may learn from the data and get better with additional training samples.

The dataset used to train the algorithm is essential to the model's effectiveness. The dataset has to be carefully managed, diversified, and population-representative. In order to guarantee the precision and dependability of the predictions, the dataset should also go through a thorough annotation and quality control procedure. The method is verified using a different dataset that was not used during training once the training phase is finished. The algorithm's performance is evaluated throughout the validation phase, and it is ensured that it generalizes effectively to new data. It is vital to remember that medical imaging AI predictions are only as accurate as the data they are trained on, therefore it is crucial to have a wide range of pictures in order to provide reliable findings. Prior to applying the AI model in a clinical context, it's crucial to exercise caution and test the results using a different dataset.

The dataset that was used to train the algorithm is essential to the model's effectiveness. A broad selection of photos that are representative of the population is necessary to get reliable findings. To guarantee the precision and dependability of the predictions, the dataset should also be well-curated and put through strict annotating and quality control procedures.

Another key stage in ensuring the algorithm's performance on untested data is the validation procedure. This is accomplished by testing the model's performance and evaluating how well it generalizes using a different dataset that was not used during the training phase. The AI model should be used with caution in a clinical environment, to sum up. Human specialists should verify the AI algorithm's predictions, and the findings should be utilised in conjunction with other diagnostic techniques. This will guarantee that the AI algorithm's predictions are accurate and trustworthy and that patients get the best care available.

Figure 4. Explaining the processes included in training the AI model.

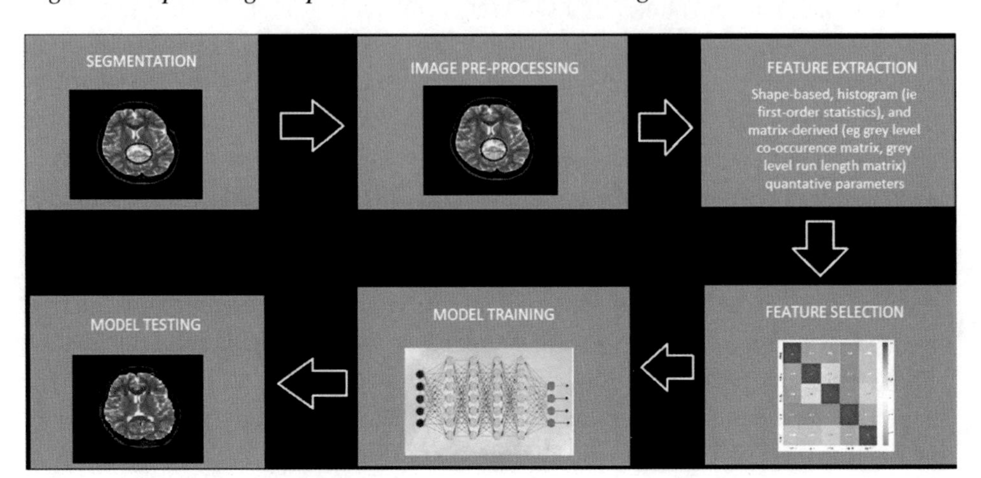

The collection of a sizable dataset of photos that represents the target population is the first stage in teaching AI to understand biological images. This dataset has to be carefully curated, diversified, and labeled with pertinent information, such as the existence of tumors, different types of illnesses, or organs. It should also include both normal and pathological photos. To guarantee that the photos are of a high standard and appropriate for training the AI model, the dataset must be preprocessed once it has been gathered. This procedure could involve deleting any unnecessary photographs, scaling them to a uniform size, or using image enhancing methods to make particular aspects in the images more visible. The subsequent stage involves extracting the important information from the photos and representing them in a way that the AI model can understand. To train the AI model, this procedure can entail converting the photos from their original format to a numerical one. An appropriate model for the job must be chosen once the dataset has been preprocessed and the features have been extracted. Depending on the objective and the dataset, this may contain a variety of models, including deep neural networks, support vector machines, and random forests. Using the retrieved characteristics from the dataset, the chosen model is trained. In order to train the model to detect the patterns in the pictures that are connected to the pertinent information, this method modifies the model's parameters. The model is then tested against a different validation dataset to determine how well it performs and how well it generalizes to new inputs. The model may be improved by changing its parameters and/or gathering more data based on the validation findings. The AI model is prepared for deployment in a real-world environment to analyze new biological pictures once the training and validation processes are finished.

CHALLENGES AND FUTURE PROSPECTS

There have been reports on the benefits of AI in a variety of healthcare fields, including the monitoring of cardiac arrhythmia, the treatment of diabetes, and aided operations. ML assists in efficiently processing large and complicated sensor data for additional analysis and enhancing decision-making skills. AI/ML also aids in the extraction of analytical data from noisy or low-resolution data sources. The AI/ML technique enables the devices to extract the concealed information based on the correlation between the sample parameters and measured signals using SML techniques. The signal strength, sensitivity, specificity, and measurement time are all enhanced using AI approaches.

Even though IoMT-integrated medical devices and healthcare practices have the potential to be revolutionized by AI/ML, a number of technological obstacles still need to be overcome in order to achieve the possibility of commercialization and adaptation in clinics and in society. The emphasis must be on gathering copious amounts of data on high-quality patient training and learning because AI/ML systems largely rely on correct data for programming and training the system. Heterogeneity in the data that have been obtained is another major issue. There are inconsistencies in the training of AI due to bias and noise present in the health records gathered from diverse clinics. The data sets may be homogenized with the use of sophisticated ML algorithms, which will increase the precision of the clinical diagnosis. The future of surgery and the medical industry will flourish with AI-supported methods.

Technology connectivity is essential for connecting people to IoMT devices. Both unidirectional and bidirectional connections are possible. Before being delivered to the microcontroller/processor, the IoMT sensor signal must be processed; this only requires digital data. By replacing the bulk electronics needed for signal conditioning, analogue front ends (AFEs) are used instead. Communication methods including I2C, SPI, and UART are typically used to link AFE to the microcontroller. The AFE and the microcontroller's communication protocols should be compatible. The primary communication options for integrating IoMT devices with the central hub are Wi-Fi and Bluetooth. Bluetooth connection links sensors to different portable devices including tablets, smartphones, and PCs across short distances of up to 10 m at a top speed of 3 Mbps. Bluetooth is particularly used for data transfer in operating rooms, intensive care units, and other places with lots of gadgets. The IoMT devices are connected to the gateway via enterprise Wi-Fi, which offers a better level of service in terms of security and performance. Internet connectivity may be lost while the measuring equipment is in motion, which might result in the loss of important data and delay patient care. Therefore, in order to sustain network persistence for mobile devices in these loud RF situations, the Wi-Fi module must offer enhanced scanning methods.

To correct for electrical and physical flaws, conventional medical gadgets for diagnostics need bulky, sophisticated electronic components. For instance, optical equipment requires a complex enclosure design to define the optical path and eliminate ambient light interference. Optical equipment intended for portable use must constantly reject system noise while detecting low-yield fluorescence. The POC or wearable biosensor devices need portable electronics, in contrast to typical electrochemical biosensors that require huge, costly electrochemical workstations. Single IC solutions, often referred to as AFEs, can be used in place of the necessary bulk electronics. The majority of AFEs come in different packages for various kinds of sensors. For example, Analog Devices Inc.'s AD5940 is exclusively suitable for electrochemical biosensors. With regard to multiplexing several sensor types, such as optical and electrochemical sensors, this AFE has limitations. For connecting with a variety of sensors, the current generation of IoMT devices needs multi-functional AFEs with numerous channels. For instance, the miniature potentiostat (M-P)(Cruz et al., 2014), created by modifying the LMP91000, enables low-power measurement and great sensitivity(Manickam et al., 2019; Manogaran et al., 2018; Gerke et al.,2020). However, the multi-channel M-P interface and subsequent smartphone operation remain difficult while having certain positive qualities.

CONCLUSION

As a result, the use of artificial intelligence in biomedical image processing has had a significant impact on how medical images are evaluated and understood. It is commonly known and well-documented that AI algorithms, such as deep learning, are capable of accurately segmenting photos, spotting anomalies, and classifying images. In fields like radiology, pathology, and ophthalmology, this has substantially increased the accuracy and speed of diagnosis and led to the development of more efficient and effective diagnostic tools. Additionally, the application of AI to biological image processing has accelerated the development of customised medicine and produced novel treatment strategies.

The topic is still in its infancy, and more work must still be done in order to fully realise AI's potential in biomedical image processing. Concerns exist regarding the ethical ramifications of AI in healthcare, including the possibility of prejudice and the lack of decision-making openness.

The manner that medical research is done could likewise be completely changed by AI-based image processing approaches. AI algorithms, for instance, can be used to quickly and accurately spot patterns in massive volumes of medical imaging data, which can substantially help in the identification of prospective drug targets and the discovery of new disease markers. Additionally, preclinical and clinical trial data interpretation can be aided by AI-based image analysis technologies, which can significantly increase the efficacy and precision of drug development.

Additionally, telemedicine greatly benefits from AI in biological image processing. Access to healthcare in rural and underdeveloped areas can be significantly improved by remote diagnosis employing AI-based picture analysis. Additionally, it enables the remote monitoring of patients with long-term diseases, which can significantly raise the standard of treatment in general.

In conclusion, the use of AI in biomedical image processing has significantly increased the timeliness, precision, and effectiveness of diagnoses, treatment regimens, and medical research. Personalized medicine and telemedicine, which have improved access to and equity in healthcare, are being developed in large part thanks to it. Although there are ethical questions about the use of AI in healthcare, the future of AI in biomedical image processing appears bright, and it is likely to play a bigger role in the healthcare sector in the coming years.

However, the integration of AI in biomedical image processing has a bright future, and it is expected to play a bigger and bigger part in the healthcare sector in the years to come.

REFERENCES

Aljamaan, I., & Al-Naib, I. (2021). Prediction of Blood Glucose Level Using Nonlinear System Identification Approach. *IEEE Access: Practical Innovations, Open Solutions*, *10*, 1936–1945. doi:10.1109/ACCESS.2021.3139578

Bellemo, V., Lim, G., Rim, T. H., Tan, G. S., Cheung, C. Y., Sadda, S., He, M., Tufail, A., Lee, M. L., Hsu, W., & Ting, D. S. W. (2019). Artificial intelligence screening for diabetic retinopathy: The real-world emerging application. *Current Diabetes Reports*, *19*(9), 1–12. doi:10.100711892-019-1189-3 PMID:31367962

Cruz, A. F. D., Norena, N., Kaushik, A., & Bhansali, S. (2014). A low-cost miniaturized potentiostat for point-of-care diagnosis. *Biosensors & Bioelectronics*, *62*, 249–254. doi:10.1016/j.bios.2014.06.053 PMID:25016332

Dörr, M., Nohturfft, V., Brasier, N., Bosshard, E., Djurdjevic, A., Gross, S., Raichle, C. J., Rhinisperger, M., Stöckli, R., & Eckstein, J. (2019). The WATCH AF trial: SmartWATCHes for detection of atrial fibrillation. *JACC Clinical Electrophysiology*, *5*(2), 199–208. doi:10.1016/j.jacep.2018.10.006 PMID:30784691

Fan, L., Huang, T., Lou, D., Peng, Z., He, Y., Zhang, X., Gu, N., & Zhang, Y. (2021). Artificial Intelligence-Aided Multiple Tumor Detection Method Based on Immunohistochemistry-Enhanced Dark-Field Imaging. *Analytical Chemistry, 94*(2), 1037–1045. doi:10.1021/acs.analchem.1c04000 PMID:34927419

Gerke, S., Minssen, T., & Cohen, G. (2020). Ethical and legal challenges of artificial intelligence-driven healthcare. In *Artificial intelligence in healthcare* (pp. 295–336). Academic Press. doi:10.1016/B978-0-12-818438-7.00012-5

Grzybowski, A., Brona, P., Lim, G., Ruamviboonsuk, P., Tan, G. S., Abramoff, M., & Ting, D. S. (2020). Artificial intelligence for diabetic retinopathy screening: A review. *Eye (London, England), 34*(3), 451–460. doi:10.103841433-019-0566-0 PMID:31488886

Hamdi, T., Ali, J. B., Fnaiech, N., Di Costanzo, V., Fnaiech, F., Moreau, E., & Ginoux, J. M. (2017, February). Artificial neural network for blood glucose level prediction. In *2017 International Conference on Smart, Monitored and Controlled Cities (SM2C)* (pp. 91-95). IEEE. 10.1109/SM2C.2017.8071825

Hasanzad, M., Aghaei Meybodi, H. R., Sarhangi, N., & Larijani, B. (2022). Artificial intelligence perspective in the future of endocrine diseases. *Journal of Diabetes and Metabolic Disorders, 21*(1), 1–8. doi:10.100740200-021-00949-2 PMID:35673469

Jiang, B., Dong, N., Shou, J., Cao, L., Hu, K., Liu, W., & Qi, X. (2021). Effectiveness of artificial intelligent cardiac remote monitoring system for evaluating asymptomatic myocardial ischemia in patients with coronary heart disease. *American Journal of Translational Research, 13*(10), 11653. PMID:34786091

Jin, P., Ji, X., Kang, W., Li, Y., Liu, H., Ma, F., Ma, S., Hu, H., Li, W., & Tian, Y. (2020). Artificial intelligence in gastric cancer: A systematic review. *Journal of Cancer Research and Clinical Oncology, 146*(9), 2339–2350. doi:10.100700432-020-03304-9 PMID:32613386

Karuppaiah, G., Velayutham, J., Hansda, S., Narayana, N., Bhansali, S., & Manickam, P. (2022). Towards the development of reagent-free and reusable electrochemical aptamer-based cortisol sensor. *Bioelectrochemistry (Amsterdam, Netherlands), 145*, 108098. doi:10.1016/j.bioelechem.2022.108098 PMID:35325786

Khanam, J. J., & Foo, S. Y. (2021). A comparison of machine learning algorithms for diabetes prediction. *ICT Express, 7*(4), 432–439. doi:10.1016/j.icte.2021.02.004

Li, J., Pan, C., Zhang, S., Spin, J. M., Deng, A., Leung, L. L., Dalman, R. L., Tsao, P. S., & Snyder, M. (2018). Decoding the genomics of abdominal aortic aneurysm. *Cell, 174*(6), 1361–1372. doi:10.1016/j.cell.2018.07.021 PMID:30193110

Liu, Z., Li, L., Li, T., Luo, D., Wang, X., & Luo, D. (2020). Does a Deep Learning–Based Computer-Assisted Diagnosis System Outperform Conventional Double Reading by Radiologists in Distinguishing Benign and Malignant Lung Nodules? *Frontiers in Oncology*, *10*, 545862. doi:10.3389/fonc.2020.545862 PMID:33163395

Manickam, P., Kanagavel, V., Sonawane, A., Thipperudraswamy, S. P., & Bhansali, S. (2019). Electrochemical systems for healthcare applications. *Bioelectrochemical Interface Engineering*, 385-409.

Manickam, P., Mariappan, S. A., Murugesan, S. M., Hansda, S., Kaushik, A., Shinde, R., & Thipperudraswamy, S. P. (2022). Artificial intelligence (AI) and internet of medical things (IoMT) assisted biomedical systems for intelligent healthcare. *Biosensors (Basel)*, *12*(8), 562. doi:10.3390/bios12080562 PMID:35892459

Manogaran, G., Chilamkurti, N., & Hsu, C. H. (2018). Emerging trends, issues, and challenges in Internet of Medical Things and wireless networks. *Personal and Ubiquitous Computing*, *22*(5), 879–882. doi:10.100700779-018-1178-6

Mercan, Ö. B., Kılıç, V., & Şen, M. (2021). Machine learning-based colorimetric determination of glucose in artificial saliva with different reagents using a smartphone coupled μPAD. *Sensors and Actuators. B, Chemical*, *329*, 129037. doi:10.1016/j.snb.2020.129037

Nakhleh, M. K., Baram, S., Jeries, R., Salim, R., Haick, H., & Hakim, M. (2016). Artificially intelligent nanoarray for the detection of preeclampsia under real-world clinical conditions. *Advanced Materials Technologies*, *1*(9), 1600132. doi:10.1002/admt.201600132

Pandiaraj, M., Benjamin, A. R., Madasamy, T., Vairamani, K., Arya, A., Sethy, N. K., Bhargava, K., & Karunakaran, C. (2014). A cost-effective volume miniaturized and microcontroller based cytochrome c assay. *Sensors and Actuators. A, Physical*, *220*, 290–297. doi:10.1016/j.sna.2014.10.018

Rigla, M., Martínez-Sarriegui, I., García-Sáez, G., Pons, B., & Hernando, M. E. (2018). Gestational diabetes management using smart mobile telemedicine. *Journal of Diabetes Science and Technology*, *12*(2), 260–264. doi:10.1177/1932296817704442 PMID:28420257

Sadasivam, M., Sakthivel, A., Nagesh, N., Hansda, S., Veerapandian, M., Alwarappan, S., & Manickam, P. (2020). Magnetic bead-amplified voltammetric detection for carbohydrate antigen 125 with enzyme labels using aptamer-antigen-antibody sandwiched assay. *Sensors and Actuators. B, Chemical*, *312*, 127985. doi:10.1016/j.snb.2020.127985

Sakthivel, A., Chandrasekaran, A., Sadasivam, M., Manickam, P., & Alwarappan, S. (2021). Sulphur doped graphitic carbon nitride as a dual biosensing platform for the detection of cancer biomarker CA15–3. *Journal of the Electrochemical Society*, *168*(1), 017507. doi:10.1149/1945-7111/abd927

Sempionatto, J. R., Montiel, V. R. V., Vargas, E., Teymourian, H., & Wang, J. (2021). Wearable and mobile sensors for personalized nutrition. *ACS Sensors*, *6*(5), 1745–1760. doi:10.1021/acssensors.1c00553 PMID:34008960

Sonawane, A., Nasim, S., Shah, P., Ramaswamy, S., Urizar, G., Manickam, P., Mujawar, M., & Bhansali, S. (2020). Communication—Detection of Salivary Cortisol Using Zinc Oxide and Copper Porphyrin Composite Using Electrodeposition and Plasma-Assisted Deposition. *ECS Journal of Solid State Science and Technology: JSS*, *9*(6), 061022. doi:10.1149/2162-8777/aba856

Tseng, P. Y., Chen, Y. T., Wang, C. H., Chiu, K. M., Peng, Y. S., Hsu, S. P., Chen, K.-L., Yang, C.-Y., & Lee, O. K. S. (2020). Prediction of the development of acute kidney injury following cardiac surgery by machine learning. *Critical Care (London, England)*, *24*(1), 1–13. doi:10.118613054-020-03179-9 PMID:32736589

Whipple, A., Bridges, M., Hanson, A., Maddipatla, D., & Atashbar, M. (2022, July). A Fully Flexible Handheld Wireless Estrogen Sensing Device. In *2022 IEEE International Conference on Flexible and Printable Sensors and Systems (FLEPS)* (pp. 1-4). IEEE. 10.1109/FLEPS53764.2022.9781499

Chapter 3
Review and Analysis of Disease Diagnostic Models Using AI and ML

Upasana Pandey
ABES Institute of Technology, India

Rakshit Singh
ABES Institute of Technology, India

Tejveer Shakya
ABES Institute of Technology, India

Tanish Mangal
ABES Institute of Technology, India

Meet Rajput
ABES Institute of Technology, India

ABSTRACT

Recently, disease prediction using diagnostic reports and images are one of the most popular applications of artificial intelligence (AI) and machine learning (ML). Several authors reported significant results in this area by combining cutting-edge hardware with AI and ML-based technologies. In this chapter, the authors present a review of different works carried for the prediction of several chronic diseases by researchers in last five years. Reported AI and ML based methodologies have been used to forecast chronic disease such as heart problems, brain tumors, asthma, diabetes, cholera, arthritis, liver diseases, kidney diseases, malaria, and leukemia. In the literature, the authors also discuss the different user interfaces which have been used to interact with real time AI and ML based disease prediction models. The authors have presented the detailed discussion of each paper including advantages, disadvantages, datasets, performance metrics such as precision, recall, accuracy and F1 score. In the final section, the survey concludes with a description of research gaps that can be addressed by future research attempts.

DOI: 10.4018/978-1-6684-6957-6.ch003

INTRODUCTION

Many organisations have been founded around the world in this digital era to supply equipment for continuous monitoring of people's health. Patients visit the clinic, and health professionals use a traditional method to advice patients based on their knowledge of the condition (Simarjeet Kaur et al, 2020; Md Manjurul Ahsan et al, 2022; Samir Malakar et al, 2022). Traditional approaches can occasionally result in subpar patient care, which can be harmful. They are also costly. As a result, technology offers an alternative to the old system, such as the introduction of a large number of computer-assisted support systems and instruments into healthcare systems (Kaustubh Arun Bhavsar et al, 2021 ; Samir Malakar et al, 2022). This bonding thus reduced treatment costs while also enhancing patient care. In this context, it's important to note that over the past six years, data mining and machine learning (ML) techniques have gained significant popularity in healthcare and patient care systems due to the increasing accessibility of digital documents and data. According to the World Health Organization's (WHO) third worldwide research on electronic health (eHealth) published in 2016, there has been a consistent increase in the usage of electronic health records (EHR) during the last 15 years, with a global increase of 46.009% in the last five years (Samir Malakar et al 2022).

A disease is an abnormal condition that primarily impacts a portion of an organ and is unrelated to damage from the outside world. There are numerous different diseases in the field of medicine, including acute, infectious, inherited, and chronic (Igor Barone de Medeiros et al, 2017). There are around 2 million people who have been diagnosed with diseases such as heart disease, brain tumours, asthma, diabetes, cholera, arthritis, chronic liver disease, renal illness, malaria, and leukaemia. This figure is very large on a global scale, demonstrating the importance of early detection of many diseases (Md Manjurul Ahsan et al 2022; Samir Malakar et al 2022). In terms of mortality, heart disease, brain tumours, asthma, diabetes, cholera, arthritis, chronic liver disease, renal illness, malaria, and leukaemia are the major diseases. Most studies in developed countries show that the number of people affected by these diseases and dying as a result of them has increased by up to 300% in the last three decades (Samir Malakar et al 2022).

The primary goal of artificial intelligence (AI) is to create algorithms and techniques for determining system's behaviour in disease diagnosis is correct or not. Machine learning (ML) is used in practically every area, from high technology. More and more industries are using machine learning, including healthcare to diagnose diseases (Md Manjurul Ahsan et al 2022; Kaustubh Arun Bhavsar et al, 2021). The potential of automatic diagnostic system which is both time and cost-effective, has been shown by several researchers and practitioner. We give a review in this paper that highlights emerging applications of ML and DL to provide some clarity on the present trend, approaches, and difficulties associated with ML in illness diagnosis, this paper describes the evolution in this subject and provides an overview of those developments (Md Manjurul Ahsan et al 2022).

The use of chatbots to speed up doctor-patient communication for disease diagnosis has emerged as a potential avenue (Sambit Satpathy et al, 2019). Such chats are more popular as synchronous text-based discussion systems are employed for remote health interventions. The use of chatbots may be most beneficial to people with long-term illnesses since they can continually keeping an eye on their health, provide accurate, information that is current and a reminder to take medication. Chatbot technology needs sophisticated reasoning abilities based on the formalisation of medical information and patient health status, as well as language vocabularies and dialogue engines, in order to be effective in the healthcare domain (Nicholas A. I. Omoregbe et al, 2020).

RELATED WORK

Disease

Heart Disease

Machine learning (ML) techniques are typically used by researchers and clinicians to detect heart problems (Ahsan et al 2022; Malakar et al 2022). For instance, Ansari et al. (2011) provided an automated method for diagnosing coronary heart disease using fuzzy logic integrated systems that offers roughly 89% accuracy (Omoregbe et al, 2020; Jatav & Sharma, 2018). The heart disease dataset from the UCI repository is one frequently used dataset. This dataset has a total of 76 attributes (one class attribute and 75 prognostic attributes) (Malakar et al 2022). In particular, the Cleveland data set is a data set that researchers use very often to predict heart disease. In the literature, we discussed works that used a single classifier to classify heart disease. Systems using a single classifier make use of NN model variations, the FS approach prior to categorization, imputation of missing values, and benchmarking research to create better models (Malakar et al 2022). Neural network framework techniques are widely used in the literature. Recent findings on the heart disease classification problem using parameter adjustment or more hidden layers in MLP with the backpropagation technique have been referenced in several studies (de Medeiros et al, 2017; Malakar et al, 2022). In addition, deep learning (DL)-based algorithms in cardiac disease detection have recently received attention (Medeiros et al, 2017). The developed model aids in the differentiation physical characteristics of those with heart disease. Their first estimates show an F score of

0.85 and an accuracy of 85.01% (Malakar et al 2022). In addition, in most cases, the explaining ability of the model is lacking during the final prediction. However, (de Medeiros et al, 2017) provides additional details on the detection of heart illness using machine learning.

Brain Tumor

For studies on brain tumors, magnetic resonance imaging (MRI) is the screening technique of choice. A single MRI scan can yield a vast amount of information and detail. The radiologist is faced with more sources of evidence but fewer testing tools when he needs to make a diagnosis (Dhaval Raval et al, 2016). The information content of the damaged organ region has been measured using multiparametric quantitative MRI data in several attempts, although these have been substantially less successful than traditional MRI studies (Ray & Chaudhuri, 2020). The majority of solutions rely on one of the opposing viewpoints: whereas the first manual delineation of the ROI is devoted to more sophisticated feature extraction techniques, segmentation approaches are conventional segmentation approaches based on many standard MRI maps (Awotunde, 2014). Through the use of image processing tools, the size of the brain tumor is calculated. Thresholding and area-increasing algorithms have drawbacks, but K-means and Fuzzy C-means effectively forecast brain regions and phase the tumor (Awotunde, 2014; Ray & Chaudhuri, 2020). The fuzzy C-Means method produces tumor margin accuracy by using the performance of the K-Means algorithm as feedback. This demonstrates how brain cancers can be identified and categorized using fuzzy logic and neural networks (Ahsan et al 2022). Other frameworks, like ANN, employ various deep learning neural networks to generate accurate results, but the yield of these schemes and systems was slower because they required a lot of hardware computation (J.B. Awotunde, 2014).

Chronic Liver Disease

Hepatology was the field that saw the introduction of AI after gastroenterology. Even so, recent developments in the field of AI research have increased. Hepatology AI can be used to diagnose non-alcoholic fatty liver disease, find focal liver lesions, forecast chronic liver disease, and detect liver fibrosis (Ray & Chaudhuri, 2020). In the end, we anticipate that AI will assist in manipulating those who have liver disease, forecasting clinical outcomes, and lowering medical errors. There are some obstacles, though, that must be surmounted. We may now briefly describe the aspects of liver disease where AI can be used (de Medeiros et al, 2017). We conducted a thorough search of the literature on hepatic fibrosis aided by AI and NAFLD diagnosis in MEDLINE, Scopus, Web of Science, and Google Scholar.

Using random-effects models, 95% confidence intervals (95% CI) might be used to calculate the aggregate sensitivity, selectivity, true positive rate, negative predictive value, and diagnostic probability value (Ray & Chaudhuri, 2020). It was for the purpose of evaluating the diagnostic efficacy of the AI-assisted system, receiver operating curve and area under the curve was constructed. There were subgroup studies by population, AI classifier, and diagnostic modality.

Leukemia

The lymphatic system and bone marrow are among the body's blood-forming components that are affected by leukaemia, a cancer. There are several different types of leukaemia. Some kinds of leukaemia are more common in children. The majority of adults who develop other kinds of leukaemia do so. Leukemia primarily affects white blood cells (Amato et al, 2013). The analysis of blood or bone marrow samples frequently reveals the presence of cancer in the lymphatic system. In 2020, a team from the University of Bonn under the direction of Prof. Dr. Peter Krawitz demonstrated how artificial intelligence can aid in treating diseases like lymphomas and leukemia diagnosis. The technology has now been refined, a big step towards clinical application, so that even smallest labs may take use of this free system. A big new feature of AI that is now being introduced is the possibility of knowledge transfer: This can be advantageous for smaller laboratories that lack the resources to construct their own AI from scratch and may also have insufficient sample sizes (Amato et al, 2013). The AI may use information acquired from tens of thousands of datasets after a brief training phase during which it learns the characteristics of a new lab.

Kidney Disease

Chronic renal disease is one of the leading causes of mortality globally and a significant public health issue. The physiological operation of numerous organs, particularly the cardiovascular system, is affected by this enigmatic, extremely complicated, and progressive disorder. CKD raises the expense of healthcare. As a cutting-edge science and technology, artificial intelligence (AI) is heavily utilised in the medical industry, primarily to increase medical treatment such early disease detection, diagnosis, and management (Arkadip Ray and Avijit Kumar Chaudhuri, 2020). Kidney disease continues to be a global health issue because of its high prevalence. Its diagnosis and therapy continue to be difficult. AI takes into account each person's circumstances when making judgments, which could result in significant improvements in the management of kidney disease. Here, we examine recent studies on AI applications for kidney disease warning systems, diagnostic assistance, therapeutic direction, and prognosis evaluation. Clinicians are aware of the promise of AI in treating kidney illness, despite the fact that the topic has received very little research (Igor Barone de Medeiros et al, 2017). Clinical settings in the future will benefit considerably from AI in terms of clinician competencies. By scanning PubMed up to 1 August 2019 (Ray & Chaudhuri, 2020), an ad hoc literature search was conducted. Use keywords like nephrology, artificial intelligence, deep learning, artificial neuron networks, chronic kidney disease, acute kidney damage, and renal disease in your searches. AI is also being researched for CKD problems early warning. According to Galloway et al., a deep learning model containing just two of his ECG leads was able to detect hypercalcemia in individuals with renal illness with an AUC.

Malaria

Parasites are the cause of the illness malaria. Through the bite of an infected mosquito, the parasite is transferred to people. Typically, malaria results in serious sickness, involving a high temperature and chills. Despite being rare in temperate climates, malaria is still widespread in tropical and subtropical countries. The creation of low-cost automated digital microscopy that can quickly photograph whole slides is necessary for the full usage of AI (Nkuma-Udah et al, 2018). Second, no local malaria slide bank that already exists has created a digital online repository. As a result, most AI studies were trained on private datasets and only used data from the National Institutes of Health's Malaria Database, which contains 27,558 images of the Plasmodium falciparum and Plasmodium vivax species. One sizable multicenter study is among these investigations. His 500-slide-trained system was evaluated using rare yet physically distinct species of Knowles, Ovalle, and malaria from 11 different countries. lacks reliable data After COVID-19, cross-border travel increases, existing malaria controls are disturbed, and due to skewed datasets, acquired non-falciparum malaria and non-vivax malaria infections are overlooked by AI. There is a chance (Nkuma-Udah et al, 2018). To supplement data on unusual malaria species, we suggest that existing regional slide banks for malaria digitise slides and make them available as publicly accessible electronic databases. An overview of image standards for training, downstream validation, and quality assurance of reliable AI solutions for malaria can be supplied by developing a global digital repository, which is the final step.

Cholera

By fusing climate data from satellites orbiting the planet with artificial intelligence (AI) technology, cholera outbreaks in coastal areas of India can be forecast for a fulfilment cost of 89 cents. They claim that by learning to identify patterns and provide testable predictions from enormous data sets, research algorithms in AI and ML can aid in resolving these issues (Ray & Chaudhuri, 2020). Infectious illness detection and early warning, trend forecasting, and public health response and assessment are all common uses for artificial intelligence (AI) technologies. These vital duties of public health surveillance and response pose special technical difficulties. B. Inadequate data. Epidemiological data are a major source of information in traditional public health. In recent years, especially in affluent nations, AI-powered methods have grown significantly, and they now complement statistical methodologies. This chapter's goal is to carefully analyse the most recent developments in using AI approaches to address the cholera pandemic and problems associated with surveillance and response (Ray & Chaudhuri, 2020). Due to poor access to clean water, sanitation, and hygiene, the bacteria that causes cholera, Vibrio cholera, still exists in impoverished nations. An estimated 4 million illnesses and 143,000 fatalities from cholera occur each year. Fecal-oral means that the disease is spread by tainted food or water. Rapid fluid and electrolyte loss from severe dehydrating cholera can cause hypovolemic shock, necessitating an IV fluid infusion very away. Without proper clinical therapy, mortality can reach over 50% but can drop to less than 1% with quick rehydration and antibiotics. During outbreaks or in places where the disease is endemic, incorporating oral cholera vaccines (OCVs) into integrated management strategies is essential. Health education, water, sanitation, and hygiene, prophylactic antibiotic therapy, and other aspects are additional components of cholera prevention and control.

Arthritis

Arthritis symptoms include one or more joints aching and swelling. The basic symptoms of arthritis are stiffness and pain in the joints, which frequently become worse with aging. The two most common forms of arthritis are rheumatoid arthritis and osteoarthritis. X-ray, MRI, and CT imaging joint detection is one of the most important and challenging processes in the automated analysis of arthritis (Omoregbe et al., 2020). The methodologies for recent ML-based joint detection that have been picked up by AI algorithms for analysing arthritis are reviewed below. The research team concentrated their studies on the metacarpophalangeal joints of the fingers, which are frequently damaged early in the course of inflammatory disorders such rheumatoid arthritis or psoriatic arthritis in patients (de Medeiros et al., 2017). High-resolution peripheral quantitative computed tomography (HR-pQCT) finger scans were used to train an artificial neural network to recognise "healthy" joints from those of people with rheumatoid or psoriatic arthritis. We are pleased with the study's findings because they demonstrate how artificial intelligence can make it easier to categorise arthritis, which may result in patients receiving speedier and more precise care (Omoregbe et al., 2020). We are aware that the network needs to receive data from additional categories, though.

Asthma

The analysis of bronchial allergies may be achieved in two ways: 1) via a questionnaire, and 2) via scientific data. Expert systems have been developed using both approaches. Through questionnaires, linguistic neural networks are used, and through clinical data, deep learning is used, which uses a mathematical approach to diagnose the disease.

For this, a convolutional neural network and an LSTM neural network were used (Ibrahim & Abdulazeez, 2021). A subset of machine learning called "deep learning" includes some nonlinear transformations. It makes use of diverse algorithms that can discover ways to view and enter statistics through the use of numerous layers of processing with complex structures. CNN is broadly hired in facial recognition, textual content analysis, organ location in the human, and organic photograph detection or recognition. The UCI repository data was found to be the database that lecturers and practitioners choose to use for creating a machine-learning-based full illness diagnostic model. However, despite the fact that modern-day datasets frequently have flaws, many researchers now rely on extra information obtained from a hospital or clinic (i.e., imbalance information, missing information) (Ahsan et al., 2022).

Diabetes

Diabetic retinopathy results from harm to the blood vessels within the tissue at the back of the eye (the retina). Poorly managed blood sugar is a danger factor. Floaters, blurriness, darkish regions of vision, and difficulty perceiving colours are early signs and symptoms of blindness (Bakator & Radosav, 2018).

To classify diabetic retinopathy, a 78,000-image dataset of the fundus is used to train a convolutional neural network. The accuracy and sensitivity were 75% and 95%, respectively.

There are presently more than 400 million diabetics worldwide, and by 2045, that number is projected to increase to 629 million, according to the International Diabetes Federation (IDF). Several studies have extensively offered ML-primarily based totally structures for diabetes patient detection. For instance, (Kandhasamy & Balamurali, 2015) examined machine learning (ML) classifiers for identifying diabetes mellitus patients. The UCI Diabetes dataset was used for the test, and the KNN (K = 1) and RF classifiers had nearly perfect accuracy. However, one drawback of this painting is that the simplest eight binary-categorized characteristics from a simplified diabetes dataset were employed. As a result, achieving 100% accuracy with a much easier dataset is not surprising. Furthermore, the test does not address how the algorithms affect the final prediction or how the outcome should be viewed from a non-technical perspective. (Ahsan et al 2022).

Graphical User Interface

To learn more about the user's or patient's fundamental individual details like gender, age, height, and weight, the system starts a dialogue or chat with them. After gathering the fundamental information, the Doctor advances to the next stage and asks the patient questions about their symptoms in accordance with the previous algorithms. The GUI design was developed with the use of the Telegram API, which also offers a custom keyboard (Omoregbe et al, 2020). Since the app is available for all mobile devices and does not require an Internet connection, the SMS text request and answer were included to facilitate communication. The Python wrapper used to conduct Telegram API communication is the python-telegram-API package (Omoregbe et al, 2020; Igor Barone de Medeiros et al, 2017). In recent years, several medical Chatbot designs have been put forth with the goal of recommending medications to the user after identifying their disease from their conversations (de Medeiros et al, 2017). Using Chatter Bean, a JAVA-based AIML interpreter, this chatbot concept was created. To use the recommended design, which employs AIML patterns to identify the illness names, the user must submit a message that must contain the illness name. When a disease is identified, the chatbot gives the user pertinent information about the problem. The earlier suggested designs did not concentrate on comprehending the severity of the ailment that the person is experiencing (Omoregbe et al, 2020; de Medeiros et al, 2017).

Table 1. Summary for Literature Survey

Reference.	Methodology	Dataset	Result with performance parameter	Conclusion	Future scope
(Kaur et al, 2020)	A systematic review	Various research paper	For a certain database, multiple models offer varying degrees of accuracy.	Manufacturing choices might be made using mathematical models. Using ML in medical diagnostics is primarily intended to increase the precision with which illnesses are identified. This thorough study emphasises the application of ML for efficient therapy diagnosis. It has been noted that ML has becoming increasingly more often used in medical diagnostics over time.	Better datasets should be used to remove data inconsistency.
(Ahsan et al 2022)	A Comprehensive Review	Cleveland dataset, chronic kidney disease dataset, BCSC, DIABIM-MUNE, Parkinson's ml dataset	Although many studies have used an unbalanced data set to conduct their experiment, one of the cited papers highlights the problems associated with unbalanced data.	75 publications were carefully chosen for in-depth research. The discussion sections have emphasised our general findings. Our key finding shows that deep learning is the most widely used approach for academics due to its outstanding effectiveness in creating a robust model.	Future research can utilise much more effective algorithms to better correctly diagnose certain diseases.
(Bhavsar et al, 2021)	A diagnostic system using fuzzy logic	Privately owned data.	The primary goal fuzzy set principle and fuzzy common sense a use the tolerance that exists in inaccurate, vague, or in part genuine facts to achieve extra sturdy and less expensive solutions	In addition to prescribing and treating, diagnosing diseases remains the primary responsibility of medical staff and creating an automated diagnostic system to support easy decision-making and rapid identification of diseases affecting a patient. In regions of the world where malaria is common, incorporating fuzzy logic into the design of such an automated system offers creative and expert ways to diagnose malaria.	Furthermore, the implementation of Fuzzy logic in medical diagnostic system will limit the work of doctors in consulting.
(Zhou et al, 2021)	An algorithm for medical diagnosis	Privately owned data	This algorithm provides 95.3% accuracy.	The only way to significantly improve the accuracy of our medical diagnoses and the speed of treatment is to use artificial intelligence to develop an intelligent medical diagnosis system, update it frequently, add classic cases and new cases, and provide adequate diagnostic tools.	More diseases should be included in the models.
(Awotunde, 2014)	Developed a diagnostic system using fuzzy logic	Privately owned data	In order to determine the most precise method for disease detection, the review assessed the eight most popular databases, which had a total of 95 articles.	On the basis of the findings of this study, we were also able to pinpoint locations and ailments that utilised AI but went unnoticed. The page also includes a quick summary of any peer-reviewed papers employing fuzzy logic, machine learning, or deep learning that are currently accessible.	The findings of this paper demonstrate that ML algorithms have a greater potential to significantly improve medical diagnostic systems.
(Omoregbe et al, 2020)	A chatbot-based diagnosis system using NLP and SVM classifier	Personal dataset prepared from a medical database	The scores are 31.56 for ROUGE-L and 25.29 for bilingual assessment understudy.	Timely access to health care without wasting patients' time is a significant issue in sub-Saharan Africa. This study was able to create a text-based medical diagnosis system based on the indicated needs that successfully suggests a disease diagnosis while providing tailored diagnoses.	Future recommendations include automating this system, treatment recommendations, medication prescribing, and medication adherence.

Continued on following page

Table 1. Continued

Reference.	Methodology	Dataset	Result with performance parameter	Conclusion	Future scope
(Aljurayfani et al, 2019)	A recommendation system that predicts cancer using MLP (Multilayer perceptron) and suggests medical services.	UCI Machine Learning Repository.	MLP classifier was selected since it offered the best accuracy.	This study suggested utilizing an artificial neural network to create a cervical cancer self-diagnosis system. In the post, a description of the system and some sample instances were provided.	In the future, more datasets from the hospital are going to be implemented.
(Uvaliyeva et al, 2018)	A differential diagnosis algorithm	Personal dataset	The resultant Accuracy is 80.90%.	The created software was evaluated using patient anamnesis data, which allowed for the diagnosis of disorders and the prescription of symptoms. The Bayesian method proved to be difficult to use for a modest sample, so a new data processing method based on the idea of the scalar product was developed.	comparing a novel approach against an established one in order to determine which sickness is most likely to exist.
(Satpathy et al, 2019)	An FPGA device that predicts pathological conditions using a fuzzy classifier.	UCI repository database.	Accuracy is 89%, sens1t1v1ty is 84%, specificity is 86.4%, and F-measure is 85.67%.	This study covers the difficulties involved in creating a smart healthcare system, such as the system's rising complexity, which raises energy costs and design expenses. Various new computational methods are proposed to overcome these shortcomings. In this study, we propose an FPGA fuzzy classifier implementation for IoT-based healthcare systems.	An IoT-based device can be deployed in the future to anticipate various pathological stages of illnesses based on the model described in this work.
(de Medeiros et al, 2017)	An inference system using fuzzy logic	Personal dataset.	The findings revealed a 9% error rate in the case of medical diagnosis. Cases without an automated diagnosis system showed an inaccuracy of 20%.	All factors were chosen from the subject's survey; which ones are pertinent for patient evaluation, concentrating on the fundamental necessity to provide a higher standard of living and a healthy existence to reduce the likelihood of developing future health issues.	The research's next phase will involve integrating this system with other artificial intelligence tools used in the instruction of medical students.
(Jatav & Sharma, 2018)	An algorithm to diagnose using SVM and random forest.	National Institute of Diabetes and University of California Irvine	This algorithm Provide 99.35% accuracy, 100% recall, 98.21% precision, and 99.1%	The relevant work investigation of several methodologies, including neural networks, naïve Bayes, SVM, K nearest neighbour, etc., is shown in this research, and it is concluded that SVM offers the highest performance now in use. The research led to the invention of the suggested method employing SVM and RF techniques.	Future data mining techniques might be used to create an improved intelligent system that delivers precise and effective outcomes.
(Park et al, 2018)	Analyses of Statistical Techniques for Calibration, Discrimination, and Performance Evaluation of Diagnostic Performance	Medical records are used as datasets.	The author of this paper uses statistical methods to measure the results. Cross-validation and ROC curve	The authors clarify crucial method factors taking part in a medical assessment of artificial intelligence to be used in drugs, specifically excessively detailed or parameterized people or predictive fashions wherein synthetic deep neural networks are used, drawing heavily on medical epidemiology and biostatistics.	This research paper does not include a demonstration of the actual algorithms that would be used to evaluate clinical performance.

Continued on following page

Table 1. Continued

Reference.	Methodology	Dataset	Result with performance parameter	Conclusion	Future scope
(Sudha, 2018)	Various microarray gene expression tools are used, such as Bioconductor, gene pattern, cytospace, BRB array tools, and Thermo Fisher Scientific All these tools are open source.	Gene Expression Omnibus, NCBI, ArrayExpress at EBI, the ImmGen database, and the GeneNetwork system	The collective accuracy of the tools is 96.75%.	This paper indicates the powerful strategies to discover remedies for inherited illnesses through the use of superior genomic and gene sequencing technologies, including microarrays, next-generation sequencing, machine learning, sample recognition, and various high-throughput computational methods.	In the future, more genetic data will be available that could help identify hereditary diseases.
(Bakator & Radosav et al, 2018)	The neural networks used for classification are CNN, DBN-NN, SDAE, CRNN, SA-SVM, CSDCNN, RBM, DL-CNN, and CAD classifiers with deep features from autoencoders.	The data sources are computed tomography, MRI, ultrasound of the lungs and breasts, CT, clinical images, and various medical datasets.	In terms of precision, sensitivity, and specificity of the complete model were 99.68%, 100%, and 99.47%, respectively.	Future traits in deep learning and gaining knowledge of promise will be added to numerous fields of medicine, particularly in scientific diagnostics. However, because it stands, it isn't always clear whether or not gaining deep knowledge can update the position of the doctor or clinician in scientific diagnosis. So far, deepening knowledge can effectively guide scientific professionals.	A foremost quandary of this paper is the dearth of a meta-evaluation of quantitative data. A theoretical introduction to destiny critiques is likewise recommended.
(Qiaoyi Li et al, 2022)	Synthesis and clinical procedures, data augmentation strategy, model comparison spectral analysis and spectral analysis using SERS measurements and applications to clinical samples	Datasets are not provided.	CNN showed the best performance in 5-fold cross-validation.	The author of this study assessed CNN's overall performance and different not-unusual facts evaluation techniques, which include PLSR, SVR, RFR, and SD on multiplexed spectral demixing SERS spectra and the use of Raman-energetic dye-categorized nanorattle probes. However, CNN's evaluation produced the most accurate and quick forecasts, which needed more processing power and memory for educating the public on the usage of large datasets.	The number of data points in the datasets could have been increased to improve the accuracy of the models.
(Kudina, & de Boer, 2021)	A philosophical evaluation using conceptual frameworks of hermeneutics and technical mediation	This paper represents a philosophical analysis of using machine learning for medical diagnosis, so no datasets were used.	Following the hermeneutic version of clinical diagnosis, the writer revisits the idea of bias and indicates that bias is a vital and efficient part of the diagnosis.	The author shows that a machine-learning system assists physicians and patients in co-designing the medical diagnostic triad. He emphasises the significance of considering the hermeneutic position of systems research.	This paper fails to account for various techniques and diseases, which may challenge its credibility.

Continued on following page

Table 1. Continued

Reference.	Methodology	Dataset	Result with performance parameter	Conclusion	Future scope
(Ibrahim & Abdulazeez, 2021)	Different algorithms were used to diagnose different diseases, and the best ones were selected, for example, CNN for COVID-19, SVM and KNN for skin cancer, and Nave Bayes, KNN, and SVM for thyroid.	All the datasets that are used are freely available, including on GitHub, Kaggle, the ISIC 2017 dataset, and the UCI data repository.	The following are the results of the models trained for COVID-19: 94%, skin cancer 97.8%, and thyroid cancer 98%.	Computational machine learning instruction sets play an extremely important role in early disease detection (achieved or won with effort). It has been used to treat numerous disorders including liver disease, long-term breast cancer, heart disease, brain tumors, and many others.	The number of data points in the datasets could have been increased to improve the accuracy of the models, and different neural networks could have been used for better results.
(Okokpujie et al, 2017)	This suggested system may be viewed using a web browser and was created using HTML, CSS, Javascript, JSON, Ajax, PHP, and MySQL for the database.	It has data set from Covenant University, Ota, Ogun State, Nigeria.	Based on the information provided by the user and patient, the designed system will assist in diagnosing symptoms and prescribing the appropriate prescription.	The engineered system will help diagnose symptoms and depending on the information given by the user or patient, prescribe the appropriate medicine. The system is robust and uses artificial intelligence	Better implementation and more datasets should be used.
(Xu et al, 2021)	Analysis of the Big Data Collection, Storage, Statistical Analysis, and Intelligent Assistant Diagnosis modules	No dataset	This study illustrates the precision of many properties in various brain wave frequency ranges.	With the new network protocol, the intelligent medical system operates more quickly and performs better while looking for common item sets.	In future, the Wave function can be used more efficiently.
(Ratawal, & Zade 2021)	Study procedures involve gathering test data including patient information, extracting the data, choosing characteristics, pre-processing the dataset, and contrasting different classifiers.	It is open problem and it does not have any data set	This Al technique for medical diagnosis provides an accuracy of around 89%.	Recent advances in AI technology have created an unbeatable applications of AI in healthcare. A hotly debated subject is whether AI data systems will someday displace human doctors.	In the future, we will be able to use a variety of AI approaches to identify any disease or to speed up the diagnosis of all diseases.

Continued on following page

Table 1. Continued

Reference.	Methodology	Dataset	Result with performance parameter	Conclusion	Future scope
(Raval et al, 2016)	A diagnosis system using DSS.	Data set of Swine Flu from the Civil Hospital Ahmadabad.	The DSS's correctness is very important in the medical system. The prospective technique gives a description of its forecast in the form of a judgment tree even though it does not achieve high accuracy, sensitivity, and specificity rates.	In this study, various data mining techniques for medical prediction are examined together with the present medical diagnosing system. With the use of network learning and data mining, the focus is on merging various techniques and goal criteria.	The proposed work will be improved upon in order to automate a more precise swine flu disease prediction.
(Faris et al, 2021)	1. Data collection and processing 2. Feature extraction 3. symptom diagnosis model 4. evaluation criteria	In this author's study on the Altibbi company information	The combination of the two modules has demonstrated strong potential for enhancing prediction outcomes and offering a more trustworthy alternative diagnosis.	The final model is the result of the late fusion of two models using a number of different methods. It obtains the maximum accuracy performance (84,9%).	In the future, we will have large-scale databases to improve machine learning models.
(Zhang, Weng, & Lund, 2022)	XAI framework for breast cancer.	Cholec80 dataset	This research suggests that various machine-learning techniques or For many medical XAI applications, deep learning methods are the best options.	We offered a paper abstract that discussed the present restrictions and potential future uses of XAI in medicine. In the multidisciplinary study of both medicine and artificial intelligence.	In the future, the author believes to provide information to lessen the discrepancy between AI and diagnostics in medicine.
(Miller, 1994)	The utilisation of simple procedures like lexical matching to produce outstanding diagnostic performance raises a philosophical question for all MDDS system developers.	There are no such datasets available like others.	Future experimental and creative implementations were made possible by the conceptual framework for MIDDS system construction that was created between 1950 and 1960.	It is well known that large-scale, generic MDDS systems can be beneficial in medical education, regardless of the extent to which they are used in actual practise.	Systems using MIDDS are becoming more varied. All of these elements will guarantee that innovative and effective MDDS applications are created, assessed, and used.
Malakar et al, 2022)	There are several methods used according to this but different for every other disease.	Breast cancer, Lung Cancer, Leukemia dataset.	One of the most rapidly expanding applications in recent years is disease prediction utilising performance parameters from diagnostic reports and pathology images.	This means that chronic illnesses typically last longer in human organs, and more crucially, there are no openings to stop this illness. As a result, this survey also aims to highlight some potential future paths that the researcher should take into account in order to make the system relevant for medical practitioners.	The dataset used in this research paper lacked numbers and a greater accuracy could be achieved with better datasets.

Continued on following page

Table 1. Continued

Reference.	Methodology	Dataset	Result with performance parameter	Conclusion	Future scope
(Ray & Chaudhuri, 2020)	This imputation-based approach uses the full set of available data to estimate and fill in the missing data with plausible values. The dataset is then imputed and used to build the classifier.	healthcare datasets, and medical datasets.	According to the article that was read and discussed, the properties of the datasets and the size between the training and testing sets affect how well ML approaches function.	In order to aid doctors in making judgments, clinical decision-making assistance systems commonly use ML and DM approaches. Additionally, our research demonstrates that different new ML algorithms have various degrees of accuracy even when using the same dataset. A new machine-learning method will be developed to offer complete and reliable forecasts for further work.	This research report emphasises the importance of timing as another crucial choice. Additionally, there is no suitable DM technique to solve all of the problems.
(Xu, Shi, & Tu et al, 2021)	To manage all forms of data processing, Hadoop is used. Map-reduce and HDFS are both part of Hadoop.	To support this investigation, no data set was used.	The huge data collecting module's superiority in this study is shown by contrasting it with the dispersed system.	The results of the simulation experiments performed on each algorithm and system module demonstrate the rationale and viability of the research on diagnostic information.	In the long run, as people's living standards continue to rise, they are paying greater attention to their health.
(Amato et al, 2013)	This suggested system was created utilising a variety of applications and is based on AI.	It is an open resource and it does not have any data set.	Findings show that methods for distilling and expounding on insightful data are ongoing and can considerably help with precise, efficient, and fast medical diagnosis.	ANN is a potent tool that can assist doctors with diagnosis and other tasks. In this aspect, ANNs have a number of benefits. The ability to digest a lot of data and a lower chance of missing important information 3 Shortening the time for diagnosis.	Authors believe that it can help us as medical professionals and in new medical applications.
(Nkuma-Udah et al, 2018)	The knowledge base for the MDES shell was created by compiling information from experts in the field of medicine that specialises in treating malaria.	There are no such datasets are provided in this research paper.	The MDES system offers suggestions for both diagnostic and therapeutic measures for malaria and related disorders, in accordance with the findings. Traditional relational databases should not be used to evaluate various possibilities for making decisions.	It is also important to emphasise that the MDES system developed here, like previous expert systems, is simply meant to be a supplemental tool and is not meant to take the role of clinician-expert activities. This includes extending the system to encompass other infectious and endemic diseases prevalent in emerging nations.	In light of the future, we are ready to increase the MDES's capabilities in next projects.

DISCUSSION

The process of deciding which disease best describes a person's symptoms is known as disease diagnosis. The most challenging issue is diagnosis since certain symptoms and indications lack specificity. Disease detection is the most important point in treating any disease. Based on prior training data, machine learning is the field that can assist in predicting illness diagnoses. To accurately identify a variety of illnesses, several scientists have created various machine-learning techniques. The ability for machines to learn without specialised programming is provided by machine learning.

In machine learning, there are many methods that can be used to predict diseases, as we can use a regressive model to predict the possibilities of disease. We can also develop a graphical user interface to create a more user-friendly medical diagnosis and use the SVM classifier as a choice for medical diagnosis. Deep learning can provide better accuracy in diagnosis, as a multi-layer perceptron provides a more accurate classification of whether a person is a cervical cancer patient or not than logistic regression and nave classification. The diseases that are hereditary can also be diagnosed at an early stage using gene expression profiling and applying various ML techniques to them.

Diseases and health conditions such as liver cancer, chronic kidney cancer, breast cancer, diabetes, and cardiac syndrome are just a few conditions that can be deadly if ignored and have major health effects. Numerous classifiers and clustering algorithms, including k-nearest, decision tree, random forest, support vector machine (SVM), Naive Bayes, and others, can offer a solution to this problem as a result of developments in machine learning and artificial intelligence.

Convolutional neural networks (CNNs) are the most widely used for deep learning and medical image analysis. It can be said that the applications of deep learning techniques are widespread; however, the majority of applications are targeted at bioinformatics, medical diagnostics, and other similar fields.

We should also keep in mind that there should be a method to classify which algorithm is better than the other for some specific diseases, as the evaluation of machine learning models that are used for medical diagnosis is also important. The methods that can be used for this evaluation are cross-validation and ROC curves.

CONCLUSION

This research looked at articles on automated disease classification between 2016 and 2022, diagnoses were published. Researchers are very curious about some conditions described using machine learning/deep learning methodologies, such as heart disease, brain tumours, asthma, diabetes, cholera, arthritis, chronic liver disease, renal disease, malaria, and leukaemia. A variety of user interfaces are also addressed. We have chosen 60 articles from the International Journal of Advanced Computer Science and Applications, Springer, IEEE Access, and Science Direct. The discussion sections emphasised our main conclusions. Our key finding shows that deep learning is the most often used academic methodology because to its exceptional effectiveness in creating a solid model.

The most popular method for automated illness detection seems to be deep learning, most research do not provide adequate explanations for the final predictions. As a result, to apply the ML model to healthcare, future automated disease diagnosis research ought to emphasise pre- and post-hoc analysis as well as interpreting the model. Future studies could aim to develop synthetic data rather of relying on data collecting and processing. Future academics and practitioners may be interested in generative adversarial networks, adaptive synthetic, synthetic minority oversampling techniques, and SVM synthetic minority oversampling techniques to develop synthetic data for the experiment. The development of secure diagnostic systems may also derive from future research into automated illness detection systems that concentrate on fusing blockchain technology with deep learning and machine learning.

REFERENCES

Ahsan, M., Luna, S. A. & Siddique, Z. (2022). *Machine-Learning-Based Disease Diagnosis: A Comprehensive Review.* MDPI: . doi:10.3390/healthcare10030541

Aljurayfani, M., Alghernas, S., & Shargabi, A. (2019). Medical Self-Diagnostic System Using Artificial Neural Networks. *International Conference on Computer and Information Sciences (ICCIS).* IEEE. doi:10.1109/ICCISci.2019.8716386

Amato, F., López, A., Peña-Méndez, E. Vaňhara, P., Hampl, A., & Havel, J. (2013), Artificial neural networks in medical diagnosis. *Journal of Applied Biomedicine.* doi:10.2478/v10136-012-0031-x

Awotunde, J. B., Matiluko, O. E., & Fatai, O. W. (2014). Medical Diagnosis System Using Fuzzy Logic. *African Journal of Computing and ICT, 7*(2), 99–106.

Bakator, M., & Radosav, D. (2018). *Deep Learning and Medical Diagnosis: A Review of Literature.* MDPI. https://dx.doi.org/10.3390/mti2030047

Barone de Medeiros, I., Machado, M., José Damasceno, J., Machado Caldeira, A., dos Santos, R., & da Silva Filho, J. (2017) A Fuzzy Inference System to Support Medical Diagnosis in Real Time. *Science Direct.* doi:10.1016/j.procs.2017.11.356

Bhavsar, K. A., Abugabah, A., Singla, J., AlZubi, A., Bashir, A., & Nikita (2021). A Comprehensive Review on Medical Diagnosis Using Machine Learning. *CMC, 67*(2).

Faris, H., Habib, M., Faris, M., Elayan, H., & Alomari, A. (2021). An intelligent multimodal medical diagnosis system based on patients' tole medical questions and structured symptoms for telemedicine. *Science Direct.* https://doi.org/10.1016/j.imu.2021.100513

Ibrahim, I. M., & Abdulazeez, A. M. (2021). The Role of Machine Learning Algorithms for Diagnosing Diseases. *JASTT.* doi:10.38094/jastt20179

Jatav S., & Sharma, V. (2018). An algorithm for predictive data mining approach in medical diagnosis. *IJCSIT, 10*(1). doi:10.5121/ijcsit.2018.10102

Karthik, S. Sudha, M. (2018). A Survey on Machine Learning Approaches in Gene Expression Classification in Modelling Computational Diagnostic System for Complex Diseases. *8*(2).

Kudina, O., & de Boer, B. (2021). Co-designing diagnosis: Towards a responsible integration of Machine Learning decision-support systems in medical diagnostics. *Journal of Evaluation in Clinical Practice.* Wiley. doi:10.1111/jep.13535

Li, J. Q., Dukes, P. V., Lee, W., Sarkis, M., & Vo-Dinh, T. (2022). Machine learning using convolutional neural networks for SERS analysis of biomarkers in medical diagnostics. *Journal of Raman Spectroscopy.* Wiley. doi:10.1002/jrs.6447

Malakar, S., Roy, S. D., Das, S., Sen, S., Velasquez, J. D., & Sarkar, R. (2022). *nComputer Based Diagnosis of Some Chronic Diseases: A Medical Journey of the Last Two Decades.* Springer. https://doi.org/10.1007/s11831-022-09776-x

Miller, R. A. (1994). Medical Diagnostic Decision Support Systems -Past, Present, and Future. *Journal of the American Medical Informatics Association, 1*(1), 8–27. https://doi.org/10.1136/jamia.1994.95236141

Nkuma-Udah, K. I., Chukwudebe, G. A., & Ekwonwune, E. N. (2018). Medical Diagnosis Expert System for Malaria and Related Diseases for Developing Countries. *Scientific Research.* https://doi.org/10.4236/etsn.2018.72002

Okokpujie, K., Orimogunje, A., Noma-Osaghae, E., Olaitan, A. (2017). An Intelligent Online Diagnostic System with Epidemic Alert. *2*(9).

Omoregbe, N. A. I., Ndaman, I. O., Misra, S., Abayomi-alli, O. O., & Damasevitius, R. (2020), Text Messaging-Based Medical Diagnosis Using Natural Language Processing and Fuzzy Logic. *Hindawi.* https://doi.org/10.1155/2020/8839524

Park, S., & Han, K. (2018). Methodologic Guide for Evaluating Clinical Performance and Effect of Artificial Intelligence Technology for Medical Diagnosis and Prediction, 286(3).

Ratawal, K. & Zade, A. (2021). Medical Diagnostic Systems Using Artificial Intelligence (AI) Algorithms. *08*(8).

Raval, D., & Bhatt, D. (2016). *Malaram K Kumhar, Vishal Parikh, Daiwat Vyas.* Medical Diagnosis System Using Machine Learning. doi:10.090592/IICSC.2016.026

Ray, A., & Chaudhuri, A. K. (2020). Smart healthcare disease diagnosis and patient management: Innovation, improvement and skill development. *Machine Learning with Applications.* https://doi.org/10.1016/j.mlwa.2020.100011

Satpathy, S., Mohan, P., Das, S., & Debbarma, S. (2019). *A new healthcare diagnosis system using an loT-based fuzzy classifier with FPGA*. Springerhttps://doi.org/10.1007/s11227-019-03013-2 doi:.

Simarjeet, K., Singla, J., Nkenyereye, L., Jha, S., Parashar, D., El-Sappagh, G. P., Islam, S., & Islam, S. M. (2020). *Medical Diagnostic Systems Using Artificial Intelligence (AI) Algorithms: Principles and Perspectives.* IEEE. doi:10.1109/ACCESS.2020.3042273

Uvaliyeva, I., Belginova, S., & Ismukhamedova, A. (2018). Development and implementation of the algorithm of differential diagnostics. *IEEE 12th International Conference on Application of Information and Communication Technologies (AICT).* IEEE. doi:10.1109/ICAICT.2018.8747116

Xu, Z., Shi, D., & Tu, Z. ((2021). Research on Diagnostic Information of Smart Medical Care Based on Big Data. *Hindawi.* doi:10.1155/2021/9977358

Xu, Z., Shi, D., & Tu, Z. (2021). Research on Diagnostic Information of Smart Medical Care Based on Big Data. *Hindawi.* doi:10.1155/2021/9977358

Zhang, Y., Weng, Y., & Lund, J. (2022). *Applications of Explainable Artificial Intelligence in Diagnosis and Surgery.* MDPI. https://doi.org/10.3390/diagnostics12020237

Zhou, H. (2021). Design of Medical Diagnostic System Based on Artificial Intelligence. *Journal of Physics: Conference Series, 2037*, 012081. doi:10.1088/1742-6596/2037/1/012081

Chapter 4
Role of AI-Based Methods in Colorectal Cancer Diagnostics:
The Current Updates

Pankaj Kumar Tripathi
https://orcid.org/0000-0002-9929-359X
Jaypee Institute of Information Technology, India

Chakresh Kumar Jain
https://orcid.org/0000-0002-9226-7719
Jaypee Institute of Information Technology, India

ABSTRACT

Colorectal cancer ranks as the second most prevalent cause of death, and proven to be a major cause of morbidity, where one in every six people worldwide dies from cancer. The early diagnostics have always been a torch bearing insight towards better and timely treatment, thus saving the life. In the recent, advanced medical technology has facilitated large amounts of variable data set for analysis, whereas artificial intelligence (AI) technology has the proven role in automatic cancer detection, enabling us to analyze more patients in less time and money hence, commonly used in oncology. The convolutional neural network based models have been quite popular to evaluate cancer imaginary data in current scenario. In this chapter, the authors summarize the computational resources, basic architecture, and applications of advanced AI based methods / soft computing methodologies; i.e. machine learning, deep learning, CNN, RNN, SVM and other machine learning methods for early and faster diagnostics of colorectal cancer with imaginary classification of patient data with challenges.

DOI: 10.4018/978-1-6684-6957-6.ch004

INTRODUCTION

The second-leading worldwide cause of mortality and one of the most prevalent cancers is colorectal cancer (Pham et al., 2018). Any sickness, whether treatable or not, must be accurately identified with enough time to take the necessary steps in a timely manner. Since early diagnosis of any disease is believed to be the key to full recovery (Saxena et al., 2021). It would save countless lives if it were discovered sooner. The categorization of medical images has been the subject of several research articles. However, the focusing area, contrast, and white balance of medical pictures collected from various sources may vary. Additionally, interior structures with various textures and pixel densities are typically present in medical pictures. It would be challenging to effectively characterize certain classes if we solely employed conventional characteristics to classify medical pictures (Lai & Deng, 2018). To stop metastases and lower the mortality rate, colorectal cancer must be detected early. One of the methods for soft tissue imaging is magnetic resonance imaging (MRI), which can clearly show distinctive anatomical features. The integrity of cell membranes and tissues may be determined using MRI and can be determined quantitatively and qualitatively (Xiao et al., 2022). AI has showed great promise in the area of diagnosis and given us a workable substitute for traditional diagnostic methods. To diagnose a disease today, a patient's samples must be taken, a series of tests must be performed on those samples, the results must be presented in a comprehensible manner, and an expert must be consulted to make decisions based on the results. Machines can now analyze samples collected from patients if they are digital or have been digitalized in some other way. These information might then provide them with a bundle of information that includes prior verdicts on analogous situations. Finally, advice on how to identify the new patient's problems must be given. Making decisions based on knowledge gleaned from previous experiences is referred to as supervised learning in the context of machine learning. Various biological signals have been classified and predicted using machine learning algorithms. As a result of deep learning algorithms, machines may now interpret data with several dimensions, for example pictures, multidimensional anatomical scans, and video. A branch of machine learning called deep describes structure-inspired learning algorithms and operation of the human mind (Tasnim et al., 2021). To increase pattern recognition skills, DL employs artificial neural networks. Above all, it is clear that AI has added a new dimension to the area of medical diagnostics and is gradually displacing conventional diagnostic procedures as a workable substitute. Now a days CNN models are being used to analyze imaginary data of cancer for the early detection (Javed Mehedi Shamrat et al., 2020 & Ghosh et al., 2021). CNNs, in particular, are commonly utilized in dynamic image classification applications and have attained notable performance. Several techniques are available for CNN-based algorithms to improve image classification performance on small datasets: Data augmentation is one approach (Frid-Adar et al., 2018). The efficiency of data augmentation in image categorization was studied by Wang and Perez (Perez & Wang, 2017).

ARTIFICIAL INTELLIGENCE AND CRC

In the 1950s, the idea of AI was initially put out (Moor, 2019) and now a days AI boom in medical science field for early detection and diagnosis of disease. In order to process all data types, AI relies on utilizing mathematical methodologies with sophisticated investigative and prognostic capacities, which enables decision-making that resembles human intelligence. Machine learning technique is a branch of AI, allow computer machine to become more proficient through the training and experience of data sets (Alizadehsani et al., 2021). There are two types of machine learning algorithms: supervised learning and unsupervised learning, depending on the sort of learning approach used. Since the objective is to anticipate a known outcome, supervised learning is the method that is most frequently used in medicine (Yu et al., 2018). Numerous disease datasets, including those related to diabetes, heart disease, and cancer, have been classified using the artificial intelligence and the To identify whether or not a patient has such disorders or disease, for this analysis Naive Bayes classification and random forest classification methods are used. Prospective AI/ML methods include multianalyte assays with algorithmic analysis (MAAA) for community screening and timely detection, as well as pattern recognition with computer vision algorithms to inform diagnostic recommendations and prognosis (Waljee et al., 2022). In classification, object detection, and segmentation tasks, AI-based methods have shown to perform well. For automatic polyp identification and classification, the benefits of AI has effectively used through interdisciplinary and collaborative effort between physicians and technologists. In order to prevent colorectal cancer, the new AI-based solutions have a higher rate of polyp identification and aid in improved clinical judgement (Viscaino et al., 2021). Since 1966, computer-aided detection/diagnosis systems (CADe/CADx) have been suggested, created, and utilized therapeutically, in the evaluation of the cancer risk (Giger, 2018).

Deep Learning Algorithms

Deep learning algorithms are a novel generation of AI-powered computer-assisted systems that may help doctors with crucial tasks like colorectal polyp identification and categorization. Deep learning-based algorithms, present promising outcomes for the processing of medical images (Viscaino et al., 2021). According to research done by a German team, a deep learning-based algorithm was able to categorize the specific tumor microenvironment and predict CRC patient survival utilizing histological images (Kather et al., 2019). Segmenting glands, classifying tumors, identifying the tumor microenvironment, and predicting prognosis are among the algorithms used in the models.

Known Deep Learning Models

1. **Multilayer Perceptrons (MLPs):** For adaptive modelling of non-linear problems in real-world systems, MLP neural networks, the most conventional and common kind of artificial neural network, have proved effective. In this models, the hidden layer receives a node's linearly weighted input vector, where its activation function transforms it. The capacity to estimate model non-linearity is provided by the activation function. MLP is perhaps the most prevalent form among all ANNs, is frequently utilised in future prediction, relation estimation, and pattern grouping simulation (Riahi-Madvar & Seifi, 2018 and Riahi-Madvar et al., 2019). An MLP is made up of three basic layers of nodes: the input layer, the hidden layer, and the output layer. Each node in the hidden and output layers may be seen as a neuron with a nonlinear activation function. The supervised learning method known as backpropagation is used by MLP. Each neuron in a neural network has its weight set when the network is first created. Backpropagation assists in altering the weights of neurons in order to provide output to be more closely aligned with expectation (Goled, 2020).

Applications of MLP: Social media platforms like Instagram and Facebook utilise it to compress image data. That considerably aids in loading the photos even when the network signal is weak. Some further uses are used for image classification issues, data compression, and voice and image recognition.

2. **Radial Basis Function Networks (RBFNs):** It is predicated on the Radial Basis Function, or approximation function, as the term RBF indicates. One of the most crucial characteristics of RBF models is the type that has a nonlinear structure in a high-dimensional space mode that may be easily fractured utilising a collection of several RBF models (Park et al., 2022).

How do the deep learning algorithms of RBFN operate:

Figure 1. A straightforward example of an RBFN is a three-layer feedforward neural network that has an input layer, a hidden layer composed of many RBF nonlinear activation units, and a linear output layer acting as a summation unit to create the final output (Top 10 Deep Learning Algorithms in Machine Learning [2022], n .d.).

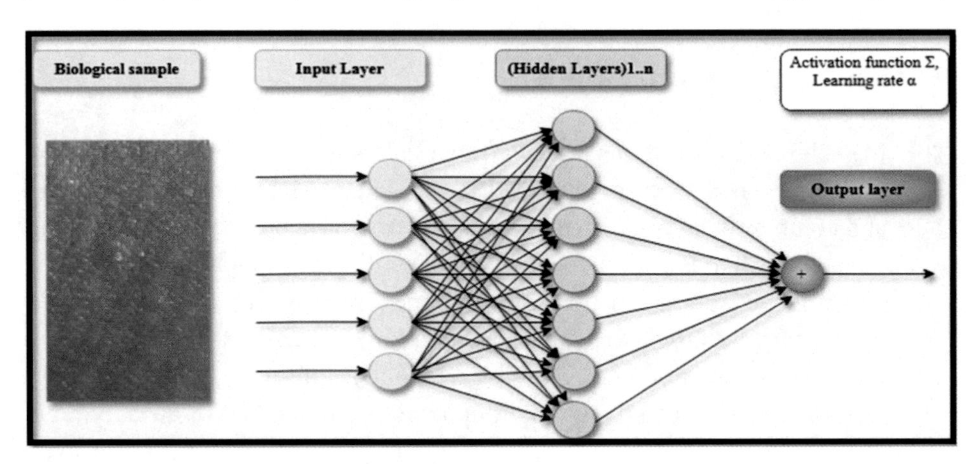

3. **Convolutional Neural Networks (CNN):** One of the most well-known deep learning method architectures is CNN.

A unique multi-layered feed-forward unsupervised neural network called a convolution neural network (CNN) was designed to handle the classification of imaginary data. It is specifically designed to extract image data without worrying about feature selection issues (Singh Gill & Singh Khehra, 2020).

The CNN is constructed over four phases once the input data is integrated into the convolutional model (Vadapalli, 2020):

a) **Convolution:** From the input data, feature maps are generated, and then an algorithm is implemented to these maps. The convolution layer of CNN is also known as the feature extraction layer.
b) **Max-Pooling:** It assists CNN in distinguishing an image from modifications.
c) **Flattering:** In this stage, data production is flattened so that CNN may analyse it.
d) **Full Connection:** A model's loss function compiler is frequently referred to as a hidden layer.

According to Mosavi, *et al.*, the back-propagation stage and the feed-forward stage are the two phases of each CNN's training procedure (Mosavi et al., 2019). The best popular CNN designs are ZFNet (Zeiler & Fergus, 2014), GoogLeNet (Szegedy et al., 2015), VGGNet (Simonyan & Zisserman, 2014), AlexNet (Krizhevsky et al., 2012), and ResNet (He et al., 2016). CNNs are capable of doing image recognition, and analysis, image classification, natural language processing and video analysis.

Application of CNN Models

CNNs are utilised by Facebook, Instagram, and other social media platforms for face detection and recognition. So we are utilising CNN models when attempting to tag our friend in a post. Other uses include forecasting, natural language processing, image identification, and video analysis.

4. **Recurrent Neural Networks (RNNs):** Recurrent Neural Networks (RNNs) are a type of neural network where the results of one phase are used as input in the subsequent phase. The most popular uses of RNNs are in sequence classification, sentiment classification, and image and video classification. A type of artificial neural network called an RNN has connections between nodes that sequentially construct a directed graph. In essence, it is a linked chain of neural network components. To the person ahead of them in line, each is communicating. While a CNN is trained to detect patterns over space, an RNN is taught to recognize patterns across time (Singh Gill et al., 2022 & Mosavi et al., 2019). Two general categories of RNN architectures exist that support issue analysis (Vadapalli, 2020) as follows:

    a) **Long Short Term Memory Networks (LSTMs):**

A unique class of RNN called LSTMs is very good at learning long-term dependencies. The LSTM network is made up of many memory units called cells. When compared to traditional RNNs, LSTMs are far more useful for simulating long-range relationships and chronological sequences. Useful for leveraging memory to forecast data in time sequences. It features the input, output, and forget gates (Vadapalli, 2020).

Application of LSTM

Some of the approaches used to discover abnormalities in IDSs (intrusion detection systems) or network traffic data include time-series predictions, auto-completion, textual and analysis of videos, and caption creation.

b) **Gated RNNs:** These would be useful for predicting data sequences from memory. The two gates are Update and Reset. (Vadapalli, 2020).

5. Restricted Boltzmann Machines (RBMs):

The Restricted Boltzmann Machine technique, used for feature selection and feature extraction, is crucial in the era of machine learning and Deep Learning for dimensionality reduction, classification, regression, and many other tasks. The Boltzmann Machine is a generative unsupervised model that relies on the learning of a probability distribution from a unique dataset and the use of that distribution to conclude unexplored data (Simplilearn, 2022). The various kinds of Boltzmann Machines are as follows:

- Deep Belief Networks (DBNs)
- Restricted Boltzmann Machines (RBMs)
- Deep Boltzmann Machines (DBMs)

The fundamental units of deep belief networks are RBMs, which are two-layer, shallow neural networks. An RBM has two layers: the visible or input layer comes first, and the concealed or hidden layer comes second. It consists of nodes, which resemble neurons and are linked to one another across layers but not inside the same layer (Xu et al., 2022).

6. Self-Organizing Maps (SOMs):

An artificial neural network called a self-organizing map was developed in the 1970s and is similarly based on biological models of brain systems. It uses a competitive learning algorithm to train its network while using an unsupervised learning methodology (Baliyan, 2020). It is utilised for high-dimensional dataset display and exploratory data analysis. SOM is used in clustering and mapping approaches to convert multidimensional data to lower-dimensional formats, which enables individuals to simplify complicated issues for simple comprehension. SOM consists of two layers: the input layer and the output layer (Bigdeli et al., 2022).

Figure 2. Data sources for CRC Polyp imaginary data and analysis of image data by using different deep learning models.

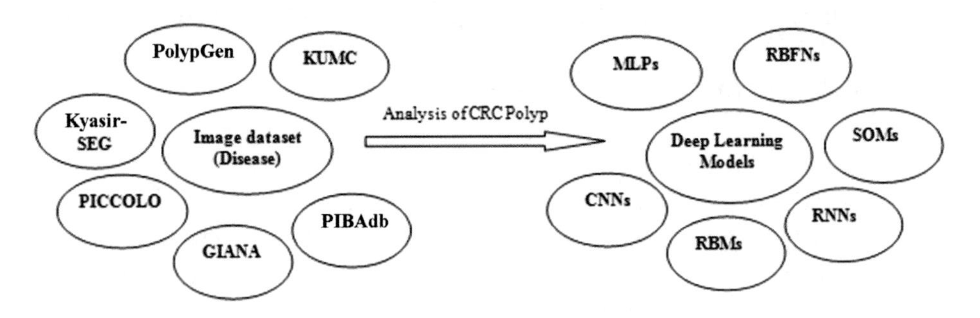

DEEP LEARNING ALGORITHMS APPLICATION IN THE DIAGNOSIS OF CRC PATHOLOGICALLY:

Gland Segmentation (GlaS)

The places where approximately 90-95 percent carcinomas can develop are glands for example salivary glands, upper and lower GI tracts, breast, exocrine pancreas, prostate, sweat glands, and biliary system. The gland structure, size and shape are important grading factors in these gland-derived malignant tumors, also known as adenocarcinomas (Fleming et al., 2012). A fully convolutional network algorithm with a three-class classification and many scales was created by Ding et al. in 2019 to lessen this problem of GlaS. (TCC-MSFCN). They used a colorectal adenocarcinoma gland (CRAG) dataset to train the model, which resulted in the model's architecture having components such as high-resolution branch, residual structure and dilated convolution (Ding et al., 2020).

Tumor Classification

In order to decrease inter- or intra-observer variance when classifying tumours into histological subtypes, additionally, a number of deep learning models have been created. These models have demonstrated extremely good performance, however they should be evaluated with caution due to the limitations of these research. In the majority of investigations, training was done using patched or cropped pictures rather than WSIs. Even many hundreds of cropped images were utilised, they all come from the same CRC patient, hence the cropped images from one WSI share comparable histological characteristics (Hosseini et al., 2019 & Kather, Pearson, et al., 2019). In a single research by Lizuka et al., epithelial tumours in biopsy WSIs of the colon and stomach were classified using deep learning applied to learning models. The models were trained using WSI that was collected from a single medical facility. Hence, future studies will need further research with a bigger variety of datasets, more recognised annotations, and the proper acceptance (Iizuka et al., 2020).

Tumor Microenvironment Analysis (TME)

The majority of TME research combined classification and segmentation, occasionally using IHC slides. A CNN model created by Shapott *et al.* to categorized epithelial, inflammatory, fibroblast, and other types of cells and they got the results averaged 65% of detection correctness and 76% of classification correctness (Shapcott et al., 2019). In a separate research, Siderska-Chadaj *et al.* trained models which are CNN-based that can spontaneously recognize and distinguish T cells using CD3 and CD8 IHC utilising 28 IHC WSIs. It demonstrated moderate robustness and high precision (Swiderska-Chadaj et al., 2019).

Prognosis Prediction

There will be a huge advantage to the clinical care of the cancer patients due to the preceision of cancer prognostic prediction. To better foresee cancer prognosis, modern statistical analysis and machine learning techniques are being incorporated, as well as translational research in biomedical is being improved. Recently, the capability to process has significantly increased and the artificial intelligence technology, especially deep learning, has advanced rapidly (Zhu et al., 2020). When dealing with vast volumes of data, it has been found that deep learning is a more general model with less amount of data manipulation, and better prediction abilities. It has been proven that the inclusion of deep learning in cancer prediction is either at par with or superior to the conventional methods like Cox proportional hazard regression (Yu, Ma, et al., 2018).

Table 1. Computational resources for Polyp Localization on Public Colonoscopy Image/video Datasets (Nogueira-Rodríguez et al., 2022)

Sr. No.	Data Resources	Data types	Reference
1.	**Gastrointestinal Image ANAlysis (GIANA)**	Image	(Bernal et al., 2021)
2.	**Polyp-CVC-CliniDB**	Image	(Bernal et al., 2015)
3.	**ETIS-Larib**	Image	(Silva et al., 2013)
4.	**ASU-Mayo Clinic Colonoscopy Video**	Video	(Tajbakhsh et al., 2016)
5.	**MICCAI**	Video	(Bernal et al., 2017)
6.	**CVC-ClinicVideoDB**	Video	(Bernal et al., 2018)
7.	**PIBAdb (Polyp Image BAnk database)**	Image	(Nogueira-Rodríguez et al., 2021)
8.	**PICCOLO**	Image	(Sanchez-Peralta et al., 2020)
9.	**Kvasir-SEG**	Image	(Jha et al., 2019)
10.	**LDPolyp Video**	Video	(Ma et al., 2021)
11.	**SUN**	Video	(Misawa et al., 2020)
12.	**KUMC**	Image	(Li et al., 2021)
13.	**PolypGen**	Image and Video	(Ali et al., 2021)

Image Classifiers

CNN Classifier: CNN Classifier: CNNs are neural networks, an algorithm for identifying patterns in data. In general, neural networks are made up of layers of neurons that are arranged in a collection, each having its own learnable biases and weights, however convolutional layers a unique kind of layer used by CNNs, provide them the ability to learn from images and image-like data (Wang et al., 2021). Convolutional neural networks (CNNs) are particularly well-liked in pathology for the automated diagnosis of numerous disorders. Fully Convolutional Networks (FCN) (Shelhamer et al., 2017), Unet (Ronneberger et al., 2015), Deeplab (Chen et al., 2018), and other commonly used CNN network designs for medical images segmentation have shown results that are superior to those of more conventional techniques. Yamada *et al.* define a method that inculcates deep learning to make colonoscopy diagnoses concurrently. They developed a system that receives video frames from the endoscopic device and used the quicker R-CNN approach to pinpoint and locate polyps in the images (Yamada et al., 2019 & Ren et al., 2017).

MobileNetV2 classifier: To classify images the MobileNet used CNN architecture framework. MobileNet design is unique, because it requires less computational processing power to function and this unique feature makes it the ideal choice for running on desktops, embedded systems, and mobile devices (Dong et al., 2020). The initial iteration of the Mobilenet models is called MobilenetV1, which are having more sophisticated features layers and settings for convolution. The Mobilenet models' second iteration is known as MobilenetV2, is has a notably lesser number of parameters in deep neural network. These types of models are quicker because to the smaller size and lower complexity of the models produced by MobilenetV2, which saves time when creating a neural network from scratch. These models also provide more lightweight deep neural networks and it works well for embedded systems due to its lightweight feature (Nganga, 2022).

SVM and RBF Kernal

SVMs (Support Vector Machines) are frequently employed to address classification issues. SVM, a well-liked machine learning technique, is supported for the both regression and classification. The goal of the SVM method is to identify a hyperplane that distinctly classifies the data points in an N-dimensional space. The number of features determines the size of the hyperplane (Roman et al., 2020). It is basically two types, simple or linear SVM and non-linear or kernel SVM.

- Linear SVM: Usually applied to classification and linear regression issues.
- Non-Linear or Kernel SVM: the one that can be more easily modified to accommodate non-linear data since more features can be added to better fit a hyperplane instead of a two-dimensional space.

Applications of SVM

In order to classify unknown data into recognised categories, the SVM algorithm relies on supervised learning techniques. These algorithms are employed in a variety of domains, some of which are covered here.

- Solving the geo-sounding problem
- Data classification
- Protein remote homology detection
- Facial detection & expression classification
- Text categorization & handwriting recognition
- Surface texture classification
- Speech recognition

SVM-Kernel: The SVM kernel is a function that takes a low-dimensional input space and transforms it into a higher-dimensional space, making it possible to separate issues that are not separable. Non-linear separation issues are where it is most helpful. The kernel, to put it simply, determines the method for separating all the data that rely on the labels or outputs provided followed by some really difficult data transformations (De Oliveira Nogueira et al., 2022)

Radial Basis Function (RBF) kernel: A sort of Artificial Neural Network (ANN) that is frequently incoporated for regression or classification is the Radial Basis Function Kernel (RBFK). Similar layers of linked neurons make up the RBFK. Its single hidden layer's neurons, however, make use of kernel functions (such the Gaussian function), which makes it possible to apply non-recursive solution methods (Anyanwu et al., 2022 and Lv & Jiang, 2021).

RBF, the default kernel in the sklearn's SVM classification algorithm, may be defined using the following formula:

$$K(x, x') = \exp(-\gamma \|x-x'\|2)$$

Where we can set gamma manually and is required to be >0. In sklearn's SVM classification method, gamma is set to the following default value:

$$\gamma = \frac{1}{n\,features * \sigma 2}$$

Random Forest: The random forest (RF) is known to be an ensemble approach that consists of a hierarchical group of basic classifiers with a tree-structure. To choose the most crucial significant characteristic, the RF algorithm utilises a straightforward predefined probability. By integrating several overfit assessors (such as decision trees) to create an ensemble learning method, RF can reduce the level of overfitting (Wang, Zhai, et al., 2021). The relevant classification decision result may be obtained for each decision tree. The RF technique was developed by Breiman who mapped a random sample of feature subspaces to sample data subsets and built multiple decision trees from those (Jackins et al., 2020).

Nalve Bayes

An artificially intelligent method founded on the comparison of specific criteria inculcated to determine if a person has cancer or not is being developed using the Naive Bayes algorithm. Utilizing a confusion matrix, the Naive Bayes method produces very accurate results to determine the proportion of true and erroneous situations. For building very large datasets and for additional analysis, the Naive Bayes model is appropriate. Even in challenging circumstances, this model, which is a very complex and easy classification algorithm, worked well (Jackins et al., 2020). By applying the Bayes theorem, use the following equation to calculate the posterior probability:

$$P(a/y) = (P(y/a)P(a))/P(y)$$

Here P(a/y) denotes the class posterior probability, P(a) denotes the prior probability of class, P(y/a) denotes the likelihood, which is the class predictor probability, and P(y) denotes the prior probability of predictor's.

K-Nearest Neighbors

K-Nearest Neighbors is one of the most fundamental but essential classification techniques in supervised machine learning and has several uses in pattern recognition, intrusion detection and data mining. The chances of a data point belonging to one group or the other based on which group it is closest to, is well calculated by the k-nearest neighbors (KNN) (Khorshid & Abdulazeez, 2021 & Joby, 2021).

CONCLUSION

Although several AI, machine learning and deep learning standard algorithms are offering the many advantages in the realm of medical sciences and using for the initial detection, diagnosis and prognosis of the ailment by using classification models in imaginary data. These models have demonstrated extremely good performance, however they should be evaluated with caution due to the limitations of these research. In the majority of investigations, training was done using patched or cropped images, even many hundreds of cropped images are utilizing, and they all come from the same CRC patient. Hence, future studies will need further research with a larger variety of original and test datasets, more verified annotations, and the proper validation. To forecast cancer prognosis more efficiently, modern statistical analysis and machine learning techniques are being used, as well as improvement in biomedical translational research is being done. In this study we concluded that, in recent years, the processing capability has significantly elevated along with the artificial intelligence technologies, especially deep learning, has evolved quickly. When dealing with vast volumes of data and large complex data, deep learning has proved to be a more general model with less amount of data manipulation, and better prediction abilities. It has been demonstrated that by using of deep learning algorithms in cancer prediction is more effective than using conventional techniques.

ACKNOWLEDGMENT

We are thankful to Department of Biotechnology, Jaypee Institute of Information Technology, Noida for providing necessary support.

Conflict of interest: The authors have no conflicts of interest to declare.

REFERENCES

Ali, S., Jha, D., Ghatwary, N., Realdon, S., Cannizzaro, R., Salem, O. E., Lamarque, D., Daul, C., Riegler, M. A., Anonsen, K. V., Petlund, A., Halvorsen, P., Rittscher, J., de Lange, T., & East, J. E. (2021). PolypGen: A multi-center polyp detection and segmentation dataset for generalisability assessment. *ArXiv:2106.04463* https://arxiv.org/abs/2106.04463

Alizadehsani, R., Khosravi, A., Roshanzamir, M., Abdar, M., Sarrafzadegan, N., Shafie, D., Khozeimeh, F., Shoeibi, A., Nahavandi, S., Panahiazar, M., Bishara, A., Beygui, R. E., Puri, R., Kapadia, S., Tan, R.-S., & Acharya, U. R. (2021). Coronary artery disease detection using artificial intelligence techniques: A survey of trends, geographical differences and diagnostic features 1991–2020. *Computers in Biology and Medicine*, *128*, 104095. doi:10.1016/j.compbiomed.2020.104095 PMID:33217660

Anyanwu, G. O., Nwakanma, C. I., Lee, J.-M., & Kim, D.-S. (2022). Optimization of RBF-SVM Kernel using Grid Search Algorithm for DDoS Attack Detection in SDN-based VANET. *IEEE Internet of Things Journal*, 1–1. doi:10.1109/JIOT.2022.3199712

Baliyan, M. (2020, July 1). *Self Organising Maps - Kohonen Maps*. GeeksforGeeks. https://www.geeksforgeeks.org/self-organising-maps-kohonen-maps/

Bernal, J., Fernández, G., García-Rodríguez, A., & Sánchez, F. J. (2021). Polyp Segmentation in Colonoscopy Images. *Computer-Aided Analysis of Gastrointestinal Videos*, *151–154*, 151–154. Advance online publication. doi:10.1007/978-3-030-64340-9_19

Bernal, J., Sánchez, F. J., Fernández-Esparrach, G., Gil, D., Rodríguez, C., & Vilariño, F. (2015). WM-DOVA maps for accurate polyp highlighting in colonoscopy: Validation vs. saliency maps from physicians. *Computerized Medical Imaging and Graphics*, *43*, 99–111. doi:10.1016/j.compmedimag.2015.02.007 PMID:25863519

Bernal, J., Tajkbaksh, N., Sanchez, F. J., Matuszewski, B. J., Chen, H., Yu, L., Angermann, Q., Romain, O., Rustad, B., Balasingham, I., Pogorelov, K., Choi, S., Debard, Q., Maier-Hein, L., Speidel, S., Stoyanov, D., Brandao, P., Cordova, H., Sanchez-Montes, C, & Histace, A. (2017). Comparative Validation of Polyp Detection Methods in Video Colonoscopy: Results From the MICCAI 2015 Endoscopic Vision Challenge. *IEEE Transactions on Medical Imaging*, *36*(6), 1231–1249. doi:10.1109/TMI.2017.2664042 PMID:28182555

Bernal, J. J., Histace, A., Masana, M., Angermann, Q., Sánchez-Montes, C., Rodriguez, C., Hammami, M., Garcia-Rodriguez, A., Córdova, H., Romain, O., Fernández-Esparrach, G., Dray, X., & Sanchez, J. (2018, June 20). *Polyp Detection Benchmark in Colonoscopy Videos using GTCreator: A Novel Fully Configurable Tool for Easy and Fast Annotation of Image Databases*. Hal.science. https://hal.science/hal-01846141/

Bigdeli, A., Maghsoudi, A., & Ghezelbash, R. (2022). Application of self-organizing map (SOM) and K-means clustering algorithms for portraying geochemical anomaly patterns in Moalleman district, NE Iran. *Journal of Geochemical Exploration*, *233*, 106923. doi:10.1016/j.gexplo.2021.106923

Chen, L.-C., Papandreou, G., Kokkinos, I., Murphy, K., & Yuille, A. L. (2018). DeepLab: Semantic Image Segmentation with Deep Convolutional Nets, Atrous Convolution, and Fully Connected CRFs. *IEEE Transactions on Pattern Analysis and Machine Intelligence*, *40*(4), 834–848. doi:10.1109/TPAMI.2017.2699184 PMID:28463186

De Oliveira Nogueira, T., Palacio, G. B. A., Braga, F. D., Maia, P. P. N., de Moura, E. P., de Andrade, C. F., & Rocha, P. A. C. (2022). Imbalance classification in a scaled-down wind turbine using radial basis function kernel and support vector machines. *Energy*, *238*, 122064. doi:10.1016/j.energy.2021.122064

Ding, H., Pan, Z., Cen, Q., Li, Y., & Chen, S. (2020). Multi-scale fully convolutional network for gland segmentation using three-class classification. *Neurocomputing*, *380*, 150–161. doi:10.1016/j.neucom.2019.10.097

Dong, K., Zhou, C., Ruan, Y., & Li, Y. (2020). MobileNetV2 Model for Image Classification. *2020 2nd International Conference on Information Technology and Computer Application (ITCA)*. 10.1109/ITCA52113.2020.00106

Fleming, M., Ravula, S., Tatishchev, S. F., & Wang, H. L. (2012). Colorectal carcinoma: Pathologic aspects. *Journal of Gastrointestinal Oncology*, *3*(3), 153–173. doi:10.3978/j.issn.2078-6891.2012.030 PMID:22943008

Frid-Adar, M., Diamant, I., Klang, E., Amitai, M., Goldberger, J., & Greenspan, H. (2018). GAN-based synthetic medical image augmentation for increased CNN performance in liver lesion classification. *Neurocomputing*, *321*, 321–331. doi:10.1016/j.neucom.2018.09.013

Ghosh, P., Azam, S., Jonkman, M., Karim, A., Shamrat, F. M. J. M., Ignatious, E., Shultana, S., Beeravolu, A. R., & De Boer, F. (2021). Efficient Prediction of Cardiovascular Disease Using Machine Learning Algorithms With Relief and LASSO Feature Selection Techniques. *IEEE Access: Practical Innovations, Open Solutions*, *9*, 19304–19326. doi:10.1109/ACCESS.2021.3053759

Giger, M. L. (2018). Machine Learning in Medical Imaging. *Journal of the American College of Radiology*, *15*(3), 512–520. doi:10.1016/j.jacr.2017.12.028 PMID:29398494

Goled, S. (2020, October 25). *Top 5 Neural Network Models For Deep Learning & Their Applications*. Analytics India Magazine. https://analyticsindiamag.com/top-5-neural-network-models-fo r-deep-learning-their-applications/

He, K., Zhang, X., Ren, S., & Sun, J. (2016). Deep Residual Learning for Image Recognition. *2016 IEEE Conference on Computer Vision and Pattern Recognition (CVPR)*, (pp. 770–778). IEEE. 10.1109/CVPR.2016.90

Hosseini, M. S., Chan, L., Tse, G., Tang, M., Deng, J., Norouzi, S., Rowsell, C., Plataniotis, K. N., & Damaskinos, S. (2019). *Atlas of Digital Pathology: A Generalized Hierarchical Histological Tissue Type-Annotated Database for Deep Learning*. Openaccess. thecvf.com. https://openaccess.thecvf.com/content_CVPR_2019/html/Hossein i_Atlas_of_Digital_Pathology_A_Generalized_Hierarchical_Hist ological_Tissue_Type-Annotated_CVPR_2019_paper.html

Iizuka, O., Kanavati, F., Kato, K., Rambeau, M., Arihiro, K., & Tsuneki, M. (2020). Deep Learning Models for Histopathological Classification of Gastric and Colonic Epithelial Tumours. *Scientific Reports*, *10*(1), 1504. doi:10.103841598-020-58467-9 PMID:32001752

Jackins, V., Vimal, S., Kaliappan, M., & Lee, M. Y. (2020). AI-based smart prediction of clinical disease using random forest classifier and Naive Bayes. *The Journal of Supercomputing*. . doi:10.100711227-020-03481-x

Javed Mehedi Shamrat, F. M., Ghosh, P., Sadek, M. H., & Kazi, Md. A., & Shultana, S. (2020). Implementation of Machine Learning Algorithms to Detect the Prognosis Rate of Kidney Disease. *2020 IEEE International Conference for Innovation in Technology (INOCON)*. IEEE. 10.1109/INOCON50539.2020.9298026

Jha, D., Smedsrud, P. H., Riegler, M. A., Halvorsen, P., de Lange, T., Johansen, D., & Johansen, H. D. (2019). Kvasir-SEG: A Segmented Polyp Dataset. *ArXiv:1911.07069* https://arxiv.org/abs/1911.07069

Joby, A. (2021, July 19). *What Is K-Nearest Neighbor? An ML Algorithm to Classify Data*. Learn.g2. https://learn.g2.com/k-nearest-neighbor

Kather, J. N., Krisam, J., Charoentong, P., Luedde, T., Herpel, E., Weis, C.-A., Gaiser, T., Marx, A., Valous, N. A., Ferber, D., Jansen, L., Reyes-Aldasoro, C. C., Zörnig, I., Jäger, D., Brenner, H., Chang-Claude, J., Hoffmeister, M., & Halama, N. (2019). Predicting survival from colorectal cancer histology slides using deep learning: A retrospective multicenter study. *PLoS Medicine*, *16*(1), e1002730. doi:10.1371/journal.pmed.1002730 PMID:30677016

Kather, J. N., Pearson, A. T., Halama, N., Jäger, D., Krause, J., Loosen, S. H., Marx, A., Boor, P., Tacke, F., Neumann, U. P., Grabsch, H. I., Yoshikawa, T., Brenner, H., Chang-Claude, J., Hoffmeister, M., Trautwein, C., & Luedde, T. (2019). Deep learning can predict microsatellite instability directly from histology in gastrointestinal cancer. *Nature Medicine*, *25*(7), 1054–1056. doi:10.103841591-019-0462-y PMID:31160815

Khorshid, S. F., & Abdulazeez, A. M. (2021). Breast Cancer Diagnosis Based On K-Nearest Neighbors: A Review. *PalArch's Journal of Archaeology of Egypt / Egyptology, 18*(4), 1927–1951. https://archives.palarch.nl/index.php/jae/article/view/6601

Krizhevsky, A., Sutskever, I., & Hinton, G. E. (2012). ImageNet Classification with Deep Convolutional Neural Networks. *Advances in Neural Information Processing Systems, 25*, 1097–1105. https://papers.nips.cc/paper/2012/hash/c399862d3b9d6b76c8436e924a68c45b-Abstract.html

Lai, Z., & Deng, H. (2018). Medical Image Classification Based on Deep Features Extracted by Deep Model and Statistic Feature Fusion with Multilayer Perceptron . *Computational Intelligence and Neuroscience*, *2018*, 1–13. doi:10.1155/2018/2061516 PMID:30298088

Li, K., Fathan, M. I., Patel, K., Zhang, T., Zhong, C., Bansal, A., Rastogi, A., Wang, J. S., & Wang, G. (2021). Colonoscopy polyp detection and classification: Dataset creation and comparative evaluations. *PLoS One*, *16*(8), e0255809. doi:10.1371/journal.pone.0255809 PMID:34403452

Lv, B., & Jiang, Y. (2021). Prediction of Short-Term Stock Price Trend Based on Multiview RBF Neural Network. *Computational Intelligence and Neuroscience, 2021*, 1–13. doi:10.1155/2021/8495288 PMID:34876898

Ma, Y., Chen, X., Cheng, K., Li, Y., & Sun, B. (2021). LDPolypVideo Benchmark: A Large-Scale Colonoscopy Video Dataset of Diverse Polyps. Medical Image Computing and Computer Assisted Intervention – MICCAI 2021, (pp. 387–396). Springer. doi:10.1007/978-3-030-87240-3_37

Misawa, M., Kudo, S., Mori, Y., Hotta, K., Ohtsuka, K., Matsuda, T., Saito, S., Kudo, T., Baba, T., Ishida, F., Itoh, H., Oda, M., & Mori, K. (2020). Development of a computer-aided detection system for colonoscopy and a publicly accessible large colonoscopy video database (with video). *Gastrointestinal Endoscopy*. doi:10.1016/j.gie.2020.07.060 PMID:32745531

Moor, J. (2019). The Dartmouth College Artificial Intelligence Conference: The Next Fifty Years. *AI Magazine*, *27*(4), 87–87. doi:10.1609/aimag.v27i4.1911

Mosavi, A. Faizollahzadeh ardabili, S., & R. Várkonyi-Kóczy, A. (2019). *List of Deep Learning Models*. Preprints. doi:10.20944/preprints201908.0152.v1

Nganga, K. (2022). *Building A Multiclass Image Classifier Using MobilenetV2 and TensorFlow*. Engineering Education (EngEd) Program. https://www.section.io/engineering-education/building-a-multiclass-image-classifier-using-mobilenet-v2-and-tensorflow/

Nogueira-Rodríguez, A., Domínguez-Carbajales, R., López-Fernández, H., Iglesias, Á., Cubiella, J., Fdez-Riverola, F., Reboiro-Jato, M., & Glez-Peña, D. (2021). Deep Neural Networks approaches for detecting and classifying colorectal polyps. *Neurocomputing*, *423*, 721–734. doi:10.1016/j.neucom.2020.02.123

Nogueira-Rodríguez, A., Reboiro-Jato, M., Glez-Peña, D., & López-Fernández, H. (2022). Performance of Convolutional Neural Networks for Polyp Localization on Public Colonoscopy Image Datasets. *Diagnostics (Basel)*, *12*(4), 898. doi:10.3390/diagnostics12040898 PMID:35453946

Park, J., Lee, W., & Huh, K. Y. (2022). Model order reduction by radial basis function network for sparse reconstruction of an industrial natural gas boiler. *Case Studies in Thermal Engineering*, *37*, 102288. doi:10.1016/j.csite.2022.102288

Perez, L., & Wang, J. (2017). The Effectiveness of Data Augmentation in Image Classification using Deep Learning. *ArXiv:1712.04621*. https://arxiv.org/abs/1712.04621

Pham, T. T., Talukder, A. M., Walsh, N. J., Lawson, A. G., Jones, A. J., Bishop, J. L., & Kruse, E. J. (2018). Clinical and epidemiological factors associated with suicide in colorectal cancer. *Supportive Care in Cancer*, *27*(2), 617–621. doi:10.100700520-018-4354-3 PMID:30027329

Ren, S., He, K., Girshick, R., & Sun, J. (2017). Faster R-CNN: Towards Real-Time Object Detection with Region Proposal Networks. *IEEE Transactions on Pattern Analysis and Machine Intelligence*, *39*(6), 1137–1149. doi:10.1109/TPAMI.2016.2577031 PMID:27295650

Riahi-Madvar, H., Dehghani, M., Seifi, A., Salwana, E., Shamshirband, S., Mosavi, A., & Chau, K. (2019). Comparative analysis of soft computing techniques RBF, MLP, and ANFIS with MLR and MNLR for predicting grade-control scour hole geometry. *Engineering Applications of Computational Fluid Mechanics*, *13*(1), 529–550. doi:10.1080/19942060.2019.1618396

Riahi-Madvar, H., & Seifi, A. (2018). Uncertainty analysis in bed load transport prediction of gravel bed rivers by ANN and ANFIS. *Arabian Journal of Geosciences*, *11*(21), 688. doi:10.100712517-018-3968-6

Roman, I., Santana, R., Mendiburu, A., & Lozano, J. A. (2020). In-depth analysis of SVM kernel learning and its components. *Neural Computing & Applications*, *33*(12), 6575–6594. doi:10.100700521-020-05419-z

Ronneberger, O., Fischer, P., & Brox, T. (2015). U-Net: Convolutional Networks for Biomedical Image Segmentation. *Lecture Notes in Computer Science*, *9351*, 234–241. doi:10.1007/978-3-319-24574-4_28

Sánchez-Peralta, L. F., Pagador, J. B., Picón, A., Calderón, Á. J., Polo, F., Andraka, N., Bilbao, R., Glover, B., Saratxaga, C. L., & Sánchez-Margallo, F. M. (2020). PICCOLO White-Light and Narrow-Band Imaging Colonoscopic Dataset: A Performance Comparative of Models and Datasets. *Applied Sciences (Basel, Switzerland)*, *10*(23), 8501. doi:10.3390/app10238501

Saxena, A., Singh Tomar, S., Jain, G., & Gupta, R. (2021). Deep learning based Diagnosis of diseases using Image Classification. *2021 11th International Conference on Cloud Computing, Data Science & Engineering (Confluence)*. IEEE. 10.1109/Confluence51648.2021.9377154

Shapcott, M., Hewitt, K. J., & Rajpoot, N. (2019). Deep Learning With Sampling in Colon Cancer Histology. *Frontiers in Bioengineering and Biotechnology*, *7*, 52. doi:10.3389/fbioe.2019.00052 PMID:30972333

Shelhamer, E., Long, J., & Darrell, T. (2017). Fully Convolutional Networks for Semantic Segmentation. *IEEE Transactions on Pattern Analysis and Machine Intelligence*, *39*(4), 640–651. doi:10.1109/TPAMI.2016.2572683 PMID:27244717

Silva, J., Histace, A., Romain, O., Dray, X., & Granado, B. (2013). Toward embedded detection of polyps in WCE images for early diagnosis of colorectal cancer. *International Journal of Computer Assisted Radiology and Surgery*, *9*(2), 283–293. doi:10.100711548-013-0926-3 PMID:24037504

Simonyan, K., & Zisserman, A. (2014). *Very Deep Convolutional Networks for Large-Scale Image Recognition.* ArXiv.org. https://arxiv.org/abs/1409.1556

Simplilearn. (2022, September 1). *What Are Restricted Boltzmann Machines? A Beginner's Guide to RBMs.* Simplilearn. https://www.simplilearn.com/restricted-boltzmann-machines-rb
ms-article

Singh Gill, H., Ibrahim Khalaf, O., Alotaibi, Y., Alghamdi, S., & Alassery, F. (2022). Multi-Model CNN-RNN-LSTM Based Fruit Recognition and Classification. *Intelligent Automation & Soft Computing*, *33*(1), 637–650. doi:10.32604/iasc.2022.022589

Singh Gill, H., & Singh Khehra, B. (2020). Efficient image classification technique for weather degraded fruit images. *IET Image Processing*, *14*(14), 3463–3470. doi:10.1049/iet-ipr.2018.5310

Swiderska-Chadaj, Z., Pinckaers, H., van Rijthoven, M., Balkenhol, M., Melnikova, M., Geessink, O., Manson, Q., Sherman, M., Polonia, A., Parry, J., Abubakar, M., Litjens, G., van der Laak, J., & Ciompi, F. (2019). Learning to detect lymphocytes in immunohistochemistry with deep learning. *Medical Image Analysis*, *58*, 101547. doi:10.1016/j.media.2019.101547 PMID:31476576

Szegedy, C., Liu, W., Jia, Y., Sermanet, P., Reed, S., Anguelov, D., Erhan, D., & Vanhoucke, V. (2015). Going deeper with convolutions. *2015 IEEE Conference on Computer Vision and Pattern Recognition (CVPR).* IEEE. 10.1109/CVPR.2015.7298594

Tajbakhsh, N., Gurudu, S. R., & Liang, J. (2016). Automated Polyp Detection in Colonoscopy Videos Using Shape and Context Information. *IEEE Transactions on Medical Imaging*, *35*(2), 630–644. doi:10.1109/TMI.2015.2487997 PMID:26462083

Tasnim, Z., Chakraborty, S., Shamrat, F. M. J. M., Chowdhury, A. N., Nuha, H. A., Karim, A., Zahir, S. B., & Billah, M. (2021). Deep Learning Predictive Model for Colon Cancer Patient using CNN-based Classification. *International Journal of Advanced Computer Science and Applications*, *12*(8). doi:10.14569/IJACSA.2021.0120880

Top 10 Deep Learning Algorithms in Machine Learning [2022]. (n.d.). ProjectPro. https://www.projectpro.io/article/deep-learning-algorithms/443

Vadapalli, P. (2020, May 29). [*Deep Learning Techniques You Should Know About*. UpGrad Blog. https://www.upgrad.com/blog/top-deep-learning-techniques-you-should-know-about/]. *Top (Madrid)*, *10*.

Viscaino, M., Torres Bustos, J., Muñoz, P., Auat Cheein, C., & Cheein, F. A. (2021). Artificial intelligence for the early detection of colorectal cancer: A comprehensive review of its advantages and misconceptions. *World Journal of Gastroenterology*, *27*(38), 6399–6414. doi:10.3748/wjg.v27.i38.6399 PMID:34720530

Waljee, A. K., Weinheimer-Haus, E. M., Abubakar, A., Ngugi, A. K., Siwo, G. H., Kwakye, G., Singal, A. G., Rao, A., Saini, S. D., Read, A. J., Baker, J. A., Balis, U., Opio, C. K., Zhu, J., & Saleh, M. N. (2022). Artificial intelligence and machine learning for early detection and diagnosis of colorectal cancer in sub-Saharan Africa. *Gut*, *71*(7), 1259–1265. doi:10.1136/gutjnl-2022-327211 PMID:35418482

Wang, X., Zhai, M., Ren, Z., Ren, H., Li, M., Quan, D., Chen, L., & Qiu, L. (2021). Exploratory study on classification of diabetes mellitus through a combined Random Forest Classifier. *BMC Medical Informatics and Decision Making*, *21*(1), 105. Advance online publication. doi:10.118612911-021-01471-4 PMID:33743696

Wang, Z. J., Turko, R., Shaikh, O., Park, H., Das, N., Hohman, F., Kahng, M., & Polo Chau, D. H. (2021). CNN Explainer: Learning Convolutional Neural Networks with Interactive Visualization. *IEEE Transactions on Visualization and Computer Graphics*, *27*(2), 1396–1406. doi:10.1109/TVCG.2020.3030418 PMID:33048723

Xiao, Y., Li, J., Zhong, J., Chen, D., Shi, J., & Jin, H. (2022). Diagnostic Performance of Diffusion-Weighted Imaging for Colorectal Cancer Detection: An Updated Systematic Review and Meta-Analysis. *Frontiers in Oncology*, *12*, 656095. doi:10.3389/fonc.2022.656095 PMID:35814462

Xu, A., Tian, M.-W., Firouzi, B., Alattas, K. A., Mohammadzadeh, A., & Ghaderpour, E. (2022). A New Deep Learning Restricted Boltzmann Machine for Energy Consumption Forecasting. *Sustainability*, *14*(16), 10081. doi:10.3390u141610081

Yamada, M., Saito, Y., Imaoka, H., Saiko, M., Yamada, S., Kondo, H., Takamaru, H., Sakamoto, T., Sese, J., Kuchiba, A., Shibata, T., & Hamamoto, R. (2019). Development of a real-time endoscopic image diagnosis support system using deep learning technology in colonoscopy. *Scientific Reports*, *9*(1), 14465. Advance online publication. doi:10.103841598-019-50567-5 PMID:31594962

Yu, K.-H., Beam, A. L., & Kohane, I. S. (2018). Artificial intelligence in healthcare. *Nature Biomedical Engineering*, *2*(10), 719–731. doi:10.103841551-018-0305-z PMID:31015651

Yu, M. K., Ma, J., Fisher, J., Kreisberg, J. F., Raphael, B. J., & Ideker, T. (2018). Visible Machine Learning for Biomedicine. *Cell*, *173*(7), 1562–1565. doi:10.1016/j.cell.2018.05.056 PMID:29906441

. Zeiler, M. D., & Fergus, R. (2014). Visualizing and Understanding Convolutional Networks. *Computer Vision – ECCV 2014*, 818–833. doi:10.1007/978-3-319-10590-1_53

Zhu, W., Xie, L., Han, J., & Guo, X. (2020). The Application of Deep Learning in Cancer Prognosis Prediction. *Cancers (Basel)*, *12*(3), 603. doi:10.3390/cancers12030603 PMID:32150991

Chapter 5
A Review of Recent Machine Learning Techniques Used for Skin Lesion Image Classification

Mayank Upadhyay
Larson and Toubro Services, India

Jyoti Rawat
DIT University, India

Kriti
DIT University, India

ABSTRACT

Skin cancer is amongst the most common forms of cancer and can become life-threatening if not detected early. Due to the rise in the number of cancer cases, there is a growing interest in using computational diagnostics for early cancer detection as the specificity rate of even an expert dermatologist is around 59%. Computer-aided diagnosis can significantly contribute to skin lesion image analysis. Skin cancer prognostication can be achieved with a classification that assigns data objects to particular classes based on extracted features. The steps for image classification are pre-processing where noise is removed and lesion features are highlighted, making it easier to classify the image, detection of the lesion on skin (i.e. segmentation), extracting useful features, and finally applying classification algorithm. This paper provides a review of the recent studies in the bailiwick of skin cancer image classification using machine learning (ML) algorithms.

DOI: 10.4018/978-1-6684-6957-6.ch005

INTRODUCTION

Cancer is defined as abnormal cell growth in an organ. It is a broad term that includes several diseases of which the prevalent forms of cancer are lung, breast, skin, colorectal, prostate, and liver cancer (WHO, 2020). Skin cancer can be defined as the unusual growth of cells on the surface of the skin and is considered to be amongst the most dangerous diseases in dermatology. There are different classes of skin lesions and in most of the research work classification between melanoma and non-melanoma is done. It is estimated that in the US alone there will be around 100,350 cases of melanoma with 6,850 deaths in 2020 (Siegel et al., 2023). Some of the external factors that contribute to the growth of cancerous cells are consumption of tobacco and alcoholic drinks, physical inactivity, age (Gelband & Sloan, 2007), prolonged exposure to UV rays, presence of arsenic in drinking water (Fabbrocini et al., 2010) Skin cancer starts in the outer region of the skin which is the epidermis. The types of cells where cancer starts in the epidermis are: 1) Squamous cells form the outer surface of the epidermis, which are periodically shed and replaced by new squamous cells. 2) Basal cells form the bottom part of the epidermis. Basal cells continuously divide to form new cells and move up in the epidermis to replace squamous cells. 3) Melanocytes produce melanin, a dark pigment that gives skin its colour and protects it from harmful UV rays. Melanoma is caused by the unusual growth of melanocytes cells (Zaidi et al., 2020). Furthermore, the majority of melanomas are first identified manually by non-specialists and or self-examination making it necessary to spread awareness regarding skin cancer (Titus et al., 2013). An accurate and early prognosis of melanoma in the initial stage increases the survival rate of the cancer patient and also decreases medical expenditure (Sabri et al., 2020).

BACKGROUND

ML techniques can play a pivotal role in the public healthcare sector, as they can give high accuracy in the prognosis of skin cancer. Typically, the steps involved in lesion image classification are as shown in figure 1. This paper presents a review of recent research performed in the area of skin lesion classification using ML algorithms.

Figure 1. Steps involved in classifying the skin lesion image dataset

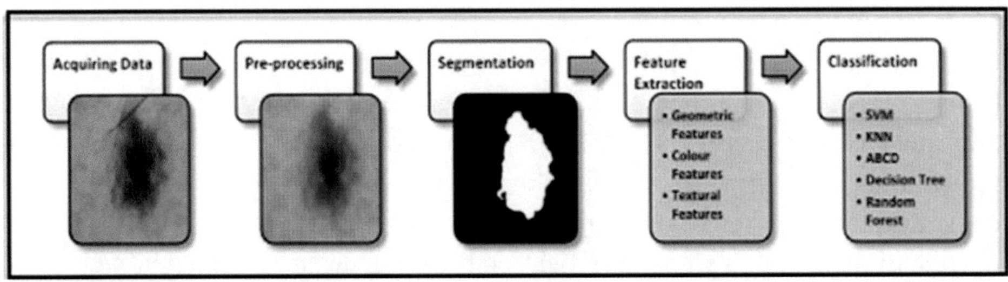

Data Acquisition

Before the pre-processing step, the image dataset needs to be collected. There are many skin cancer image repositories available online which are widely used in cancer image classification research. The dataset used for training the model should be sufficiently large (Petrellis, 2018) and if the dataset is imbalanced then techniques like data augmentation (Vidya & Karki, 2020) and SMOTE (Chakravorty et al., 2016) can be used. However, one of the limitations in the reviewed literature was the small size of the dataset used. Figure 2 shows the size of the dataset used in the reviewed literature, as 59% of the literature used dataset containing no. of images only between 1 to 200.

Pre-Processing

The first step of skin lesion classification is pre-processing. The images acquired may contain noise and poor contrast. So pre-processing is done to improve the image and highlight important attributes of the image, the steps involve image resizing, denoising the image, adjusting poor brightness and contrast, and removal of artefacts like skin lines, hairs, air bubbles, and blood vessels (Filali et al., 2018). The goal of pre-processing is to make skin lesion detection easy. This step highlights the lesion features making it easier to classify the image. Poor pre-processing techniques can result in a loss of useful knowledge about the dataset and adversely affect the outcome of segmentation (Sabri et al., 2020).

Figure 2. Illustration of dataset size used in the literature

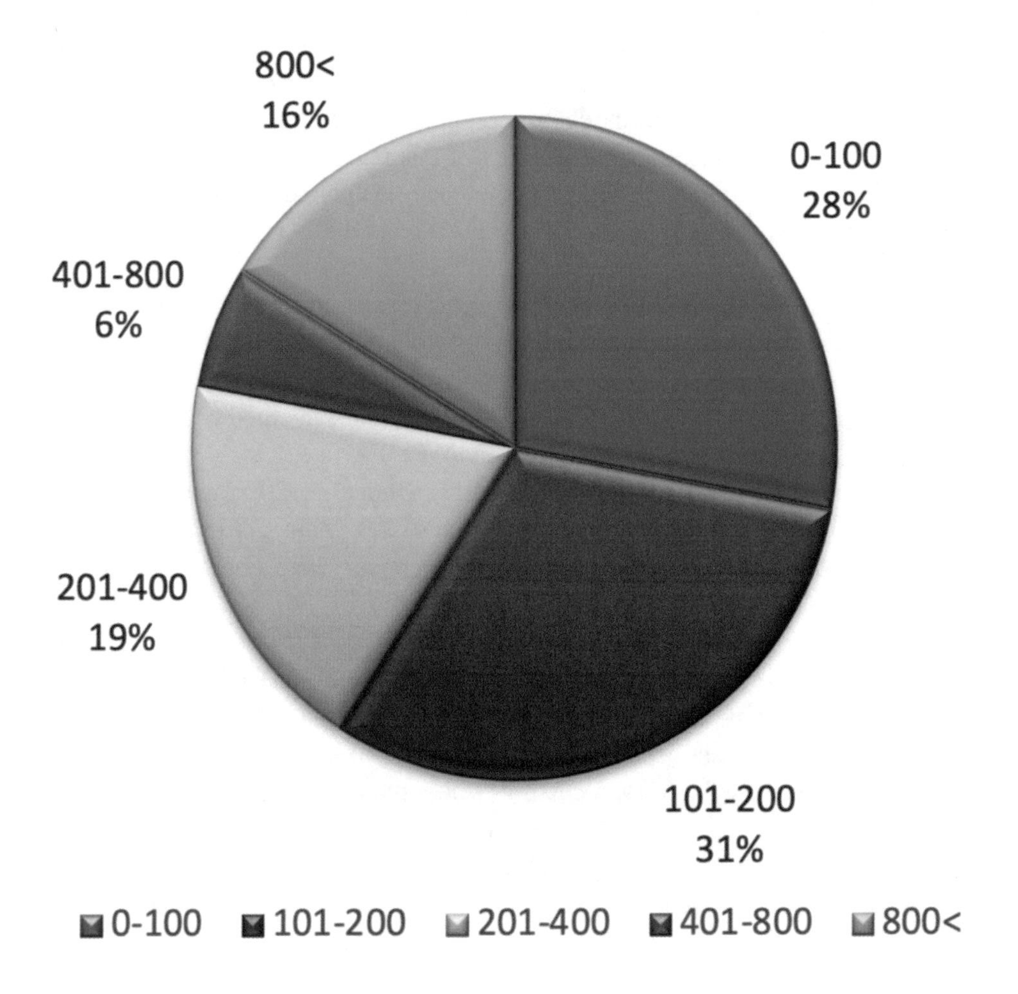

The input skin lesion image may not be properly illuminated because of the surrounding environment, or the quality of the photographic device used to capture the images. These images might require correction in different aspects like contrast, tonal adjustment, sharpness, and saturation. Hence researchers used image enhancement techniques (Amirjahan & Sujatha, 2016) like:

(a) *gamma correction.* To deal with poor contrast and brightness in images *(Jain & Pise, 2015).* It is used to calibrate the image in such a way that they are easy to be perceived by the human eye.

(b) *histogram equalization.* Alquran et al. (2018) and Rawat et al., (2017) used histogram equalization for contrast enhancement of images. In histogram equalization, each pixel intensity is improved globally. It is useful for images with very high brightness or very low brightness.

(c) *Contrast Limited Adaptive Histogram Equalization (CLAHE). Used f*or correcting the contrast of the input image (Suganya, 2016). CLAHE is a modified adaptive technique where the contrast is improved locally i.e. contrast is adjusted according to the neighbourhood pixels of that region and the maximum value of histogram is clipped. This technique can be applied for grayscale as well as coloured images.

For noise removal in lesion image use of dull razor (for thick hair) which uses closing operation to detect hair and bilinear interpolation to replace hair pixels, and median filter (for thin hair) where a mask of given size slides over every pixel of the input image and the value of the pixel being processed is updated with the median value of the pixels within the mask (Alquran, 2017; Vidya & Karki, 2020) were the techniques used by many researchers (Gulati & Bhogal, 2020; Shalu & Kamboj, 2018; Suganya, 2016). Morphological operations like opening, closing (Lattoofi et al., 2019), a top-hat filter (Korjakowska & Tadeusiewicz, 2015) for removal of thick black hair and bottom-hat filter (Vidya & Karki, 2020; Viknesh et al., 2019) are image processing technique that updates pixel values based on structuring elements, also Gaussian filter (Amirjahan & Sujatha, 2016; Korjakowska & Tadeusiewicz, 2015; Linsangan et al., 2019) and low pass filter (Razazzadeh & Khalili, 2015) for blurring images were used in pre-processing. AUJOL model for image decomposition is also a technique used in pre-processing, where the lesion image is split into two components which are texture component with possible noise from the original image and object component (Filali et al. 2017; Filali et al., 2018; Sabri et al., 2020).

Ruela et al., (2013) manually selected 177 images out of 169 images from the dataset that satisfied the selection criteria of lesion boundary staying within the captured image.

Segmentation

The second step of skin lesion image classification is segmentation. Segmentation means splitting the image into several parts with the aim being the representation of the original image into something more relevant for the feature extraction phase. Segmentation is done for the detection and separation of the region of interest (ROI) (Rawat et al. 2022). In skin cancer classification segmentation is performed to obtain the lesion part from the image.

Segmentation is an essential step in image processing as the essential features required for classification are extracted from the segmented lesion. A skin cancer image might contain small blobs that are not skin lesions making it difficult to identify the skin lesion. Jain & Pise (2015) proposed considering the biggest blob as a skin lesion from the resultant segmented image.

A comparison between manual segmentation by experts and automatic thresholding showed that manual segmentation gave better results (Ruela et al., 2013).

However, for the advancement of a CAD (Computer-Aided Diagnosis) system, automatic segmentation is crucial. Segmentation can be performed by use of techniques like Otsu's thresholding (Alquran et al., 2017; Filali et al., 2018; Jain & Pise, 2015; Kharazmi et al., 2017; Lattoofi et al., 2019; Linsangan et al., 2019; Sabri et al., 2020; Vidya & Karki, 2020), K-means (Amirjahan & Sujatha, 2016; Kharazmi et al., 2017; Suganya, 2016; Sundar & Vadivel, 2016), Seeded region growing (Korjakowska & Tadeusiewicz, 2015; Viknesh et al., 2019), Expectation-Maximization (Filali et al., 2017), Active Contours (Gulati & Bhogal, 2020; Shalu & Kamboj, 2018; Vidya & Karki, 2020), edge detection (Abbas et al., 2019; Linsangan et al., 2019) and GrabCut.

Feature Extraction and Selection

The subsequent step after segmentation in lesion image classification is feature extraction. The outcome of segmentation is the skin lesion minus the background. In the feature extraction phase, the relevant information or features from the segmented lesion are extracted, these features uniquely describe the lesion and are utilized to categorize the lesion image as malignant or benign. Feature extraction is used to reduce information that needs to be processed from the image while keeping the important information about the image needed for accurate classification which results in reduced processing time (Nie, 2011). In literature, numerous features of a segmented lesion like geometric features (Jain & Pise, 2015; Linsangan et al., 2019; Moussa et al., 2016), textural features (Amirjahan & Sujatha, 2016; Filali et al., 2017) and color features (Ruela et al., 2013; Shalu & Kamboj, 2018) were extracted.

Several features extraction techniques were used in literature like GLCM (Gray Level Co-occurrence Matrix) method used to obtain textural features (Abbas et al., 2019; Amirjahan & Sujatha, 2016; Filali et al., 2017; Gulati & Bhogal, 2020; Rawat et al., 2018; Sundar & Vadivel, 2016), ABCD rule to extract texture, shape and colour features (Filali et al., 2018; Moussa et al., 2016; Vidya & Karki, 2020; Viknesh et al., 2019), Gabor filter.

After feature extraction, the selection of relevant and useful features is important as it can reduce the computational complexities making the model more efficient. Methods like Information gain (Sabri et al., 2020), RELIEF (Filali et al., 2018),

Genetic optimization (Amirjahan & Sujatha, 2016), Wikis lambda (Suganya, 2016) and PCA (principal component analysis) (Razazzadeh & Khalili, 2015), can be used for feature selection. In the lesion classification process, several features are extracted during the feature extraction phase which are rarely used.

CLASSIFICATION

This is the final step in skin cancer image classification where the information obtained from the previous steps are used for skin cancer prognosis. In this phase, the images are categorized into predefined labels i.e. malignant or benign based on the detected object and extracted features. In combination with extracted features from the segmented lesion, several ML algorithms were applied for labelling the image as cancerous or benign.

Support Vector Machine (SVM)

SVM is a supervised machine learning algorithm used for classification and regression which uses hyperplane to separate the dataset.

The data points lying on the margin are support vectors and an optimal hyperplane has the maximum margin. Although the SVM algorithm is a linear classifier, kernel functions like sigmoid, radial basis function (RBF), and polynomial can be used for non-linear classes.

Several ML techniques were applied for the classification of skin lesion images in recent studies and amongst all the techniques SVM was the most extensively used one (Filali et al., 2017). Figure 3 shows the algorithms used in the literature.

Figure 3. Illustration of classification algorithms used in the literature

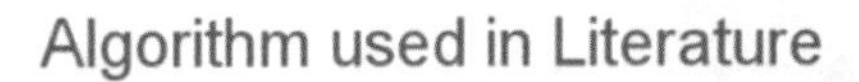

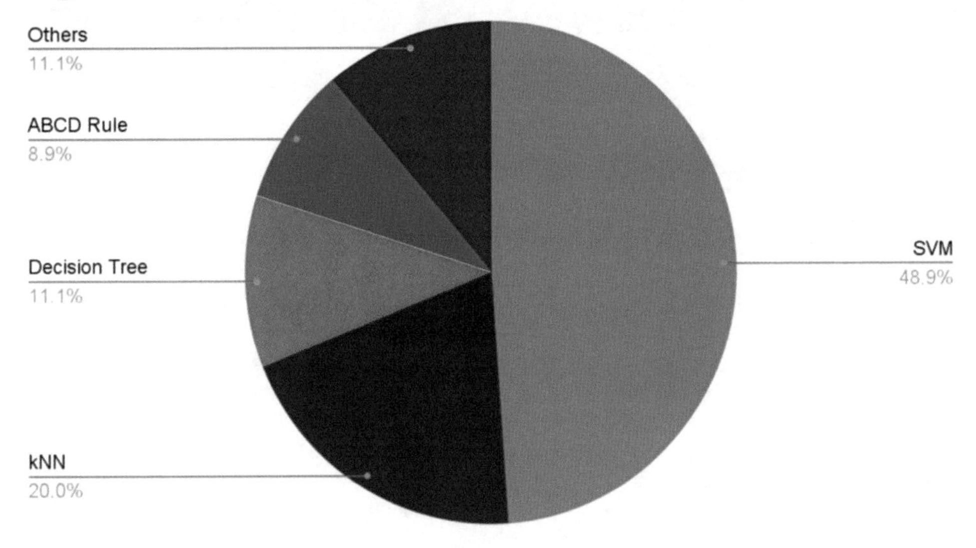

Detection of skin cancer in the early stages is crucial to increase the survival rate of patients. Filali et al., (2018) evaluated different approaches for skin lesion image classification. Logistic regression, Tree, SVM and KNN were compared and SVM with quadratic kernel gave the best result.

Many researchers only focus on classifying the image as malignant or benign. The studies that classified images further into lesion classes are mentioned. In the research by Suganya, (2016) four skin cancer classes were taken in the dataset. They were classified first as malignant or benign and then further classified into Melanocytic Nevi or Melanoma if malignant, or into Seborrheic keratosis (SK) or Basal cell carcinoma (BCC) if benign. Figure 4 shows the highest accuracy achieved by each classifier in the literature.

Figure 4. Highest accuracy achieved by each classifier in the literature

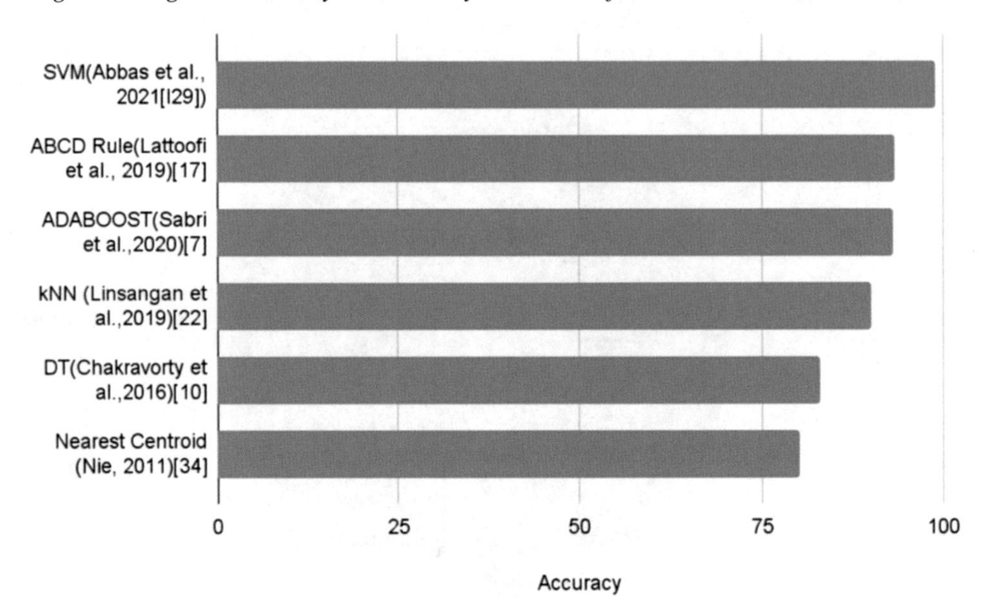

K-Nearest Neighbour (KNN)

It is a simple and easy classification algorithm, which is a non-parametric method of classification. Where the classification is done based on neighborhood voting. K nearest neighbors of the input data are retrieved then input data is assigned to the class based on majority voting by neighborhood data. In the KNN algorithm, K is the only parameter that can be changed, and there are several methods for choosing the value of K. However, the easiest technique is to run the model multiple times with different K values and choose the value that gave the best result (Linsangan et al., 2019).

ABCD Rule

ABCD rule is one of the most common techniques to identify the malignant lesion and is used in CAD for feature extraction (Moussa et al., 2016; Razazzadeh & Khalili, 2015; Viknesh et al., 2019) and classification. ABCD rule is defined as **Asymmetry** (Chakravorty et al., 2016) that is if the lesion is divided into two-part then both parts will have a different structure, **Border irregularity** (Korjakowska & Tadeusiewicz, 2015) that is the lesion peripheral is uneven, **Colour** as a malignant lesion has more than one colour, and **Diameter** a lesion is generally classified as malignant if it is equal or greater than 6mm. **Evolving** as a parameter can also be used to classify the lesion image (Navarro et al., 2019). In ABCD classification total dermatoscopy score (TDS) of the lesion is calculated and if the score is less than 4.75 then the lesion is categorized as benign and if it is greater than 5.45 the lesion is classified as malignant. Equation 1 is used to calculate the TDS value.

$$TDS = 1.3*A + 0.1*B + 0.5*\sum C + 0.5*D \quad (1)$$

where A is asymmetry score, B is border irregularity score, C is no of colours and D is the diameter of the lesion.

Examining the ABCD features of the skin lesion is one of the methods dermatologists used to identify melanoma. Lattoofi et al., (2019) used CAD and the segmented lesions overall dermoscopic score was calculated using the ABCD rule and the skin lesion image was classified as benign or malignant. Korjakowska & Tadeusiewicz, (2015) used border shape to identify malignant from benign.

Decision Tree

The decision tree is a supervised ML algorithm that splits dataset multiple times based on criteria forming a structure that resembles a tree structure with decision nodes and leaf nodes. The measure of the purity of the split is given by entropy and lower entropy means a better split. Table 1 shows the classification algorithms used in literature, and in research with multiple classifiers, the one with the best overall performance is shown in the table.

Table 1. Feature extraction and classification methods used in literature

Reference	Feature Extraction & Selection		Classification			
	Method	*Features used*	*Classifier*	*SE*	*SP*	*ACC*
Sabri et al. (2020)	Information gain	5 features	AdaBoost	93	63	93
Chakravorty et al. (2016)	N/A	Geometric, Colour, Structural features	DT	67	89	83
			KNN	63	90	82
Suganya (2016)	Wikis lambda	Text, Subregion, Colour features	SVM	95.4	89.3	96.8
Gulati & Bhogal (2020)	GLCM	Texture, shape and colour features used	SVM	82.50	97.50	94.50
Shalu & Kamboj (2018)	Statistical measures were extracted	24 Colour features	DT	74.2	88	82.3
Lattoofi et al. (2019)	N/A	Structural and Colour features	ABCD rule	90.1	92.5	93.2
Razazzadeh & Khalili (2015)	ABCD rule and GLCM	119 Texture, Shape and Colour features	SVM with RBF kernel	79.8	90.0	84.0
Filali et al. (2017)	GLCM	Textural features	SVM	96.3	94.9	83
Abbas et al. (2019)	GLCM	10 features used	SVM	99.1	98.6	99.0
Note: SE: Sensitivity, SPE: Specificity, ACC: Accuracy, DT: Decision tree, KNN: K-nearest neighbour, SVM: Support vector machine, GLCM: Gray level co-occurrence matrix.						

Analysis

The dataset used for training and testing the accuracy of the classifiers should be sufficiently large. For the imbalanced dataset, data augmentation techniques can be applied. An imbalanced dataset hampers the training and testing process of the classification model. The input images might require correction in different aspects like contrast, tonal adjustment, sharpness, and saturation which can be achieved by image pre-processing. Techniques like information gain, PCA can be used to select necessary features for better classification. Furthermore, multi-class classification of lesion images should be done rather than binary classification allowing to immediately start treatment for that type of skin cancer.

CONCLUSION

A large number of melanoma cases are detected through self-diagnosis thus making it imperative to raise awareness towards skin cancer. A key factor determining the survival rate of skin cancer patients is to identify the disease early. Several image processing methods are suggested to help dermatologists in skin lesion image diagnosis. This can be more useful in rural areas with a lack of expert dermatologists. By using Machine Learning it's possible to detect and classify skin cancer with higher accuracy than expert dermatologists. To attain high accuracy, it is essential to choose a correct classifier as every classifier doesn't work for all types of datasets. Furthermore, the classifier to be chosen depends on the quality of the input dataset and its environment. Sometimes more than one algorithm can be taken, and an ensemble of multiple models can be used. Some limitations include classifying lesions as malignant or benign is not sufficient; they need to be further classified into lesion types for better treatment. Also, if the lesion is cancerous then determining the stage of cancer is another aspect that needs to be further explored.

REFERENCES

Abbas, Z., Rehman, M. U., Najam, S., & Rizvi, S. D. (2019, February). An efficient gray-level co-occurrence matrix (GLCM) based approach towards classification of skin lesion. In *2019 amity international conference on artificial intelligence (AICAI)* (pp. 317-320). IEEE.

Alquran, H., Qasmieh, I. A., Alqudah, A. M., Alhammouri, S., Alawneh, E., Abughazaleh, A., & Hasayen, F. (2017, October). The melanoma skin cancer detection and classification using support vector machine. In *2017 IEEE Jordan Conference on Applied Electrical Engineering and Computing Technologies (AEECT)* (pp. 1-5). IEEE. 10.1109/AEECT.2017.8257738

Amirjahan, M., & Sujatha, D. N. (2016). *Comparative analysis of various classification algorithms for skin Cancer detection. PG & Research Department of Computer Science, Raja Doraisingam Govt.* Art College.

Chakravorty, R., Liang, S., Abedini, M., & Garnavi, R. (2016, August). Dermatologist-like feature extraction from skin lesion for improved asymmetry classification in PH 2 database. In *2016 38th Annual International Conference of the IEEE Engineering in Medicine and Biology Society (EMBC)* (pp. 3855-3858). IEEE.

Fabbrocini, G., Triassi, M., Mauriello, M. C., Torre, G., Annunziata, M. C., Vita, V. D., & Monfrecola, G. (2010). Epidemiology of skin cancer: Role of some environmental factors. *Cancers (Basel)*, *2*(4), 1980–1989. doi:10.3390/cancers2041980 PMID:24281212

Filali, Y., Ennouni, A., Sabri, M. A., & Aarab, A. (2017, May). Multiscale approach for skin lesion analysis and classification. In *2017 International Conference on Advanced Technologies for Signal and Image Processing (ATSIP)* (pp. 1-6). IEEE. 10.1109/ATSIP.2017.8075545

Filali, Y., Ennouni, A., Sabri, M. A., & Aarab, A. (2018, April). A study of lesion skin segmentation, features selection and classification approaches. In *2018 International Conference on Intelligent Systems and Computer Vision (ISCV)* (pp. 1-7). IEEE. 10.1109/ISACV.2018.8354069

Gelband, H., & Sloan, F. A. (Eds.). (2007). *Cancer control opportunities in low-and middle-income countries*. Academic Press.

Gulati, S., & Bhogal, R. K. (2020). Classification of melanoma from dermoscopic images using machine learning. In *Smart Intelligent Computing and Applications: Proceedings of the Third International Conference on Smart Computing and Informatics*, Volume 1 (pp. 345-354). Springer. 10.1007/978-981-13-9282-5_32

Jain, S., & Pise, N. (2015). Computer aided melanoma skin cancer detection using image processing. *Procedia Computer Science*, *48*, 735–740. doi:10.1016/j.procs.2015.04.209

Jaworek-Korjakowska, J., & Tadeusiewicz, R. (2015, August). Determination of border irregularity in dermoscopic color images of pigmented skin lesions. In *Annual International Conference of the IEEE Engineering in Medicine and Biology Society*, (Vol. 2015, pp. 2665-2668). IEEE.

Kharazmi, P., AlJasser, M. I., Lui, H., Wang, Z. J., & Lee, T. K. (2016). Automated detection and segmentation of vascular structures of skin lesions seen in Dermoscopy, with an application to basal cell carcinoma classification. *IEEE Journal of Biomedical and Health Informatics*, *21*(6), 1675–1684. doi:10.1109/JBHI.2016.2637342 PMID:27959832

Lattoofi, N. F., Al-Sharuee, I. F., Kamil, M. Y., Obaid, A. H., Mahidi, A. A., & Omar, A. A. (2019, December). Melanoma skin cancer detection based on ABCD rule. In *2019 First International Conference of Computer and Applied Sciences (CAS)* (pp. 154-157). IEEE. 10.1109/CAS47993.2019.9075465

Linsangan, N. B., Adtoon, J. J., & Torres, J. L. (2018, November). Geometric analysis of skin lesion for skin cancer using image processing. In *2018 IEEE 10th International Conference on Humanoid, Nanotechnology, Information Technology, Communication and Control, Environment and Management (HNICEM)* (pp. 1-5). IEEE. 10.1109/HNICEM.2018.8666296

Moussa, R., Gerges, F., Salem, C., Akiki, R., Falou, O., & Azar, D. (2016, October). Computer-aided detection of Melanoma using geometric features. In *2016 3rd Middle East Conference on Biomedical Engineering (MECBME)* (pp. 125-128). IEEE. 10.1109/MECBME.2016.7745423

Navarro, F., Escudero-Vinolo, M., & Bescós, J. (2018). Accurate segmentation and registration of skin lesion images to evaluate lesion change. *IEEE Journal of Biomedical and Health Informatics*, *23*(2), 501–508. doi:10.1109/JBHI.2018.2825251 PMID:29993849

Nie, D. (2011, March). Classification of melanoma and clark nevus skin lesions based on Medical Image Processing Techniques. In *2011 3rd International Conference on Computer Research and Development* (*Vol. 3,* pp. 31-34). IEEE.

Petrellis, N. (2018, July). The Effect of the Training Set Size in a Skin Disorder Classification Application. In *2018 41st International Conference on Telecommunications and Signal Processing (TSP)* (pp. 1-5). IEEE. 10.1109/TSP.2018.8441474

Rawat, J., Singh, A., Bhadauria, H. S., Virmani, J., & Devgun, J. S. (2017). Classification of acute lymphoblastic leukaemia using hybrid hierarchical classifiers. *Multimedia Tools and Applications*, *76*(18), 19057–19085. doi:10.100711042-017-4478-3

Rawat, J., Singh, A., Bhadauria, H. S., Virmani, J., & Devgun, J. S. (2018). Leukocyte classification using adaptive neuro-fuzzy inference system in microscopic blood images. *Arabian Journal for Science and Engineering*, *43*(12), 7041–7058. doi:10.100713369-017-2959-3

Rawat, J., Virmani, J., Singh, A., Bhadauria, H. S., Kumar, I., & Devgan, J. S. (2022). FAB classification of acute leukemia using an ensemble of neural networks. *Evolutionary Intelligence*, *15*(1), 99–117. doi:10.100712065-020-00491-9

Razazzadeh, N., & Khalili, M. (2015, May). A high performance algorithm to diagnosis of skin lesions deterioration in dermatoscopic images using new feature extraction. In *2015 IEEE 28th Canadian Conference on Electrical and Computer Engineering (CCECE)* (pp. 1207-1212). IEEE. 10.1109/CCECE.2015.7129449

Ruela, M., Barata, C., & Marques, J. S. (2013). What is the role of color symmetry in the detection of melanomas? In Advances in Visual Computing: 9th International Symposium, ISVC 2013, Proceedings, *9*(Part I), 1–10. IEEE.

Sabri, M. A., Filali, Y., El Khoukhi, H., & Aarab, A. (2020, June). Skin cancer diagnosis using an improved ensemble machine learning model. In *2020 International Conference on Intelligent Systems and Computer Vision (ISCV)* (pp. 1-5). IEEE. 10.1109/ISCV49265.2020.9204324

Shalu, K., A. (2018, December). A color-based approach for melanoma skin cancer detection. In *2018 First International Conference on Secure Cyber Computing and Communication (ICSCCC)* (pp. 508-513). IEEE. 10.1109/ICSCCC.2018.8703309

Siegel, R. L., Miller, K. D., Wagle, N. S., & Jemal, A. (2023). Cancer statistics, 2023. *CA: a Cancer Journal for Clinicians*, *73*(1), 17–48. doi:10.3322/caac.21763 PMID:36633525

Suganya, R. (2016, April). An automated computer aided diagnosis of skin lesions detection and classification for dermoscopy images. In *2016 International Conference on Recent Trends in Information Technology (ICRTIT)* (pp. 1-5). IEEE. 10.1109/ICRTIT.2016.7569538

Sundar, R. S., & Vadivel, M. (2016, March). Performance analysis of melanoma early detection using skin lession classification system. In *2016 International Conference on Circuit, Power and Computing Technologies (ICCPCT)* (pp. 1-5). IEEE. 10.1109/ICCPCT.2016.7530182

Titus, L. J., Clough-Gorr, K., Mackenzie, T. A., Perry, A., Spencer, S. K., Weiss, J., Abrahams-Gessel, S., & Ernstoff, M. S. (2013). Recent skin self-examination and doctor visits in relation to melanoma risk and tumour depth. *British Journal of Dermatology*, *168*(3), 571–576. doi:10.1111/bjd.12003 PMID:22897437

Vidya, M., & Karki, M. V. (2020, July). Skin cancer detection using machine learning techniques. In *2020 IEEE international conference on electronics, computing and communication technologies (CONECCT)* (pp. 1-5). IEEE.

Viknesh, C. K., Kumar, P. N., & Seetharaman, R. (2019, January). Computer aided diagnostic system for the classification of skin cancer using dermoscopic images. In *2019 Third International Conference on Inventive Systems and Control (ICISC)* (pp. 342-345). IEEE. 10.1109/ICISC44355.2019.9036327

World health organization. (n.d.). *Cancer*. WHO. https://www.who.int/health-topics/cancer#tab=tab_1 (Accessed July, 06, 2020)

Zaidi, M. R., Fisher, D. E., & Rizos, H. (2020). Biology of melanocytes and primary melanoma. *Cutaneous Melanoma*, 3-40.

Chapter 6
A Medical Assistant for the Visually Impaired

Kavita Pandey
https://orcid.org/0000-0003-2613-4800
Jaypee Institute of Information Technology, India

Dhiraj Pandey
https://orcid.org/0000-0001-5969-6071
JSS Academy of Technical Education, India

Rijwan Khan
https://orcid.org/0000-0003-3354-3047
ABES Institute of Technology, India

ABSTRACT

A visually impaired individual loses vision when a part of the eye or the brain that processes images becomes diseased or damaged. Visually impaired people face many problems during their daily activities such as walking around places, identifying objects, identifying people's feelings or emotions, detecting obstacles, etc. Several solutions work around these problems. The area that needs the attention of researchers is helping the visually impaired people in reading the medical reports, a product's name, and a device's reading. To make them independent, this paper proposed a medical assistant "M.A.V.I" which helps a visually impaired person to read medical blood reports, products, normal reports, and LED screens of inaccessible medical devices like a glucose monitor, BP machine, and weighing machine, etc.

DOI: 10.4018/978-1-6684-6957-6.ch006

INTRODUCTION

The importance of vision in our daily lives cannot be underestimated. Vision is used by humans to navigate through highways, find items, and so on. Blind people, on the other hand, are not blessed with vision, which makes life tough for them. The rate of blindness in our society has been steadily rising. According to the survey in the article (Pandey, 2021 ; Pandey, 2021), this number is expected to triple from its current level by 20. As per the World Health Organization report (World, 2022), at least 2.2 billion individuals worldwide will suffer from near or far vision impairment. Vision impairment may have been avoided or managed in at least 1 billion – or nearly half – of these cases. Uncorrected refractive errors and cataracts are the major causes of visual impairment and blindness. The majority of persons who suffer from vision impairment or blindness are over the age of 50; however, vision loss can affect persons of any age. The annual global costs of productivity losses related to visual impairment from untreated myopia and presbyopia are estimated to be US$ 244 billion and US$ 25.4 billion, respectively, due to vision impairment (Ani, 2017).

A visually impaired person faces several obstacles while living their life such as navigation, shopping, identifying objects, streets, products, recognizing human expression etc. Similarly, they face a lot of difficulties when they need to see their medical reports, medical products and devices. Thus, to make smart technological advancements in this regard, this paper is intended to provide a solution by proposing and developing a cross-platform mobile application for visually impaired people, which can help them in reading the medical blood reports, medical product's name, and digital medical device's reading. From the proposed application in this article, the visually impaired can easily access and take information written in their medical documents or devices without any help from others. The rear camera will capture images in front of the blind person in real-time after the application is opened. Then with the help of optical character recognition (OCR), the application will identify the object and be able to read it out with the help of text-to-speech (TTS). The application also has a voice assistant to guide the user.

We've seen how the visually impaired encounter obstacles in their daily lives and various assistive technologies based on sensors, IoT, and computer vision have been launched to help blind people. These systems have their advantages and limitations. So, after going through many research papers it has been decided that there is no such work that focuses on medical reports, product's name and medical devices reading. This paper proposed a medical assistant "M.A.V.I" which would help a visually impaired person to read medical blood reports, product details, normal reports and LED screens of inaccessible medical devices like a glucose monitor, BP machine and weighing machine etc.

The research work of this article is further divided into various sections. Section 2 discusses the work that has already been done in this direction and this section, further, we have materials and methods in section 3 which discuss the technology and system requirements used in this paper. In section 4, we have discussed the proposed work in detail in this research paper. In section 5 we have discussed the implementation of our work. Section 6 discusses the results which are followed by a conclusion and references.

RELATED WORK

A visually impaired person faces a lot of difficulties in their daily life activities like navigation, shopping, identifying objects, streets, products, recognizing human expression etc. Similarly, they feel a lot of difficulties when they need to see their medical reports, medical products and devices. In (Rajput, 2017), authors presented a solution that proposes an aid to assist disabled individuals in reading text labels in their daily lives, which can be implemented by isolating the object via busy backdrops or by enclosing the object in the camera view. By shaking the object in the image, this research establishes a productive and efficient motion-based methodology for establishing a region of interest (ROI) in the video.

In (Deshpande, 2016), authors proposed a solution to assist blind people in reading text labels on a variety of patterns with complicated backgrounds that can be found on a variety of everyday products such as hand-held objects. The work in (Shenoy, 2017) describes the collection of images from medical reports, the display of digital metres, the detection of text, and the recognition of seven-segment numbers from gathered samples, all of which may be useful for visually impaired people. The dataset presented offers enormous promise for completely automated optical character recognition (OCR)-based electricity billing. A variety of digital energy metre photos is included in the dataset. The photographs were taken in both day and nighttime lighting settings. Our dataset was used to research detecting text from a seven-segment display in energy metres under difficult text recognition settings such as tilted position, hazy, and daytime. The labeling approach based on the OCR algorithm, image processing and TTS method has been used for text detection and recognition. The whole application is built using flutter which is a cross-platform for mobile apps. An Alan voice-based assistant for smooth accessibility and an IoT device for capturing the photos of LED screens, reports, and medical products are used in our project(Chang, 2020).

In (Finnegan, 2019), authors developed a method for detecting and reading seven-segment numerals on medical equipment using a smartphone camera. They used a dataset from a real-world scenario to train and evaluate a digit classifier. They created a method that used retinex with two bilateral filters and adaptive histogram equalization to pre-process the input image. Two algorithms work in tandem to locate the digit segment inside the image: MSER (Maximally Stable External Region) and connected components of the binarized image. Filtering and clustering algorithms produce seven-segment digits.

The HOG feature set and a neural network trained on the synthetic digits are used to classify the generated digits. On digits detected on the medical gadget, the model was 93 per cent accurate. In (Kanagarathinam, 2019), authors proposed a review of the literature, dataset collection, text detection and recognition, findings, and a conclusion, as well as the 'Yuva EB dataset' collection, detection, and recognition. The goal was to use the 'Label box' tool to build a raw picture dataset and common objects in a context (coco) annotation JSON file to help with energy consumption billing by using OCR to extract the value and implement MSER.

In (Popayorm, 2019) provided a framework based on a predetermined HSV colour slicing methodology that achieves precision, recall, and accuracy rates of 94.46 per cent, 92.24 per cent, and 87.17 per cent, respectively. They use HSV colour slicing and digit detection and identification. Authors of (Peng, 2012) made a proposal to locate and detect seven-segment displays on digital energy meters. On a dataset of 175 photos of digital energy meters recorded with a mobile camera, they devised a system that can handle photos with uneven light, shadows, poor contrast, and blur and achieves an identification accuracy of 97 per cent.

In the past, researchers had proposed several methods regarding the use of OCR, SSOCR (seven-segment OCR), Machine learning, IoT, and TTS for aid to the visually impaired (Gong, 2021) (Filteau, 2018), (Musale, 2018). These technologies as an individual or a combination of two or more technologies were not useful and interactive for visually impaired people. From what we have researched we have realized that most of these research papers do not have voice assistive technology and cross-platform benefit. Most of these mentioned approaches are just have complex methods and also not given any solution for the visually impaired. In this paper, we have proposed a simple way or application for blind people to help them read medical reports and devices.

MATERIALS AND METHODS

Technology Used

- Flutter Framework (Flutter, 2021): To scan and read the medical reports for visually impaired people, we need some platform. So we have used Flutter to build an application where they can use it from their Android or IOS device to scan the medical report(Batista, 2021).

- Alan (Alan, 2021): Alan provides the complete conversational platform to let you add a voice interface to your app. Alan offers easy-to-integrate SDKs for different platforms: Web, iOS, Android, Flutter, Ionic, React Native, Cordova.
- Flutter TTS (Flutter_tts, 2021): This flutter TTS plugin was designed to work with native functionality. TextToSpeech for Android and AVSpeechSynthesizer for iOS are used behind the scenes. In this article, we'll look at the flutter TTS plugin's functions.
- Flutter mobile vision (Flutter_mobile_vision, 2021): Google Mobile Vision implementation in Flutter. Mobile Vision is an API that uses real-time on-device vision technologies to assist us to find items in photographs and videos. Objects in photographs and movies can be detected using this framework.
- OCR.space API (Get, 2021), (Jitss, 2020): Optical Character Recognition (OCR) is used by the OCR.space OCR service to convert scans or (smartphone) photographs of text documents into editable files (OCR).
- Nanonet's custom model API (Nanonets, 2022): Nanonet has a custom model on their server that we train and further uses as an API for OCR purposes. We use it for the digital medical machine's seven-segment number's training.

System Requirements

- Hardware Requirements: Disk Space for Flutter SDK is 1.32 GB (doesn't include disk space for IDE/tools).
- Software Requirements: Flutter SDK requires Windows 7 SP1 or later (64-bit), x86-64 based and VS Code uses Windows 7 (with .NET Framework 4.5.2), 8.0, 8.1 and 10 (32-bit and 64-bit) Operating systems. Flutter depends on these tools being available in your environment, Windows PowerShell 5.0 and Git for Windows 2. x, with the Use Git from the Windows.

PROPOSED WORK

This prototype system presents text reading from the camera captured image and converts it into voice to get information that the blind person wants to know. This system is divided into 4 sections.

1. A wake-up call from the user wakes up the Alan voice assistant, the intent to click the blood report button from the user's voice will be picked up by Alan and it will call the parsethetext() function which will send the image to OCR API and receive the parsed text which will be spoken by TTS function.
2. A wake-up call from the user wakes up the Alan voice assistant, the intent to click the medical report button from the user's voice will be picked up by Alan and it will call the _read() function which will use flutter_mobile_vision to extract the medical product's name which will be spoken by TTS function.
3. A wake-up call from the user wakes up the Alan voice assistant, the intent to click the normal text button from the user's voice will be picked up by Alan and it will call the parsetext() function which will send the image to OCR API and receive the parsed text which will be spoken by TTS function.
4. A wake-up call from the user wakes up the Alan voice assistant, the intent to click the BP machine button from the user's voice will be picked up by Alan and it will call the parsethebp() function which will send the image to Nanonet's API and receive the parsed text which will be spoken by the TTS function.

Architecture

Figure 1 presents an architectural view for blood report, medical button and normal medical test report and Figure 2 is an architectural view for BP machines.

Figure 1. Step-by-step diagram to recognize blood and text report and medical product

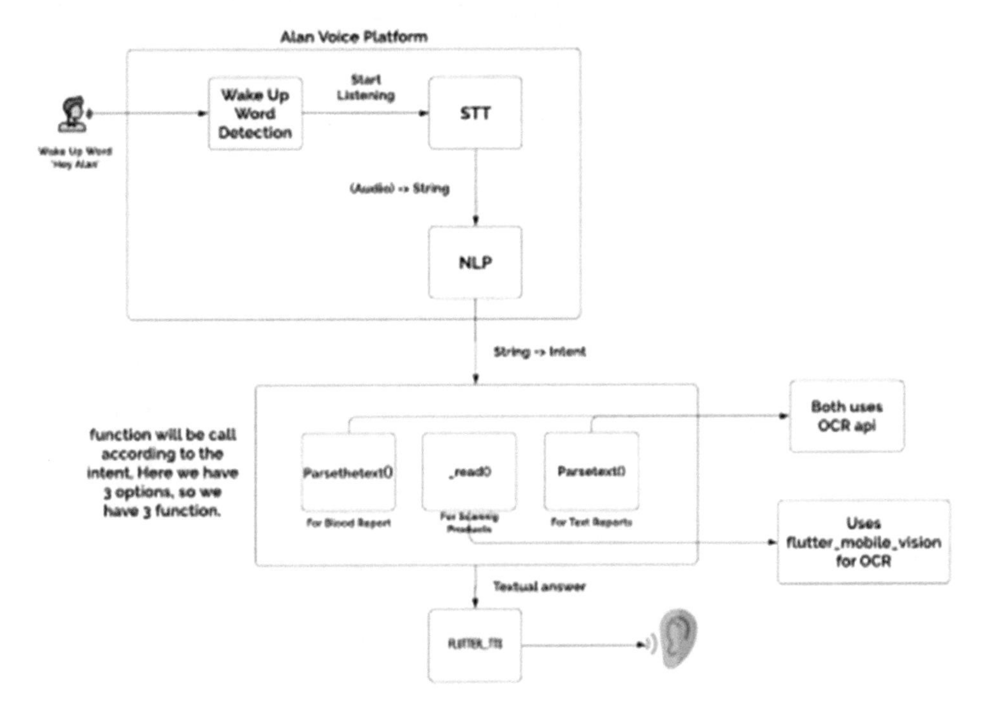

Figure 2. Step-by-step diagram to recognize the digital medical devices

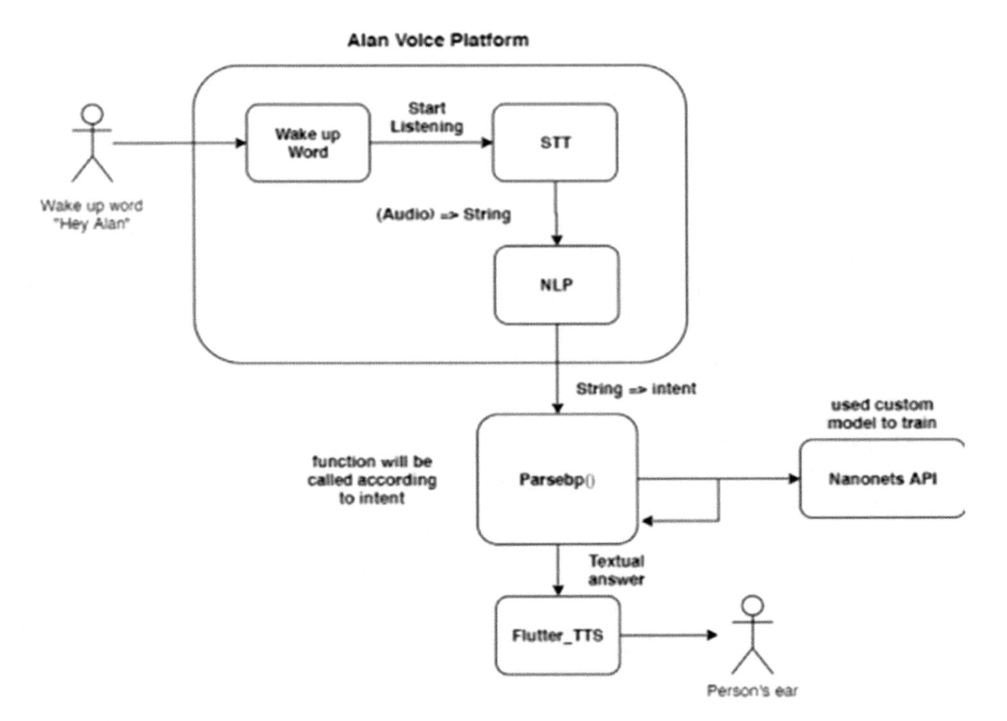

IMPLEMENTATION

In flutter, everything is a widget so we created a widget containing a header with an app's name "M.A.V.I", three buttons with different functionalities, and Alan's floating button and a container to show parsed text. The first button is for recognizing blood reports. The second one is for detecting medical products names or brands. The last one is for recognizing normal text reports,

- **Blood Report's Button**

When a user clicks this button, a function will be called and the user has to pick an image from the gallery. Then in function image will be prepared and sent to OCR API and OCR API will give the result object containing our text. Then we extract that text and apply some logic to it to get a logical solution. The parsed text we extracted will be sent to the Flutter_TTS function for this button to speak out the text to the user.

```
final imagefile = await ImagePicker().getImage(source:
ImageSource.gallery, maxWidth: 670, maxHeight: 970);
```

This will prepare the image

```
var bytes = Io.File(imagefile.path.toString()).
readAsBytesSync(); String img64 = base64Encode(bytes);
```

This will send the image to api

```
var result = jsonDecode(post.body);
```

This will get back result from API

```
var url = 'https://api.ocr.space/parse/image'; var payload =
{"base64Image":"data:image/jpg;base64,${img64.toString()}"};
var header = {"apikey": '3abb227f0b88957'};
var post = await http.post(url, body: payload, headers:
header);
```

- **Medical Product's Button**

When the user clicks this button or calls it to click through Alan voice, it will call a function and use Flutter_Mobile_Vision to initialize the camera and scan a product to recognize a text from it. Flutter_Mobile_Vision will use all OCR, Image processing and ML methods behind the scenes.

- **Normal Text Report's Button**

This button's code is the same as the blood report's button except it doesn't have the logic to extract blood report's information. It will recognize text reports easily,

- **BP machine Button**

When a user clicks this button, a function will be called and the user has to click an image. Then in function, the image will be prepared and sent to nanonet's API and the API will give the result object containing our text. Then we extract that text and apply some logic to it to get a logical solution. The parsed text we extracted will be sent to the Flutter_TTS function for this button to speak out the text to the user.

- **Alan Voice Button**

When a user says a wake-up word "Hey Alan" or simply clicks it, it will wake up to listen. Then it will hear whatever the user's intent was and do the specific job, for example, it will open up the gallery, open the camera to scan, give the current visual of the page and also some information about the page. To make all this happen, we have to add a package known as Alan_voice and add an Alan button, then to do the specific job we have to code in Alan studio on the server and specify intents, this intent will be handled in our code to perform a certain task.

RESULTS

When the user says, "Hey, Alan," the Alan voice platform starts listening to the user's intent. When the user says to upload a blood report, it will open a gallery and when we click an image, it will parse the text like shown in Figure-4 and TTS will speak the parsed text. When the user says to scan a product, it will open a camera and start scanning as visualized from Figure-3 but when the user clicks the box which is formed around text it will parse the text as shown in Figure-6 and TTS will speak the parsed text. When the user says to upload a text report, it will recognize text and parsed text like Figure-5 will be spoken by TTS.

Figure 3. Image samples applied for text reading

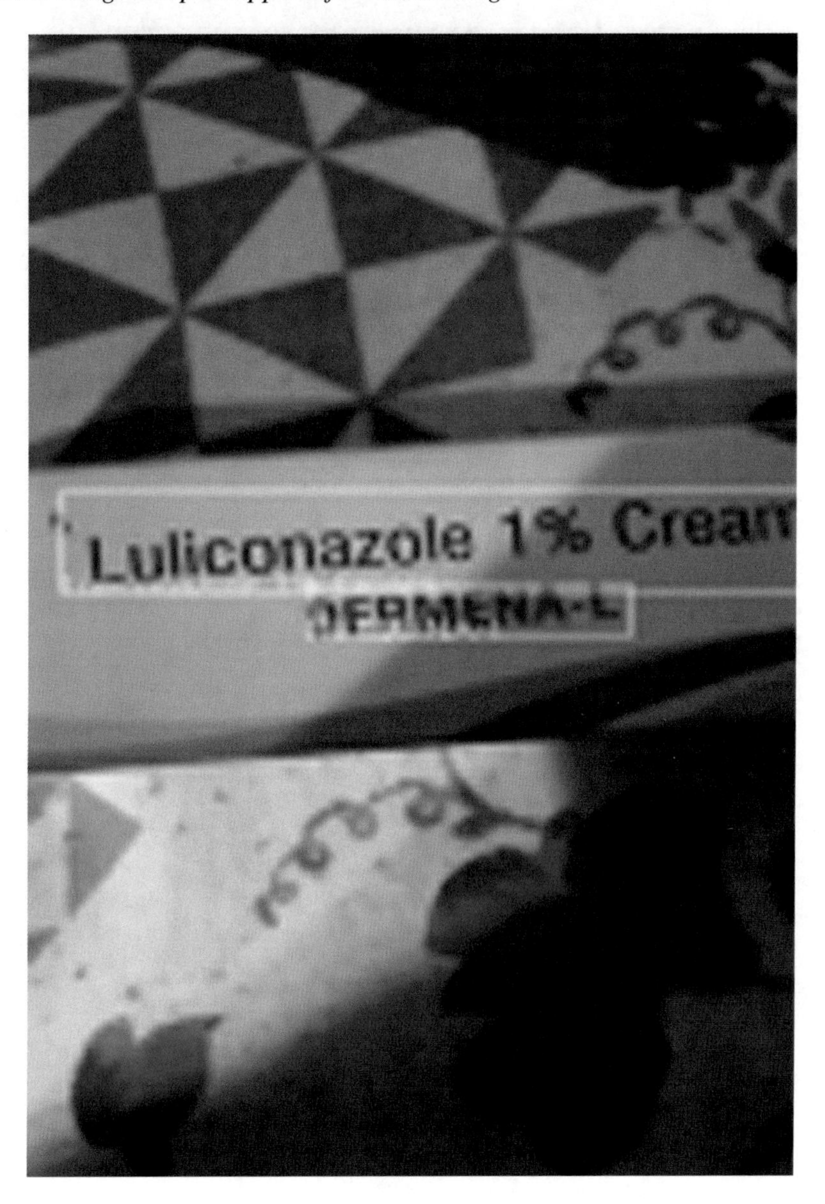

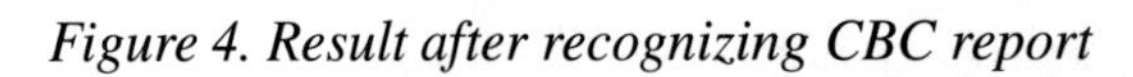

Figure 4. Result after recognizing CBC report

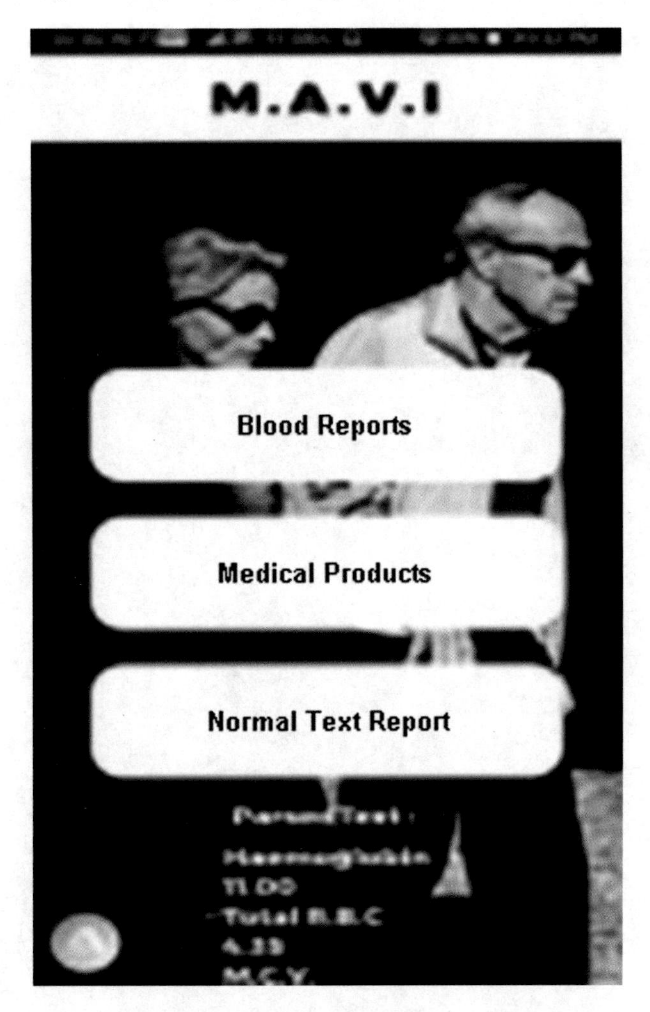

Figure 5. Result after recognizing CBC report

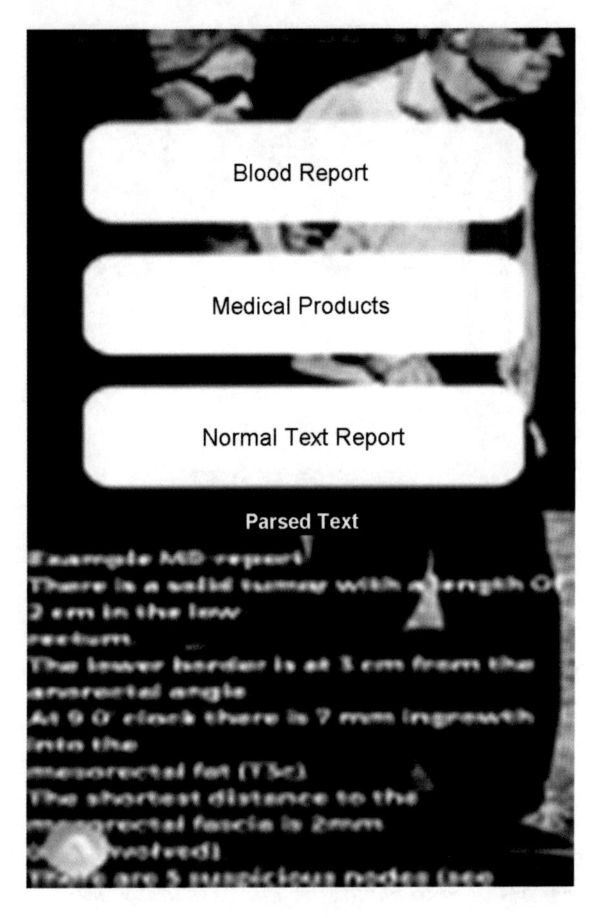

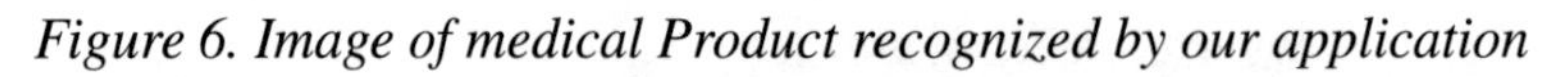

Figure 6. Image of medical Product recognized by our application

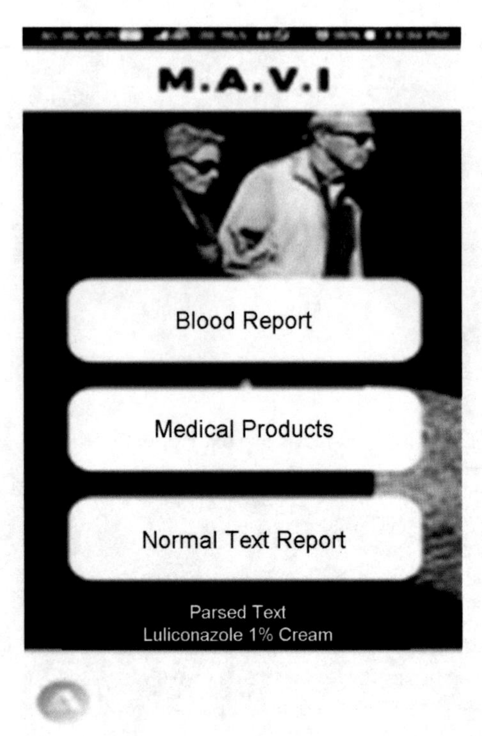

Figure 7. CBC reports used to make sure our assistant works

TEST	RESULT	UNIT
BLOOD COUNTS & INDICES		
Haemoglobin	11.00	gm%
Total R.B.C.	4.35	mill/cmm
P.C.V.	33.10	%
M.C.V.	76.09	fL
M.C.H.	25.29	pg
M.C.H.C.	33.23	%
R.D.W.	15.60	%
Total W.B.C.	5100	/cmm
Platelet Count	265,000	/cmm

Test Name	Result
COMPLETE BLOOD COUNT (EDTA Blood)	
WBC Count (Impedence)	6840
RBC Count (Impedence)	5.75
Haemoglobin (SLS Method)	17.4
Haematocrit (PCV)	47.2
(RBC Pulse Height Detector Method)	
MCV (Calculated)	82.1
MCH (Calculated)	30.3
MCHC (Calculated)	36.9
Platelet Count (Impedence)	298000
RDW-CV (Calculated)	11.8
DIFFERENTIAL COUNT	
Neutrophils (Flowcytometry)	53.9
Lymphocytes (Flowcytometry)	35.2
Monocytes (Flowcytometry)	9.2
Eosinophils (Flowcytometry)	1.3
Basophils (Flowcytometry)	0.4
IG	0.10

We have tested some cases:

1. For Blood Report

So, in this section we have firstly scanned the blood report then it will be uploaded in our application then, our application will be able to read out the entire data of the blood report and thus, it will be easy for the blind people to listen to it.

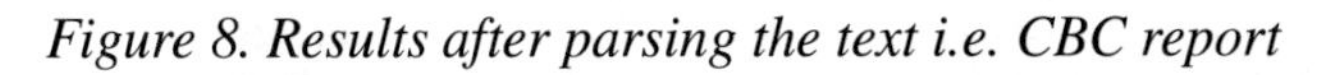

Figure 8. Results after parsing the text i.e. CBC report

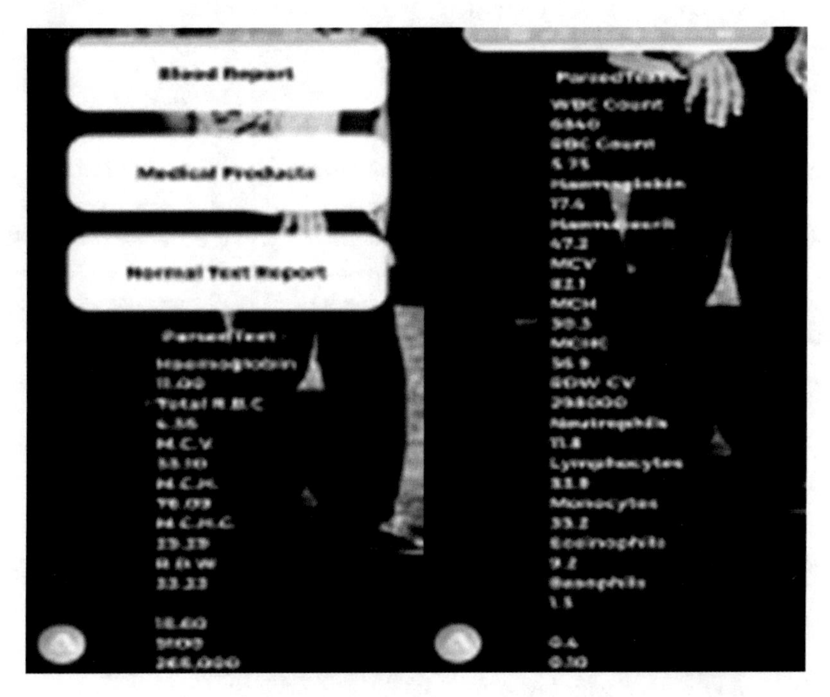

Figure 9. Medical product samples for text read

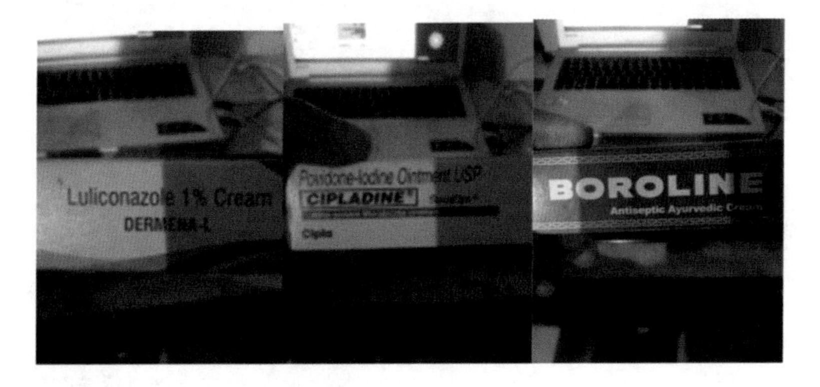

2. For Medical Products

Figure 10. Results after recognizing the medical product samples

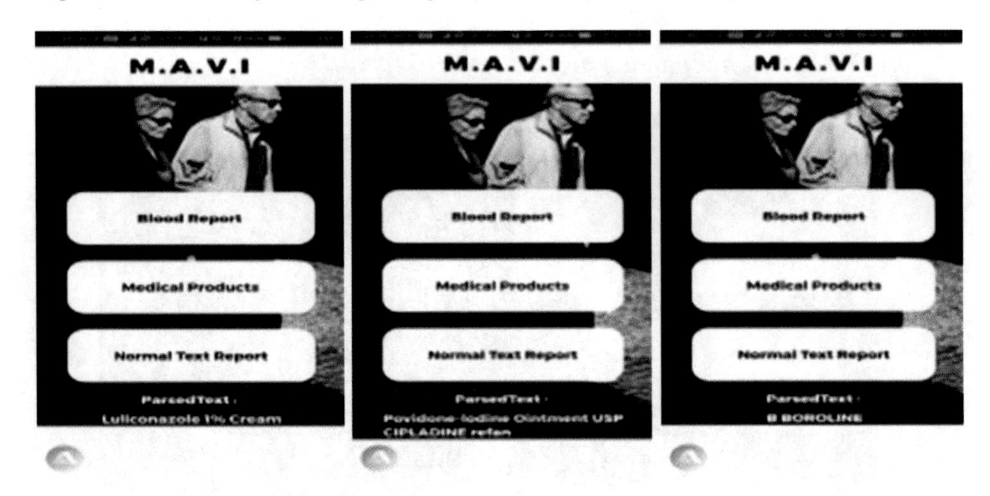

3. For Text Reports

we have taken some samples for text reading of the reports, so here are some examples given below

Figure 11. text report samples to read

Example MR-report

There is a solid tumor with a length of 2 cm in the low-rectum.
The lower border is at 3 cm from the anorectal angle.
At 9 o' clock there is 7 mm ingrowth into the mesorectal fat (T3c).
The shortest distance to the mesorectal fascia is 2mm (not involved).
There are 5 suspicious nodes (see image no....).

Conclusion:
cT3c-N2 tumor with 2mm distance to MRF at 9 o' clock.

Abdomen CT without contrast adminstration with scanning from liver dome tothe pelvis at 10mm intervals is performed. The result showed:

1.The liver is normally positioned and has normal size and smooth borderd.Its internal structure and attenuation values are normal. The intrahepatic and extrahepatic bil ducts and gallbladder are unremarkable.
2.The spleen is orthotopic and of normal size. .
3.The pancrease is normal in size,position, and internal structure with smooth,lobulated outer contours.The pancreatic duct is unobstructed.
4.Both kidneys show normal size and position. The renal parenchyma show normal width and structure. The renal pelvis and calies show a normal configuration.The urinary tract is unobstructed.
5.The adrenal glands are unremarkable.
6.Major blood vessels appear normal,and there is no evidence of lymphoadenopathy.
7.There are no ascites or pleural effusion.

Imp:Normal picture in upper abdomen CT study

Figure 12. Result showed after parsing the text

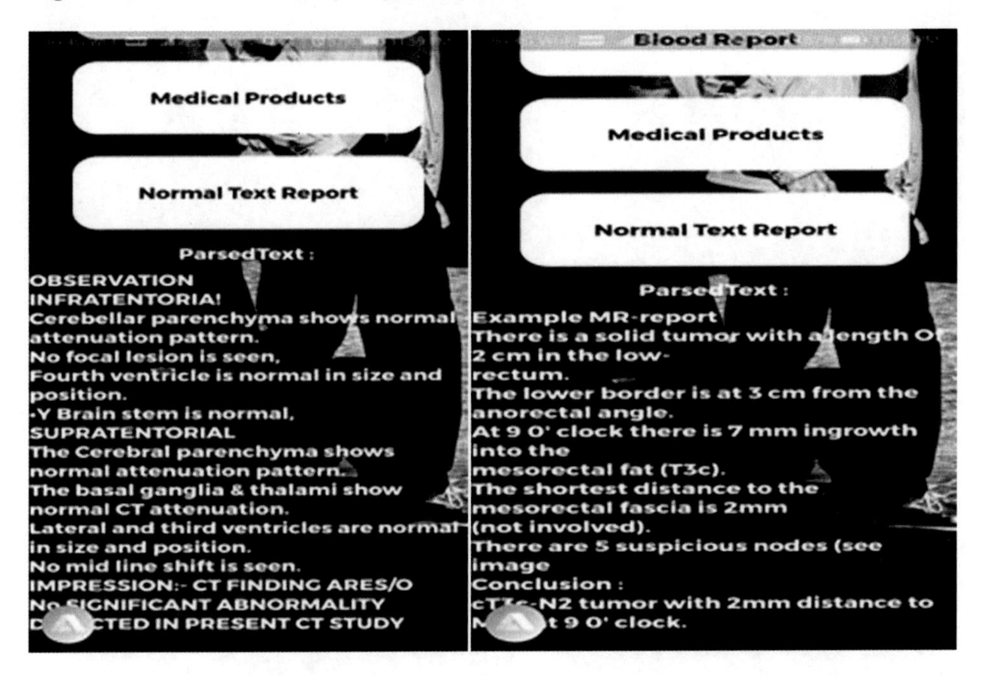

These are the images on which nanonets, machine learning custom model applied and model recognized the required information on this image. So, You can see the boxes around the required information in these images.

Figure 13. Screenshots from ML model

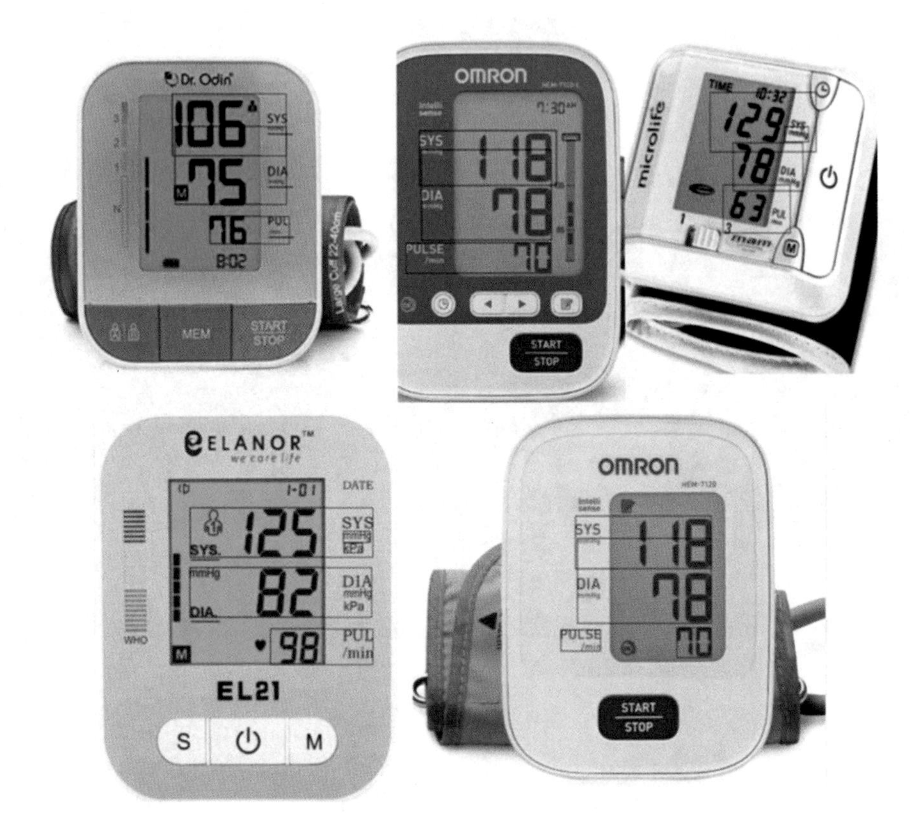

CONCLUSION

In the present research work, a framework is designed and executed to proposed a medical assistant "M.A.V.I" with the help of several technologies which would help a visually impaired person to read medical blood reports, products, normal reports and LED screens of inaccessible medical devices like a glucose monitor, BP machine and weighing machine etc. The system will transform the text to the audio output for blind people in the medical area. In, this system we tried to build an efficient system for the blind as in today's world various diseases and pandemics are occurring in the world so the people are affected day by day so people are going to the hospitals for the blood reports or medical reports so, seeing this problem we made an application which helps the blind people to read their medical reports without any help from others. The findings show that employing OCR and TTS for text detection and recognition, great performance may be achieved.

REFERENCES

Alan, A. I. (2021). Conversational Voice AI Platform. Alan. https://Alan.app/

Ani, R., Maria, E., Joyce, J. J., Sakkaravarthy, V., & Raja, M. A. (2017, March). Smart Specs: Voice assisted text reading system for visually impaired persons using TTS method. In *2017 International Conference on Innovations in Green Energy and Healthcare Technologies (IGEHT)* (pp. 1-6). IEEE., 10.1109/IGEHT.2017.8094103

Batista, E. D. (2021), Building Voice-First Flutter apps. [Video] Flutter Europe, Youtube. https://www.youtube.com/watch?v=L-c-ZyX-KtY

Chang, W. J., Chen, L. B., Hsu, C. H., Chen, J. H., Yang, T. C., & Lin, C. P. (2020). MedGlasses: A wearable smart-glasses-based drug pill recognition system using deep learning for visually impaired chronic patients. *IEEE Access: Practical Innovations, Open Solutions*, *8*, 17013–17024. doi:10.1109/ACCESS.2020.2967400

Deshpande, S., & Shriram, R. (2016, September). Real time text detection and recognition on hand held objects to assist blind people. In *2016 International Conference on Automatic Control and Dynamic Optimization Techniques (ICACDOT)* (pp. 1020-1024). IEEE. 10.1109/ICACDOT.2016.7877741

Filteau, J., Lee, S. J., & Jung, A. (2018, December). Real-time streaming application for IoT using Raspberry Pi and handheld devices. In *2018 IEEE Global Conference on Internet of Things (GCIoT)* (pp. 1-5). IEEE.10.1109/GCIoT.2018.8620141

Finnegan, E., Villarroel, M., Velardo, C., & Tarassenko, L. (2019). Automated method for detecting and reading seven-segment digits from images of blood glucose metres and blood pressure monitors. *Journal of Medical Engineering & Technology*, *43*(6), 341–355. doi:10.1080/03091902.2019.1673844 PMID:31679409

Flutter Beautiful native apps in record time. (2021). Flutter. https://flutter.dev/

Flutter_mobile_vision (2021), Flutter. https://pub.dev/packages/flutter_mobile_vision

Flutter_tts (2021). Flutter. https://pub.dev/packages/flutter_tts

Gong, L., Thota, M., Yu, M., Duan, W., Swainson, M., Ye, X., & Kollias, S. (2021). A novel unified deep neural networks methodology for use by date recognition in retail food package image. *Signal, Image and Video Processing*, *15*(3), 449–457. https://doi.org/10.1007/s11760-020-01764-7

Kanagarathinam, K., & Sekar, K. (2019). Text detection and recognition in raw image dataset of seven segment digital energy meter display. *Energy Reports*, *5*, 842–852.

Mohite, J. (2020). OCR Using Flutter. Optical character recognition is a Flutter World. *The Medium.* https://medium.com/flutterworld/ocr-using-flutter-6f5765af49a6#:~:text=Optical%20character%20recognition%20is%20a%20process%20of%20conversion%20of%20typed,images%20that%20contains%20the%20text

Musale, S., & Ghiye, V. (2018, January). Smart reader for visually impaired. In *2018 2nd International Conference on Inventive Systems and Control (ICISC)* (pp. 339-342). IEEE. doi:10.1109/ICISC.2018.8399091

Nanonets: Intelligent document processing with. (2022). Nanonets. https://nanonets.com/

Pandey, D., & Pandey, K. (2021, September). An Assistive Technology-based Approach towards Helping Visually Impaired People. In *2021 9th International Conference on Reliability, Infocom Technologies and Optimization (Trends and Future Directions)(ICRITO)* (pp. 1-5). IEEE.

Pandey, K., Yadav, V., Pandey, D., & Vikhram, S. (2021). MAGIC-I as an Assistance for the Visually Impaired People. *Recent Advances in Computer Science and Communications (Formerly: Recent Patents on Computer Science), 14*(9), 3012-3024.

Peng, E., Peursum, P., & Li, L. (2012, December). Product barcode and expiry date detection for the visually impaired using a smartphone. In *2012 International Conference on Digital Image Computing Techniques and Applications (DICTA)* (pp. 1-7). IEEE. doi:10.1109/DICTA.2012.6411673

Popayorm, S., Titijaroonroj, T., Phoka, T., & Massagram, W. (2019, July). Seven segment display detection and recognition using predefined HSV color slicing technique. In *2019 16th International Joint Conference on Computer Science and Software Engineering (JCSSE)* (pp. 224-229). IEEE. doi:10.1109/JCSSE.2019.8864189

Rajput, R., & Borse, R. (2017, August). Alternative product label reading and speech conversion: an aid for blind person. In *2017 International Conference on Computing, Communication, Control and Automation (ICCUBEA)* (pp. 1-6). IEEE. doi:10.1109/ICCUBEA.2017.8463923

Shenoy, V. N., & Aalami, O. O. (2017). Utilizing smartphone-based machine learning in medical monitor data collection: Seven segment digit recognition. *AMIA ... Annual Symposium Proceedings - AMIA Symposium. AMIA Symposium, 2017*, 1564.

World Health Organization. *(2022). Visual impairment and blindness.* WHO. https://www.who.int/news-room/fact-sheets/detail/blindness-and-visual-im payment

Chapter 7
Opportunities and Applications of Blockchain for Empowering Tele-Healthcare

Inderpreet Kaur
Galgotia College of Engineering and Technology, India

Renu Mishra
Sharda University, India

Mamta Narwaria
G.H. Patel College of Engineering and Technology, India

Sandeep Saxena
https://orcid.org/0000-0001-7879-5286
GNIOT Group of Institutions, India

ABSTRACT

With the progressive growth in the adaptability of the Blockchain technology with flexible solutions, various industries, academicians and researchers are paying attentions in such area to explore Nobel opportunities. Due to its qualities like decentralization, immutability, and encryption, block chain has the potential to shift the hierarchy of healthcare also. This area has observed many benefits of Blockchain technology, but still people have hesitations to adapt it due to lack of standardization, high cost, lack of awareness, and lack of technical knowledge to implement it. This chapter aimed to showcase the potential for block chain technology in the tale care system. Various BC based models and frameworks are discussed to cover various stages of secured data transfer for patient empowerment. This covers all technological issues in storing medical records in the various application areas where block chains will provide secured and authenticated transfers of patient personal data.

DOI: 10.4018/978-1-6684-6957-6.ch007

INTRODUCTION TO DISTRIBUTED LEDGER TECHNOLOGY (DLT)

Finding ways to secure medical data and safeguard online privacy is essential in a digital age that is constantly changing. Healthcare security attack might be in the form of compromising the privacy of patient data,misuse of medical records for misguiding the patients and other frauds related to different players in healthcare.blockchain is a cutting-edge distributed technology that has been welcomed into the healthcare environment to secure and protect medical data. One essential requirement in the medical field is that patients have the ability to manage their health information. Global users will be able to store their health records using blockchain, decide how to use the data, and get individualised health advice.latest involved research project in such domain, look at a wide range of blockchain applications, including identity management, supply chain management, inventory management, and a concept known as zero-knowledge proof, which describes how to uniquely identify a person without revealing any personal information.the idea of using blockchain to underpin the well-known cryptocurrency bitcoin was first put forth (Clauson, Breeden, Davidson, & Mackey, 2018). Block chain, however, has recently been embraced in a number of new industries such as healthcare, Smart transportation and IoT (Dash, Gantayat, & Das, 2021). It may improve transparency and fairness which help businesses economically and space. Blockchain technology is incorporated in various modern applications such as financial activities, healthcare,internet of things, military and defense and other governmental services (Langer, 2022) (Cason, 2017).

To welcome the advent of new paradigms for supporting smart and secure healthcare, we must have some basic idea ofvarious steps involved in blockchain technology to support the smart and secure functioning of the any application(Agrawal & Kumar 2020).Blockchain is a particular type of database as shown in the Figure1,where every new data is stored in the block which blocks are then chained together.since each block contains its own mathematical hash, blockchains are immutable, unless the majority reached a consensus to do so.

Figure 1. Basic flow of the blockchain technology

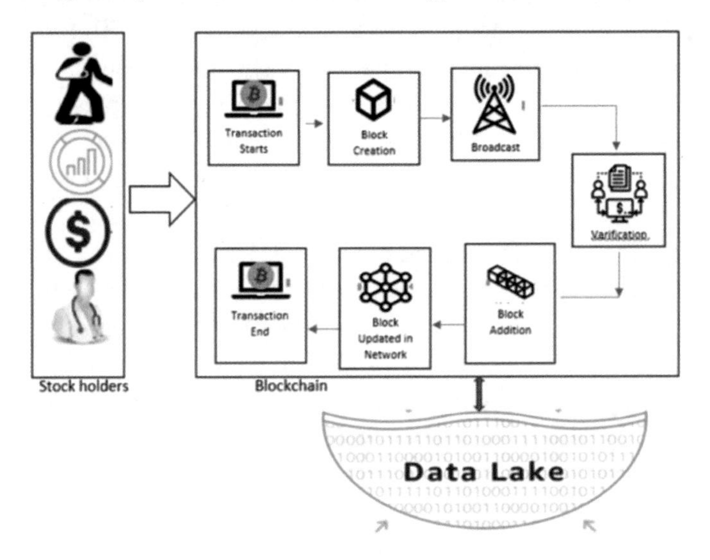

Innovative technology like blockchain makes it feasible to develop reliable applications(Radanović & Likić, 2018). Blockchain technology's global, immutable repositories guarantee reliable storage and other security controls(Langer, 2022). The chapter provided a comprehensive overview of the benefits that blockchain technology can provide to healthcare (Agrawal & Kumar 2020). The second segment covers a wide range of Usecases of healthcare sector and specially talemedicine where blockchain technology can be used. The further sections proposed two different architecture approaches for implementaingBlockchain in Tele-Healthcare.At last the chapter is concluded by stating that the medicare environment may see new value as a result of the confluence of blockchain.

HEALTHCARE BLOCKCHAIN AND ITS USECASES

There are numerous stakeholders in the area of healthcare, such as pharmaceutical firms, medical device oems, suppliers, insurers and healthcare workers, needs to authenticate themselves as organisations, log contracts, and tracking of various goods and services transactions, and their payment clearance details.Healthcare systems typically require patients to gather and transmit their health information with professionals, electronically on some storage devices, notwithstanding the importance of sharing health data. This technique of sharing medical records is ineffective since it is sluggish, unsafe, and lacking in information. In addition, it is "provider oriented" rather than "patient centric." this technique of sharing is ineffective mostly because healthcare organisations lack trust in one another and their various it platforms do not communicate with one another (Dash, Gantayat, & Das, 2021) asserts that the three basic levels of healthcare interoperability should be foundational, structural, and semantic.in order to achieve data privacy, private healthcare data is stored using blockchain as a trusted ledger database(Thierry Awesso, Zolla, & Marke, 2022). The patient has the ownership of healthcare data who is capable of sharing (or not sharing) his personal data at will securely.blockchain and smart contract keep track of the transactions in the blockchain ledger to avoide any disputes.the system must also provide assurances regarding the veracity of each user's identity to ensure system security and avoid malicious attacks.Healthcareblockchain despiteof exchanging medical statistics, health institutions typically require a patient to gather and ex blockchain technology may be used to address this interoperability problem (Clauson, Breeden, Davidson, & Mackey, 2018).In fact, with the usage of blockchain technology, patient recordsgot to share with the appropriate authorizations via smart-contracts that regulate actions like the modification of viewing privileges or formulation of new records(Radanović & Likić, 2018). The key benefits includes improved prescribing; preventing medical identity fraud and standardised identity that is verifiable towards safe, fast, and high-quality care of patient.according to the group from asublockchain research lab,several instances like patient identity management and their health records management are identified, where blockchain technology being used in the global healthcare industry (Clauson, Breeden, Davidson, & Mackey, 2018). Areas where blockchain can be used is shown in the Figure 2.

Figure 2. Blockchain For Healthcare Applications

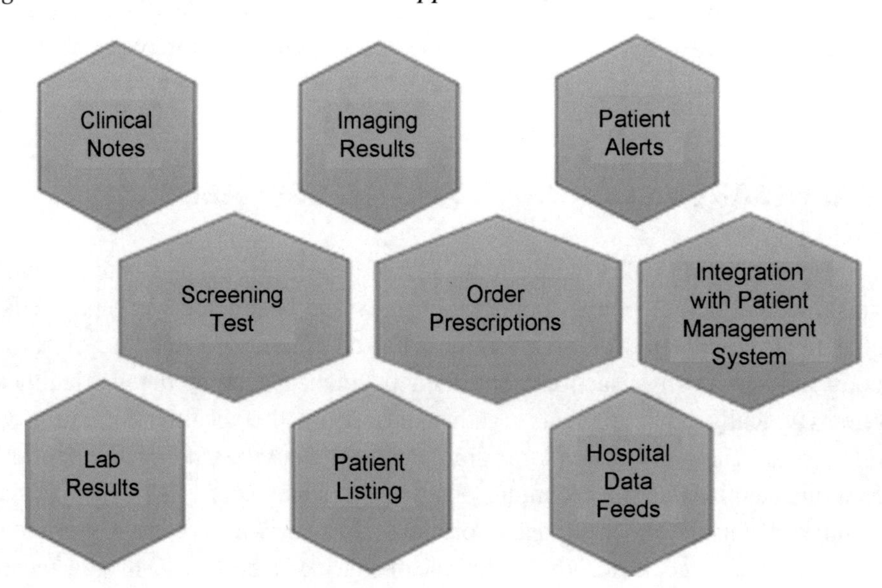

Patient identity: A crucial part of the transmission of health information is patient identification claim that medical errors result in 195,000 fatalities annually in the usa, with identification issues making up 57% of all errors. A shared wide-ranging patient index database that is accessible to all healthcare facilities, blockchain technology can enforce a provable, uniform identity for every patient in such a situation (Dash, Gantayat, & Das, 2021).health records: typically, the traditional computerised centralized systems do not deal with the underlying issue of patient data sharing. However, with the use of blockchains, a patient may now easily gather their medical history without requesting copies from each physician they have consulted(Radanović & Likić, 2018). Thus, the blockchain technology enables the development of broadly accessible, secure data distribution services that integrate with various current healthcare systems. Additionally, using a blockchain makes it simpler and more secure for patients and doctors to share data (Dixit, Bansal, Singh Rathore, & Payal, 2020).

Telemedicine: patients who have internet access can avoid waiting in line at the hospital and get quick care for minor but serious issues. However, remote medical specialists might not be able to constantly access health information acquired during telemedicine therapy episodes, leading to an inadequatemedicinal history and jeopardising the standard of care as a whole(Radanović & Likić, 2018). Thus, in current scenario, the blockchain technology can close the communication gap between various stakeholders by doing away with the requirement for third-party authorities and enabling active members to communicate directly (Dixit, Bansal, Singh Rathore, & Payal, 2020).

Blockchainbased Digital Health Records Management

Digital health records (DHRs) are the real time digital record of patient's medical history including mri reports, previous medical investigation, immunizations records, lab reports, and any allergies the patientmay have, kept overtime by hospital or a practitioner(Mishra, Kaur, Sharma, & Bharti 2022). They can be shared across number of health care firms for significant research purposes by authorized users only. DHRs are accessed automatically anytime and anywhere through various interfaces for monitoring continued progress of healthcare (Ribeiro & Vasconcelos, 2020). DHRS can be useful for accessing health information with improved precision and clarity of information, which decreases potential delays in treatment and allows for better and quicker decision-making. However, due to the enormous improvement in technology, these records are now more open to illicit use. Documented medical histories can help doctors in case of emergencies (by telling them about drug allergies, for instance) and even vary the course of therapy for enduring diseases, for the patient.

Figure 3. Different Parameters in the DHRS

Frauds
P2P Insurance
Policy Creation & Claims Processing
Challenges Of The Insurance System
Non-Proper Remote Interaction
Lack of on-demand insurance
Reinsurance

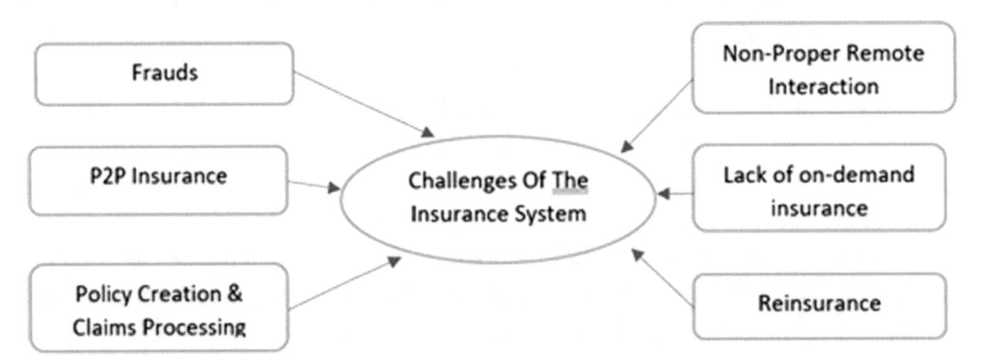

Since the DHRS contains information on the patient's medical history, demographics (such as age and weight), lab test results, and other personally identifiable information, it is crucial to protect its security and privacy (Tian & Li, 2021). The different parameters in the digital health management are shown in the figure 3.The difficulties in developing and putting into use healthcare systems, such as single-point assaults and malicious insider attacks against centralised server models that put patient data in dhr systems at danger of being leaked by malicious insiders to another organisation, require further attention(Mishra, Kaur, Sharma, & Bharti 2022). Meanwhile, sharing data can enhance the delivery of medical services by utilising the interconnection across various healthcare companies. Data redundancy, bureaucracy, and privacy issues are all a result of the "information and resource island" (information silo).

The privacy, security, and standardised way of transactions standards are framed in health insurance portability and accountability act (HIPAA). (Mishra, Kaur, Sharma, & Bharti 2022) These laws are for ensuring the privacy and security of sensitive health information. Personal health information must be kept private, hence a collaborative and transparent data exchange system is used. This aids in auditing, post-incident investigation, or forensics in the event that any data is leaked. It is important to address the security issues surrounding how the medical business distributes, stores, and retrieves patient health records. To assure the validity, integrity, and confidentiality of the records, document encryption and the usage of digital signature standards should be used.

Genomic Data Protection Through Blockchain

It is now possible to instantly transport anonymous genetic information throughout the globe using genomic data and the blockchain network. Meet the businesses that aim to assist us in protecting and managing our own genetic information. Data ownership has been a topic of discussion as the cost of sequencing a single genome declines and more people gain access to their genomic data (Pankova, 2018). Specifically, whose data is created by genetic tests owned or ought to be owned.personal genome sequencing becoming commonplace is what genetic cryptocurrency entrepreneurs are counting on because it will increase the value of the "tokens" in their systems. Additionally, there will be a rise in demand for programmes that analyse genetic data, which they will be well-positioned to create and offer access to genetic data is a useful resource for pharmaceutical companies working on novel treatments and diagnostics in the era of personalized medicine (Halid, 2022).Blockchain is the technology that makes the digital currency bitcoin powerful, is being used by zenome and other businesses in this field, like the california-based nebula genomics, to help establish a fair market for genetic data. Blockchain is a type of information technology that forms a "decentralised" server that is considerably more secure since it does not rely on a single central server. Instead, all users are a member of the network. It makes it possible for two parties to exchange new information in a secure and private manner.in order to enable others to access the code and further improve it, both zenome and dnatix have made some of their technology available as open source on the developer site github.

Block Chain Enabled SCM And Drug Traceability

It is challenging to guarantee product safety in the supply chain because of the increased accessibility to drugs through online pharmacies and illegal distribution channels. Also because of the limited data marketing in inventory and stock levels along the supply chain, there are more chances for counterfeit items to reach the marketplace (Tian & Li, 2021).The process of determining the authenticity and originality of a product, known as drug traceability.This enables all partners to follow the transactions at every important point in the supply chain (Ribeiro & Vasconcelos, 2020) .USA drug supply chain security act (dscsa) which will be implemented in different phases by the year 2023 which enable all supply chain participants to install trustworthy actions that enhance product traceability.

Medical Staff Credential Verification Using Blockchain

Blockchain technology can be used to follow medical practitioners' experience in the similar manner as following the provenance of a medical good. Best healthcare organisations& academies can record their staff's credentials, which streamlines the organisation's hiring process (Mishra, Kaur, Sharma, & Bharti 2022). Procredex,a us based organization has built such a system for medical credential verification using the R3 corda blockchain protocol to provide quicker credentialing for healthcare organisations during the hiring process ad ensuring the transparency due to its ability to share provider data in a transparent and safe manner, other businesses promote it as the solution for provider credentialing and primary source verification blochealth to create a network for exchanging credentials of healthcare professionals (Tian & Li, 2021).Procredex, its exchange in 2019. Every firm that uses credentials data confronts different difficulties. Procredex is specifically designed to meet these unique needs and maximise the value and insights concealed in credentials data. it uses distributed ledger technology(DLT) to make data immutable, identify its origin,and guarantee its ongoing traceability.

Blockchain Transforming The Insurance Industry

This area has a long list of challenges to look upon which include improper health data mangement and lack of proper health insurance claim lead to low customer satisfaction. The various challenges are shown in the Figure 4.This particular issue can be dealt with the use of blockchain, which enables proper healthcare data exchange and ensure fast claims processing.reinsurance-the process of reinsurance is inefficient and takes time to process but utilizing blockchain for creating online contracts and automate a lot of different processes related to reinsurance is very benefitial (Halid, 2022).

Blockchain-based systems enables insurance providers in the healthcare domain to function based on contract terms digitally.manufacturers, distributors, and healthcare organisations can utilize shared digital contracts considerably help in settle disagreements around chargebacks for prescription medications and other things kept on a blockchain ledger. Managing patient medical insurance contracts can be done with shared smart contracts.with the exception of blockchain, which is still in the proof-of-concept phase, the majority of technologies have progressively made their way into the insurance industry.

Figure 4. Challenges of the Insurance System

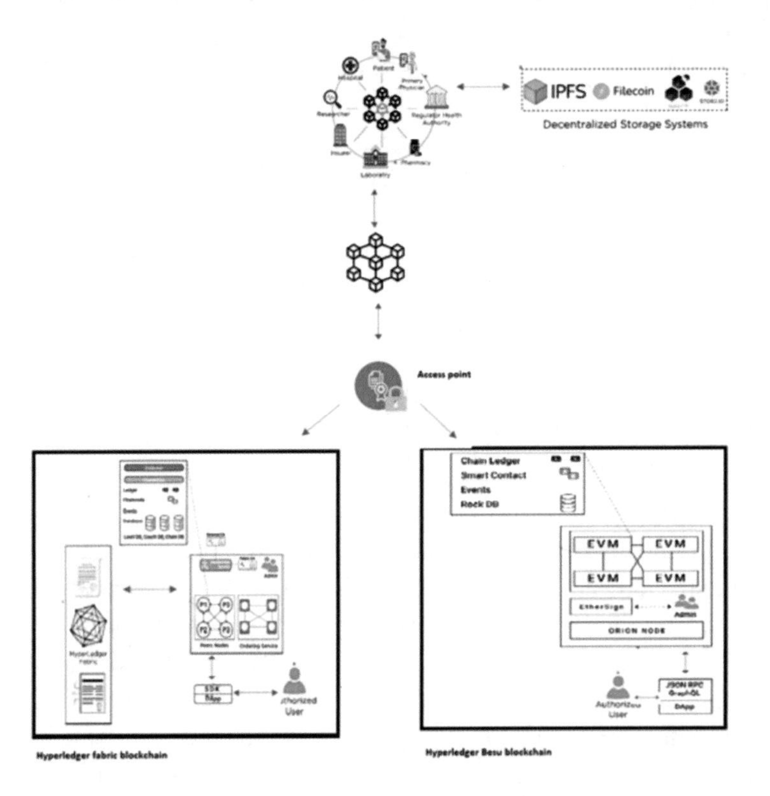

Insurance providers can employ more advance analytic tools to optimise health outcomes and costs as the data is digitalized. Insurance sector can benefit immensely from the blockchain technology(Thierry Awesso, Zolla, & Marke, 2022). The blockchain features which help in dealing with the current challenges of insurance include interoperability, data integrity, date security and universal access of data. There is certain step to be adopt blockchain for insurance such as customer centric processes, internal proof of concept, iot enablement. Blockchain technique has significantly solved various problems in insurance domain like preventing frauds & risk, policy creation & claim processing, rationalization routine interactions,reinsurance, p2p coverage and microinsurance.

Block Chain In Telemedicine

Patients who have internet access can avoid waiting in line at the hospital and get quick care for minor but serious issues. However, remote medical specialists might not be able to constantly access health information acquired during telemedicine therapy episodes, resulting to an incomplete medical history and jeopardising the standard of care as a whole (Hameed et al., 2021). Thus, the blockchain technology can part the communication slit among various benefactors by doing away with the requirement for third-party authorities and enabling active members to communicate directly. Medical data protection is one of the key issue in telemedicine. Added efforts are required to prevent unauthorized access to patients' medical information used via public network or an unencrypted channel, to access telemedicine (Thierry Awesso, Zolla, & Marke, 2022). The challenges is to secure the blockchain. Such that, in order to perform the computations necessary to verify data on the blockchain, bitcoin miners use their electricity-consuming processing equipment. In exchange, they get a reward in the form of virtual money.

BLOCKCHAIN ARCHITECTURES FOR TELE-HEALTHCARE

In this section, two popular blockchain-based designs are discussed in order to meet crucial requirements for medication. In contrast to other blockchain frameworks like ethereum, quorum, bigchain, etc., the proposed architecture is based on hyperledger fabric and hyperledgerbesu because they offer a improved level of trust, decentralisation, data transparency, data confidentiality & privacy, data integrity, deployment, and scalability(Thierry Awesso, Zolla, & Marke, 2022). These architectures may be essential building blocks for developing private permissioned blockchain ecosystems in which regulatory authorities or a set of regulatory authorities and stakeholders will register, control, and regulate pharmaceutical investors and their end-users.

Figure 5. Hyperledger Fabric And Hyperledgerbesu Architecture For Drug Traceability

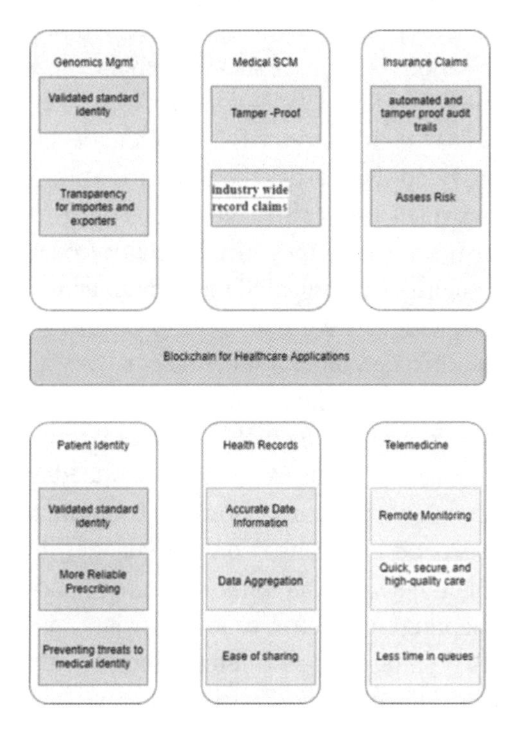

Hyperledger Fabric Architecture

Hyperledger fabric platform offers the solution for distributed ledger.The steps are shown in Figure 5. It is fortified segmental design that provides extensive level of privacy, reliability, adaptability, as well as scalability. It is a blockchain-based distributed ledger technology (dlt) designed for businesses based on smart contracts to uphold trust between several parties. Hyperledger fabric still has many of the benefits of a traditional cryptocurrency blockchain (like bitcoin or ethereum), including block immutability, determining the order of events, the avoidance of double spending etc., despite eliminating the concept of mining. Hyperledger fabric are capable to process up to several of hundreds and thousands of additional transactions per second. Due to all the above features, hyperledger fabric is an ideal choice for usage in complex supply chain systems that involve a lot of logical and physical processes and parties.

Major components of fabric are: membership service provider(msp), client, peer, orderer.Hyperledger fabricnecessitates the use of an local or external msp.Various stakeholders (identities) are governed, authenticated, validated, and given access to blockchain resources after the rules and regulationsestablished by this framework, necessary to setup trusted environment between untrusted participants. The authority uses msp element of the proposed hyperledger fabric notion to identify and register all participating organisations (pharmaceutical stakeholders) and their end customers, creating a permissioned private blockchain network. In order for clients to join the network, the msp handles user ids and verifies their identity, to propose transactions, credentials must be provided. The certificate authority, a pluggable interface used by the msp, verifies and revokes user certificates upon confirmation of identification. Both an external certificate authority and the default (local) certificate authority given by hyperledger fabric are pluggable msp components such as using openssl certificates, integration with active directoryetc (Thierry Awesso, Zolla, & Marke, 2022).This ensures the confidentiality and privacy of every network user and makes activity tracing forthright (e.g. Malicious transaction).

The hyperledger fabric architecture includes the ordering service and peer nodes as well.Peers operate smart-contracts (referred as chaincode in hyperledger fabric), keep copies of the ledger, endorse transactions, and commit them. The transactions must be added to the shared ledger in a constant manner in a blockchain enabled network. The blockchain network's committed peers are notified these blocks via broadcast after the accepting endorsed transactions from client application, grouping them into chunks with cryptographic signatures from the ratifying peers, andfuther broadcasts these for endorsement policy confirmation. There are some steps to perform, initiallya registered organisational user (client app)submit a transaction proposal report(Thierry Awesso, Zolla, & Marke, 2022) .The transaction proposal report is a request which invokes a parameterized chaincode functions to read and/or update the ledger .Futher, a number of endorsing peers are selected from all ratifying peers to execute the proposal as per chaincode endorsement rules.A smart contract specifies the transaction logic that manages a business object's lifespan within the world state. The chaincode is subsequently packed and sent to the blockchain enabled network. The smart contracts are demarcatedin chaincode,. In a single chaincode, multiple smart contracts can be defined. The smart contracts in chaincode are made accessible to the application when it is deployed.

The transaction proposal is responded to the client app by encrypting the results (or endorsements) and recorded with signatures and read/writesets ofendorsing peers. This is referred as the endorsement phase.The ledger has no updates in this phase.The client app inspect endorsement responses to check whether rw sets and chaincode ledger are restructured during proposal and endorsement phases. Itbroadcasts transaction message from the proposal and respond accordingly to the ordering service .A transactional message comprehends read/writesets, ratifying peer signatures, and a channel proof of identity which is then managed by the decentralised ordering service for its execution order using a pluggable consensus system. The ordering service streamline the hashes of consequent blocks to former blocks and sequentially arranges several drug transactions into blocks(Thierry Awesso, Zolla, & Marke, 2022).

Leading peers of hyperledger fabric network acquire the most recent blocks via os broadcast in the execution phase.The ordering service is aware of these top peers,responsible for allocating the chunks to other promising peers in the system using the gossip protocol .peers verify whether the endorsements are legitimate in line with the endorsement guidelines of the chaincodes and confirm that the rw sets haven't updated since the last check.in case of invalid endorsement or the unmatchread/writesetswith current world state, the transaction is noted as invalid. In turn,to ensure determinism, the ledger updates itself and the transactions to the channels' ledgers are added by all peers (Hameed et al., 2021) .Global state is framed with valid transactions andeach peer in the network notified to the client app for valid transaction proposal while invalid/not true ones are recorded on the ledger .

HyperledgerBesu Architecture

The projected hyperledger besu architecture offers a fullyappropriate open source distributed ledger result for businesses using blockchain .hyperledgerbesu enables the development of networks using private transaction processing as well as combination with public blockchains (like ethereum) and preserving high transaction throughput and architectural flexibility .

The proposed hyperledgerbesu system allows supply chain of pharmaceutical firms to build high performance and more scalable applications over peer-to-peer private networks as Itfillthe gap between private and public blockchains to achieve data confidentiality and complex authorizing management. Hyperledgerbesu supports solidity in blockchain based smart contracts and supports the use of tokens and the cryptocurrency ether.

A signed private transaction request is first shared by an organisational user (client) via a distributed application to a hyperledgerbesu**ethereum virtual machine (evm)** node in order to accomplish a transaction (to run a somesmart contract function or transfer some assets).

To transmit transactions to orion using the private transaction handler, the distributed application user interface employs *JSON-RPC* 2.0, which is a simple and lightweight transport-agnostic protocol that allows remote procedure calls and notifications between two systemsusing the recipient addresses or privacy group ids to identify the recipients.Orion dispenses the transactions to more orion nodes. Orion sites will store the transactions from the state/base database and send the transaction calculated hash value back to the pmt.Theptm is privacy marker transactions (pmt) .Alongside private transactions which are further mined into blocks and broadcasted.

The transactions are carried to the contract for execution on the nodes with private precompiled smart contract, after being processed by the mainnet transaction processor on each hyperledgerbesu node. This contract book searches the orion for the private transaction using the calculated transaction hash value, and sends it to the private processor, which executes it and commits the operations(read-write) to the private world state to update all of the coordinating nodes.

CONCLUSION

By putting the patient at the centre of the health care ecosystem and enhancing security, privacy, and interoperability, blockchain technology has come up with the potential to transform health data.massive amounts of patient data can be managed by healthcare organisations using the blockchain platform in a safe and secure manner. various drawbacks of telemedicine including false and unauthorized participation can be resolved by involving blockchain technology, as a trust building mechanism by using effective technology solutions in blockchain. Decentralized ledgers are invulnerable to cybercrime by their design, as there is a need to simultaneously target every copy stored throughout the network in order to be successful.

REFERENCES

Agrawal, R. Chatterjee, J. M., Kumar A., & Rathore P. S. (2020). Blockchain technology and the internet of things: Challenges and applications in bitcoin and security. Taylor & Francis. doi:10.1201/9781003022688

Agrawal, R., Chatterjee, J. M., Kumar, A., & Rathore, P. S. (2020). *Blockchain technology and the internet of things: challenges and applications in bitcoin and security.* Routledge.

Cason, J. (2017). Telehealth is face-to-face service delivery. *International Journal of Telerehabilitation*, *77-78*, 77–78. doi:10.5195/ijt.2017.6225 PMID:28814997

Clauson, K. A., Breeden, E. A., Davidson, C., & Mackey, T. K. (2018). *Leveraging blockchain technology to enhance supply chain management in healthcare*. Blockchain in Healthcare Today. doi:10.30953/bhty.v1.20

Dash, S., Gantayat, P. K., & Das, R. K. (2021). Blockchain technology in Healthcare: Opportunities and challenges. *Intelligent Systems Reference Library*, 97-111. doi:10.1007/978-3-030-69395-4_6

Dixit, P., Bansal, A., Singh Rathore, P., & Payal, M. (2020). An overview of blockchain technology: Architecture, consensus algorithm, and its challenges. *Blockchain Technology and the Internet of Things*, 21-46. doi:10.1201/9781003022688-2

Halid, K. (2022). *Pharmaledger: Blockchain-Enabled Healthcare: Privacy-enhancement with Blockchain.* Blockchain in Healthcare Today., doi:10.30953/tmt.v7.226

Hameed, K., Bajwa, I. S., Sarwar, N., Anwar, W., Mushtaq, Z., & Rashid, T. (2021). Integration of 5G and block-chain technologies in smart telemedicine using IOT. *Journal of Healthcare Engineering, 2021*, 1–18. doi:10.1155/2021/8814364 PMID:33824715

Kumar, S., Lim, W.M., & Sivarajah, U. (2022). . Artificial intelligence and blockchain integration in business: trends from a bibliometric-content analysis. *Inf syst front* doi:10.1007/s10796-022-10279-0

Langer, T. (2022). IND02-01 overview of the innovative medicines initiative neuoderisk project. *Toxicology Letters, 368*, S81. doi:10.1016/j.toxlet.2022.07.235

Mishra, R., Kaur, I., Sharma, V., & Bharti, A. (2022). Computational Intelligence and Blockchain-Based Security for Wireless Sensor Networks. In A. Tyagi (Ed.), *Handbook of Research on Technical, Privacy, and Security Challenges in a Modern World* (pp. 324–336). IGI Global. doi:10.4018/978-1-6684-5250-9.ch017

Nair, M. M., & Tyagi, A. K. (2021). Privacy: history, statistics, policy, laws, preservation and threat analysis. *Journal of information assurance & security, 16*(1).

Padalkar, N. R., Sheikh-Zadeh, A., & Song, J. (2020). Business value of smart contract: case of inventory information discrepancies. *Scholars.*

Pankova, N. (2018). Blockchain for advancing precision medicine and drug discovery through genomic data storage and analysis. *Journal of Pharmacogenomics & Pharmacoproteomics, 09*. doi:10.4172/2153-0645-C1-021

Radanović, I., & Likić, R. (2018). Opportunities for use of blockchain technology in medicine. *Applied Health Economics and Health Policy, 16*(5), 583–590. doi:10.100740258-018-0412-8 PMID:30022440

Ribeiro, M., & Vasconcelos, A. (2020). Medblock: Using Blockchain in health healthcare application based on Blockchain and smart contracts. *Proceedings of the 22nd International Conference on Enterprise Information Systems*. ScitePress. 10.5220/0009417101560164

Tandon, A., Dhir, A., Islam, A. N., & Mäntymäki, M. (2020). Blockchain in Healthcare: A systematic literature review, synthesizing framework and future research agenda. *Computers in Industry*, *122*, 103290. doi:10.1016/j.compind.2020.103290

Thangamuthu, P., Ranganathan, I., Mani, K., Shanmugam, S., & Palanimuthu, S. (2020). Blockchain technology and its relevance in Healthcare. *Blockchain and Machine Learning for E-Healthcare Systems,* 1-24. doi:10.1049/PBHE029E_ch1

Thierry Awesso, D. E., Zolla, M., & Marke, A. (2022). Potential interaction among artificial intelligence, internet of things and distributed Ledger Technology. *Governing Carbon Markets with Distributed Ledger Technology,* 33-60. doi:10.1017/9781108919166.005

Tian, H., & Li, Y. (2021). Pharmaceutical anti-counterfeiting traceability system based on block chain double chain. *2021 International Conference on Computer Engineering and Application (ICCEA).* IEEE. 10.1109/ICCEA53728.2021.00016

Chapter 8
Applications of Machine Learning Models With Medical Images and Omics Technologies in Diabetes Detection

Chakresh Kumar Jain
https://orcid.org/0000-0002-9226-7719
Jaypee Institute of Information Technology, India

Aishani Kulshreshtha
Jaypee Institute of Information Technology, India

Avinav Agarwal
Jaypee Institute of Information Technology, India

Harshita Saxena
Jaypee Institute of Information Technology, India

Pankaj Kumar Tripathi
https://orcid.org/0000-0002-9929-359X
Jaypee Institute of Information Technology, India

Prashant Kaushik
Jaypee Institute of Information Technology, India

DOI: 10.4018/978-1-6684-6957-6.ch008

ABSTRACT

Diabetes mellitus is a long-term condition characterized by hyperglycaemia resulting in the emergence of a variety of health problems, such as diabetic retinopathy, kidney failure, dental problems, heart disease, nerve damage, etc.; and is governed by several factors, i.e. biological, genetics, food habits, sedentary lifestyle choices, poor diets and environments, etc. According to the recent morbidity figures, the global diabetic patient population is anticipated to reach 642 million by 2040, implying that one out of every ten people will be diabetic. The data generation and AI based methods—i.e., SVM, kNN, decision tree, Baysian method in medical health –have facilitated the effective prediction and classification of voluminous size of biological data of different types of BMI, skin thickness, glucose, age, tongue and retinal images apart from Omics data, for early diagnostics. The chapter summarizes the basic methods and applications of machine learning and soft computing techniques for diabetes diagnosis and prediction with limitations of integrative approaches.

INTRODUCTION

Healthcare is one of the most major concerns for the world in this day and age. Health is a measure of an individual's well-being. A healthy lifestyle is one of the crucial goals of any person, and access to proper healthcare forms an essential aspect of every individual's life. Due to increasing sedentary lifestyle choices and poor diets, people are getting diagnosed with Diabetes at an alarming rate. A whopping figure of 422 million people, according to the World Health Organisation (WHO) have been diagnosed with diabetes, which adds up to about 1.5 million deaths annually. It is estimated that this number will increase rapidly in the coming years, affecting primarily India, China and the USA (World Health Organization, 2022).

Diabetes is an incurable condition wherein the glucose level in the blood is more elevated than usual. One of the reasons for this can be inadequate secretion of insulin by the body, or it's improper response to it (Thakkar et al., 2021). Diabetes can both be due to inadequate lifestyle as well as certain genetic factors. There are primarily two types of diabetes; Type 1 and Type 2 diabetes as depicted in figure I. Typically type 1 diabetes patients are younger and have to be treated with insulin therapy. Due to this, this type is commonly known as insulin-dependent diabetes. Comparatively type 2 diabetes patients are usually middle-aged and above, and can be effectively treated with oral medication. This type is often associated with other complications such as obesity and hypertension amongst others (Robertson et al., 2011). Apart from these two, another type of diabetes known as gestational diabetes primarily affects pregnant women. This type of diabetes is resolved after birth, but results in greater chances of patients developing type 2 diabetes later on in life. Apart from this, Diabetes can lead to more dangerous medical conditions such as eye, kidney and dental problems, heart disease, and nerve damage (National Institute of Diabetes and Digestive and Kidney Diseases, 2016). Such a disease therefore demands efficient treatment and control, especially since a significant portion of patients still remain undiagnosed (Kaul et al., 2012).

Traditionally, diabetes is diagnosed on the basis of laboratory test reports and the assessment of the doctor. This constitutes clinical data. While it is still a common and effective diagnostic technique, it is time-consuming and bias prone. The diagnosis is entirely dependent upon the experience of the medical practitioner, and quality of the laboratory tests, which may fluctuate (Choubey et al., 2018). Clearly, there is a need for early detection of this disease for effective treatment. With the advent of soft computing techniques, the diagnosis and prediction of diabetes has become less time-consuming. Soft computing enables the incorporation of methods that aim to quickly design answers to challenging real-world problems. A variety of strategies can be combined to create soft computing techniques, which are used to solve complicated real-world problems (ex. in management, agriculture, economics, and other fields) that were otherwise insurmountable (Agarwal & Mehta, 2014).

This chapter aims to provide a comprehensive review on the current updates in various advanced soft computing techniques that have been employed for diabetes classification and prognosis. Various techniques such as logistic regression, naïve bayes, and decision tree have been discussed.

Figure 1. Pathophysiology of Diabetes Mellitus (a) Type 1 Diabetes (b) Type 2 Diabetes

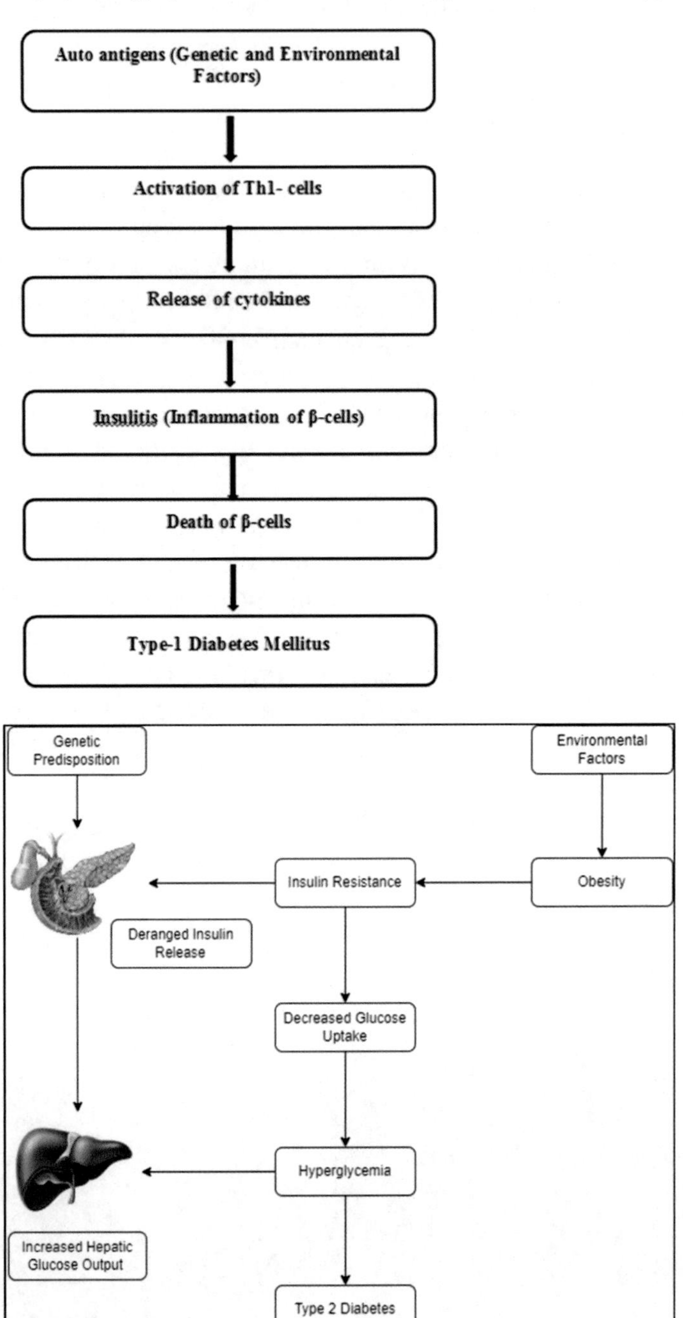

RELEVANCE OF BIOLOGICAL DATA

Before discussing various integrative biology and soft computing techniques used for diabetes detection and classification, it is important to put emphasis on the type and quality of biological data used for these studies. Despite being so prevalent, unfortunately only a minimal number of datasets are available and utilised for prediction of diabetes, and amongst those only one or two datasets are available for public use (Liaw & Wiener, 2002). One of the most commonly used datasets available for studies is the PIMA Indians diabetes dataset. It has about 768 instances and 8 attributes. It is a reliable and versatile dataset consisting of only females above the age of 21 years (Mirza et al., 2018). It had been used in numerous studies (Kumari et al., 2021; Bukhari et al., 2021; Permana et al., 2021).

Table 1. PIMA Diabetes Dataset Description

S.no.	Features	Description	Range
1.	Skin Thickness (ST)	Triceps skin fold thickness (mm)	0-99
2.	Body Mass Index (BMI)	Weight (kg) divided by height (m^2)	0-67.1
3.	Age	Age in years	21-81
4.	Insulin (I)	2 hr serum insulin (mu U/ml)	0-846
5.	Blood Pressure (BP)	Diastolic blood pressure (mmHg)	0-122
6.	Pregnancies (P)	Number of times a participant is pregnant	0-17
7.	Glucose (G)	2 hr glucose concentration in an oral glucose tolerance test	0-199
8.	Diabetes Pedigree Function (DPF)	Genetic history of diabetes	0.08-2.42

Attributes and features listed in the datasets are considered significant factors for disease prediction, and their quantity can alter precision (Liaw & Wiener, 2002). Therefore, for studies using new diabetes datasets, deciding which ones and how many features should be included is an important task. A significant number of studies construct their own datasets (Choubey et al., 2018), or choose datasets according to their local regions (Derevitskii & Kovalchuk, 2020; Maulana et al., 2018). Generally, these datasets contain attributes such as BMI, skin thickness, glucose, age amongst others. However, in cases such as that of (Posonia et al., 2020), instead of these attributes, tongue pictures were used for classification. In another instance, a survey was conducted that considered many more variables such as smoking, physical activity, marital status, occupation etc in order to inculcate lifestyle attributes for prediction as well (Wang et al., 2021).

Integrative biology studies generally do not use this kind of data, however. The biological data used in these studies comprises microarray and omics data. Numerous studies have used microarray expression data to identify differentially expressed genes (DEGs) that can help in tracking and understanding pathogenesis of diseases (Ding et al., 2019; Cui et al., 2017; Wang et al., 2016). GEO (https://www.ncbi.nlm.nih.gov/geo/) database is one of the most widely used sources for microarray data. It is a worldwide public repository that houses and openly disseminates high-throughput functional genomics data from sources like microarrays, next-generation sequencing, and other research community-contributed sources. Users can download curated gene expression profiles and experiment results using tools that are provided (geo, 2019). Datasets contain vast information, including organism, summary of dataset information, citation of paper, and date of publishing. For instance, a study used microarray dataset GSE20966, which consisted of pancreatic beta cells. 10 diabetic and 10 non-diabetic samples were utilised in the microarray (Ding et al., 2019). This dataset was curated originally by (Marselli et al., 2010). Microarray data is then further subjected to analyses such as GO function, KEGG pathway, and PPI networks are constructed. This process helped in gaining further insight into type 2 diabetes mellitus pathogenesis.

As omics branches, different classes including genomics, proteomics, metabolomics and metagenomics provide a refined assessment by examining both quantitative and qualitative biomolecular characteristics. Omics methods in human models have made it possible to identify brand-new, alluring therapeutic approaches for a variety of metabolic illnesses, including Type 2 Diabetes. These methods have in fact improved our understanding of the molecular pathogenic alterations underlying Diabetes and related comorbidities.

Systems biology is the integration of various techniques, whereas an omics-based approach uses technologies to identify genes, RNAs, proteins, and metabolites at a universal level (Horgan & Kenny, 2011). It is envisaged that an omics approach will help researchers earn more comprehensive understanding of chemicals and how they alter both healthy and diseased processes. The main advantage of using omics-based technologies is that researchers can now investigate several molecules, including as genes, proteins, and metabolites, at the same time and swiftly collect a large amount of data as opposed to just a limited amount of specific data. (Karahalil, 2016). This helps researchers to better understand the molecular components linked to the cellular processes that underlie them and how they change over time, under different settings, such as disease states compared to healthy persons (Karahalil, 2016). Additionally, it aids in illuminating their relationships and dynamic functions. As a result, a gene, protein, or metabolite's expression profile must ideally distinguish between cases and controls for a sick state in order for it to be used as a diagnostic biomarker.

By mining clinical 'omics' data, another study intends to repurpose commercially available medications and clinical candidates for novel indications in the treatment of diabetes (Zhang et al., 2015). A total of 992 proteins have been identified as possible anti-diabetic targets in humans after data from genome wide association studies (GWAS), proteomics, and metabolomics investigations were analysed. The Therapeutic Target Database (TTD) was searched for information on the medications that target these 992 proteins, and 108 of them include information on drug programmes. 35 out of the 108 proteins were chosen as druggable proteins after research and potential drug targets were removed. Five of them were recognised targets for the treatment of diabetes. Twelve protein targets of 58 medications were discovered to have new indications for the treatment of diabetes based on the pathogenesis data acquired from the OMIM and PubMed databases. Additionally, it aids in illuminating their relationships and dynamic functions. Therefore, a gene, protein, or metabolite's expression profile should ideally be able to distinguish between cases and controls for a sick state in order for it to be used as a diagnostic biomarker (Chuang et al., 2010).

Omics technologies are high-throughput biochemical tests that simultaneously and thoroughly measure similar-type molecules from a biological sample. One of the thorough omics databases with information on several datasets, including genomic, transcriptomic, proteomic, and metabolomic data is the Phytozome and OmicsDI database. In order to facilitate biological comprehension, there is one key tool called ODG (Omics database generator), which is used for creating, searching, and analysing multi-omics comparative databases. Datasets produced with omics technology, whether on a small or large scale, are often required to be made publicly available in order to be published in scientific journals (Horgan & Kenny, 2011; Chuang et al., 2010).

Overall, depositing data in openly accessible databases improves science's quality and greatly facilitates analysis of diabetes. Further the role of machine learning based list of algorithms in biological data analytics is indispensable as mentioned in fig II.

Figure 2. Classification of Machine Learning Algorithms

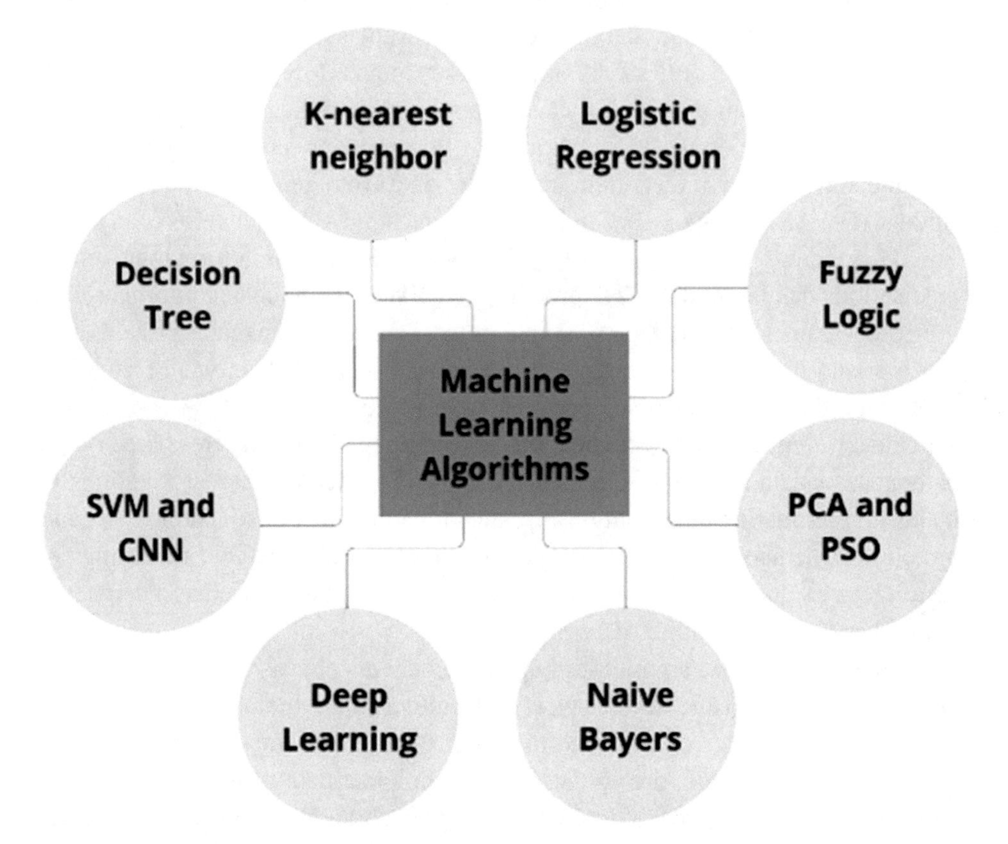

Comparison of Data with K-Nearest Neighbour

A supervised machine learning algorithm is the KNN algorithm. This supervised machine learning approach may be applied to both regression and classification issues. As it uses all of the data for training while classifying the data, it is also known as a lazy learner.

KNN searches for similarities between newly supplied data and data that has previously been collected in the past. It assesses how similar the new data is to the previous data. The algorithm takes immediate action on the dataset rather than learning from taught data. New data is categorised into the category that is the most comparable to the stored dataset when it is fed to the algorithm (Saxena & Al, 2021). The distance function between the samples comes in a variety of forms. Below example shows finding the distance using Euclidean Distance Function with k being no. of values and X1, X2 input samples (Ali et al., 2020).

$$d = \sqrt{\sum_{k=1}^{n} \left(X_{1k} - X_{2k}\right)^2}$$

Prediction of diabetes by the KNN Algorithm starts with the simple procedure of loading the dataset in the tool as the first task. K-nearest Classifier is applied on the dataset to get the accuracy, precision from the dataset. By selecting significant features through co-relation-based feature selection method, irrelevant data can be filtered out and replace the values that are missing by mean of the data. Optimise few parameters and then again K- nearest neighbour classifier is applied to check the accuracy. There will be an improvement in accuracy using the parameters as a result. Thus, it is concluded that accuracy has increased by 8.48 percent, from 70.1% to 78.58%, following the deployment of the method. (Saxena & Al, 2021).

The KNN algorithm's simple working principle is to calculate the Euclidean distance between each changing sample and each set of predefined classes. The minimum nearest neighbours for each category are then selected by the KNN algorithm. The samples are categorised on the basis of nearest K-neighbours. Values of both Fasting Plasma Glucose (FPG) and the 2-hour Plasma Glucose (2-h PG) after a 75-gram oral glucose tolerance test are used to diagnose diabetes (FPG). The results of both suggests that the Fine KNN classifier is favoured above all, since it provides 100 percent accuracy (Ali et al., 2020).

If results from the two algorithms are compared, that is of logistic regression and KNN, it is clearly seen that the KNN results have a higher sensitive value than the Logistic Regression findings. This indicates that KNN performs better in classification than Logistic Regression. KNN has a drawback, too, in that it is unable to determine whether parameters or predictors have a significant impact on predicting targets.

However, it is wise to utilise KNN if we concentrate more on the outcomes of the predictions rather than the percentage of predictors' influence on the model.

Naive Bayesian Algorithm in Complex Analysis

Naive Bayesian Algorithm is a supervised learning optimal classifier algorithm that is based on the concept of Bayes' theorem. This algorithm is helpful in extremely large datasets because of its easy parameter valuation (Das et al., 2018). It converts prior probability to posterior probability and is used to carry out intricate classification tasks (Das et al., 2018).

Naive Bayesian theorem gives a method to find out the value of posterior probability P(X|Y), from the values of P(X), P(Y), and P(Y|X), represented in the equation,

$$P(Y) = \frac{(P(X)P(X))}{P(Y)}$$

Reduction Methods

Presence of redundant or irregular features in the dataset can lead to less accurate results. Use of reduction methods such as PCA and PSO give best features which can be used for classification and have more accurate results when compared with only classification methods (Choubey et al., 2019). The methods are explained in brief below,

Principle Component Analysis (PCA)

PCA is an example of unsupervised dimensional-reduction method, which removes the correlated set of variables. Through the vectors of Principle components, a large vector can be represented as a low-dimension representation (Choubey et al., 2019).

PCA can find patterns in data, reduce the number of dimensions, and visualise the data. It is used to identify the relevant features of linearly dependent features (Choubey et al., 2019).

PCA Algorithm

Assume $x_1, x_2, \ldots\ldots, x_m$ are vectors of dimensions N × 1,

Step 1: $\underline{x} = \frac{1}{M}\sum_{i=1}^{M} x_i$

Step 2: Subtracting the mean:

$\phi_i = x_i - \hat{x}$ (Center at zero)

Step 3: Create matrix A = [ϕ1 $_,$ ϕ2, ……, ϕm] $_o$f (N x M), then compute:

$$C = \frac{1}{M}\sum_{i=1}^{M} n\phi_n\phi_n^T = \frac{1}{M}AA^T$$

Step 4: Eigenvalues for,

C: $\lambda 1_> \lambda 2 > \ldots, \lambda N$

Step 5: Eigenvectors for,

C: u*1*, u2, ..., u*N*

$$x - \underline{x} = b_1u_1 + b_2u_2 + \ldots + b_Nu_N = \sum_{i=1}^{N} b_iu_i$$

Where, $b_i = \dfrac{(x - \underline{x}).u_i}{(u_i.u_i)}$

Step 6: Highest K eigenvalue terms are kept,

$$\hat{x} - x = \sum_{i=1}^{k} b_iu_i$$

Where, K << N

The linear transformation $R^N \times R^K$ which does the dimensionality or feature reduction is:

$$[b_1, b_2 \ldots b_k] = \left[u_1^T, u_2^T \ldots u_K^T\right](x - \underline{x}) = U^T(x - \underline{x})$$

PCA has been utilised in a number of studies. A study compared PCA with SpO_2 measurement on the prediction of diabetic foot ulcer. At optimum threshold, the sensitivity prediction of healing using PCA was 87.5% whereas that of SpO_2 was 50%. The positive predictive value of PCA was 0.91 and oxygen saturation was 0.86. This study concluded that better prediction of healing can be done when analysed with PCA than by SpO_2 (Thakkar et al., 2021).

In another case, a CNN architecture model RUnet-PCA was proposed, and compared it against the well-known CNN models such as AlexNet, VggNet-s, VggNet-16, GoogleNet and ResNet model. The proposed model of RUnet-PCA showed the highest diagnosis accuracy of 98.44% which was more promising when compared with the other methods (Mohammedhasan & Uğuz, 2020).

Simulation of Behaviour Using Particle Swarm Optimization (PSO)

Particle Swarm Optimization (PSO) is an optimization technique which is inspired by the social behaviour and movement of birds, fish, insects, etc (Choubey et al., 2019). PSO replicates the behaviour of a group of birds randomly searching for food in an area. It begins with a set of random particles and then finding of the optimal value by updating groups. During every iteration, the particles are updated by following the concept of two "best" values (Choubey et al., 2019).

One "best" value is the best result the particles have so far. It is termed as global best or G_{best}. The other "best" value is the value obtained by any individual particle of the population. This value is termed as P_{best}. P_{best} value which is closest to the solution is known as G_{best}. The velocity and the position of particles is updated after the computation of P_{best} and G_{best} values, where each feature represents a direction in which the particle can move (Choubey et al., 2019).

A study applied PSO algorithm with decision tree classification to access the risk factors involved in type II diabetes. Using the aforementioned model, risk factors for the disease were recognized with a higher accuracy than the pre-existing approaches and procedures (Sheik Abdullah & Selvakumar, 2018).

A hybrid algorithm of modified PSO and LS-SVM for classification of type II diabetes mellitus patients was performed in (Soliman & AboElhamd, 2014). LS-SVM was used for classification which separates various categories. Modified PSO was used as optimizer for LS-SVM parameters. The experimental results showed the superiority of the proposed algorithm which achieved the classification accuracy of 97.83%.

Classification of Data With Decision Tree

A fundamental method for classification and regression is decision trees. The selection tree model's tree structure describes the method of classifying instances of supported features (Quinlan, 1986). This method is a collection of if-then rules, a category space, and a probability distribution that's specified by the function. The selection tree is an organized tree that starts with one node to symbolize the academic program (Habibi et al., 2015; Zou et al., 2018). The category may be accustomed to determining whether a node could be a leaf and whether the samples are members of the identical class if they're members of a minimum of one. Within the absence of such information, the algorithm chooses the identification characteristic supported by the present node of the choice tree. The training pattern is split into various subsets, each producing a branch, with various values forming numerous branches, counting on this decision node attribute value (Liaw & Wiener, 2002; Quinlan, 1986). Every subset within the previous step is repeated within the previous stage, recursively creating a call tree for every partitioned sample (Quinlan, 1986; Habibi et al., 2015).

$$Entropy = -\sum_{i1=1}^{n1} p_{i1}^{*} log\left(p_{i1}\right) Gini\ Index = 1 - \sum_{i1=1}^{n1} p_{i1} 2$$

A study involving the choice Tree J48 classification method made use of the Pima Indians Diabetes dataset for Diabetes prediction. This dataset was also analysed using the Weka tool. Overall, this study showed that the developed model had an efficiency of 91.2% (Posonia et al., 2020).

Yet again using the PIDD dataset, other authors established a unique prediction model for Diabetes Mellitus Classification using Synthetic Minority Oversampling Technique, Decision Tree, and Genetic Algorithm. With an astounding accuracy of 82.1256%, the suggested PMSGD algorithm easily outperformed its rivals. The suggested system's highest values were CA (82.1256%), CE (17.8744%), accuracy (0.8070%), sensitivity (0.8598%), FM (0.8326%), and AUROC (0.8511%) (Azad et al., 2021).

In another study, a retrospective cross-sectional methodology was applied. Between January and July of 2017, 10,436 persons were enlisted for a health examination. These facts along with the J48 method are enough to create a choice tree model. The dataset's primary features, including some input variables and a couple of output variables, were revealed by the choice tree model to be highly related to the event of diabetes and also modifiable. Additionally, the model used in the study demonstrated 90.3% classification accuracy, 89.7% precision, and 90.3% recall (Pei et al., 2020).

Another study used six different decision tree-based (DTB) classifiers to perform bagging and boosting operations on trial data to predict diabetes. The accuracy rates of DTB classifiers employing specific implementation, bagging, and boosting were also examined during this study. With the use of Naive Bayes Tree (NBTree) and Adaptive Boosting (AdaBoost) bagging, the study achieved an accuracy score of 98.65%. In addition, individual DTB classifiers outperformed boosting and bagging methods (Taser, 2021).

The initial stage diabetes risk prediction dataset is accustomed created a choice tree using the c4.5 technique as published in the article (https://www.kaggle.com/singhakash/early-stage-diabetes-riskp rediction-datasets.) The trial data indicated that polydipsia has the most impact on diabetes. This study achieved an accuracy value of 90.38% from its algorithm model's performance results (Permana et al., 2021).

In a different model, SMOTE and a choice tree classifier were utilized by the authors to predict diabetes prognosis. The clinical dataset employed in this study contained information on 734 patients of various ages. SMOTE was utilized to correct data imbalances within the start, and a call tree classifier was used to diagnose diabetes within the second stage. The accuracy of the categorization that was obtained was 94.7013% (Mirza et al., 2018).

CLINICAL ANALYSIS THROUGH LOGISTIC REGRESSION

A machine learning classification model, logistic regression is widely utilised in clinical analysis. The association between one or more independent variables and a binary dependent variable is estimated using this algorithm, which utilizes probabilistic estimations to do so (Rajendra & Latifi, 2021; Joshi & Dhakal, 2021).

Binary logistic regressions determine the likelihood that an attribute of a binary variable is present based on the values of the covariates. Assume Y to be a binary variable with independent values [Y1, Y2, ..., Yn] and Yi=1 for the character's presence and Yi=0 for its absence. Consider the set of variables x = (x1, x2, ..., xp) as either continuous, discrete, or a combination of both, with serving as the parameter to be evaluated (Permana et al., 2021).

Logistic Regression can be carried out via below formula:

$$logit(\pi_i) = loglog\left(\frac{\pi_i}{1-\pi_i}\right) = \beta_0 + \beta_1 x_{i1} + \beta_2 x_{i2} + \ldots + \beta_p x_{i,p};$$

Where,

$$\pi_i = \frac{expexp\left(\beta_0 + \beta_1 x_{i1} + \beta_2 x_{i2} + \ldots + \beta_p x_{i,p}\right)}{1 + expexp\left(\beta_0 + \beta_1 x_{i1} + \beta_2 x_{i2} + \ldots + \beta_p x_{i,p}\right)} = \frac{expexp\left(x_i^{'}\beta\right)}{1 + expexp\left(x_i^{'}\beta\right)} = \Delta\left(x_i^{'}\beta\right)$$

Logistic Regression is methodical approach for analysing an information where at least one aspect affects the outcome. A machine learning order calculation known as calculated relapse is used to predict the possibility of a subordinate variable with a high degree of clarity. Calculated relapse's goal is to find the best-fitting model to show the relationship between a number of unrelated, independent variables. The dependent variable in strategic relapse is a paired variable with data coded as 1 or 0. Logistic relapse is used to resolve the arrangement challenges, and direct regression is used to address regression-related concerns. Instead of fitting a relapsing line in the case of logistic regression, one fits a "S" shaped computed work that anticipates the two most extreme characteristics (0 or 1). Thus, if the outcome turns out to be 0 then it means that the patient is not diabetic and if it turns out to be 1, then he is diabetic.

With data gathered from numerous sources, the logistic regression algorithm can be used as a way to predict and analyse diabetes. By applying the validation Method in (Maulana et al., 2018), the accuracy level shown is about 94%. The use of logistic regression methods to predict and analyse diabetes can be determined to have a good discrimination score. The logistic regression methods' key benefit is their nearly perfect ROC score of 100% in it (the Logistic Regression method) (Maulana et al., 2018).

Support Vector Machine (SVM)

An approach for statistically supervised learning used for classification is called the Support Vector Machine (SVM), which searches for a separating hyperplane by translating data from the input space into a high-dimensional feature space using sets of mathematical operations known as kernels. Kernel functions are paramount for conversion of input space into the required feature space (Sun & Zhang, 2019). Using the right kernel function, SVM can perform effectively with unstructured and semi-structured datasets like photos and text. Despite being a robust technique, it has some drawbacks. Choosing the appropriate kernel function might be challenging at times. Additionally, it takes a long time to train when using large datasets. Although the weights of the variables of the final model are challenging to comprehend, it can nonetheless produce reliable and accurate results (Larabi-Marie-Sainte et al., 2019).

SVM classification (Jakkula, n.d.):

$$\|f\|_K^2 + C\sum_{i=1}^{l} \xi_i$$

Where,

$$y_i f(x_i) \geq 1 - \xi_i, \ \ for\ all\ i \ \ \xi_i \geq 0$$

SVM classification, Dual formulation:

$$\sum_{i=1}^{l} \alpha_i - \frac{1}{2}\sum_{i=1}^{l}\sum_{j=1}^{l} \alpha_i \alpha_j y_i y_j K(x_i, x_j)$$

Where,

$$0 \leq \alpha_i \leq C, \ \ for\ all\ i; \ \sum_{i=1}^{l} \alpha_i y_i = 0$$

Use of SVM models is extensive in the classification of diabetes. A recent study proposed a non-linear prediction model based on SVM for detecting people at high risk of developing type 2 diabetes (T2DM). They demonstrated that plasma glucose concentrations served as an optimal feature subset for prediction. The model reached a mean accuracy of 96.80% after 100 iterations (Abbas et al., 2019). In another case, authors used tongue images of a total of 827 subjects and extracted features from them such as colour and texture. They then developed a genetic SVM algorithm that displayed an accuracy of 83.06% after normalizing parameters of the images and cross validation (Zhang et al., 2017).

Fuzzy SVM has been used for classification and detection of diabetes (Lukmanto et al., 2019). To find the useful characteristics in a dataset, feature selection was utilised. The output was then categorised using a fuzzy inference technique after the dataset was trained using SVM to provide fuzzy rules. This methodology was thus applied to the Pima Indian Diabetes (PID) dataset. The findings indicated an encouraging accuracy of 89.02% in identifying patients with Diabetes.

Computational Approach with Fuzzy Logic

Fuzzy logic was initiated by Zadeh. Not only did he discover this concept, he also developed the infrastructure of today's popular forms of use such as relations of similarity, decision making and fuzzy programming in a short time (Zadeh, 1965). Fuzzy logic is a computation-based approach to the truth of the real-world problems, which is far more than true-false or 0-1 in Boolean logic. In logic, only two answers can be found for each proposition: True and False. When the set theory is defined, the characteristic function of the membership of an x element of set A is being talked about. For each element of universal set X, the function generates the values 0 and 1 is called the characteristic function.

FL has become applicable to medical science together with the first article expressing its applications in biology (Zadeh, 1969). Fuzzy logic has a wide range of applications in medicine, for instance, to calculate the volume of brain tissue using magnetic resonance imaging (MRI) system, to analyse functional MRI data, to detect breast cancer, to visualize nerve fibres in the human brain, amongst others (Murat Kirisci et al., 2019).

A study introduced a fuzzy expert system that supported the diabetes decision application. They developed a 5-layerontology based model. The accuracy of this model depending on the age attribute like slightly old, slightly young, more or less young, young, and very young was found to be 91.2%, 90.3%, 85.9%, 81.7%, and 77.3% respectively (Chang-Shing Lee & Mei-Hui Wang, 2011).

In 2018, researchers created an expert decision support system for early diagnosis of diabetes using fuzzy logic. The variables used were BMI, diabetes pedigree function, blood pressure, glucose concentration and whether person is pregnant. The data was processed using Mamdani's fuzzy inference system (FIS). The system was found to have 96% accuracy. Apart from the aforementioned studies, table II contains additional studies incorporating fuzzy logic methods for diabetes prediction (Deshmukh & Fadewar, 2018).

Table 2. Some Fuzzy Logic Methods along with their Accuracies for comparison

S. No	Methods	Accuracy	References
1	Fuzzy Logic excluding Genetics Algorithm	69.42%	(Ephzibah, 2011)
2	Fuzzy Inference System	75.51%	(Choubey et al., 2018)
3	Adaptive Neuro Fuzzy Interference System	78.79%	(Rahman & Afroz, 2013)
4	Fuzzy logic and Artificial Neural Network	83.3%	(Rajeswari et al., 2011)
5	PSO Algorithm and Fuzzy Classifier	85.6%	(Sahebi & Ebrahimi, 2015)
6	Fuzzy Logic and Genetics Algorithm	87.4%	(Ephzibah, 2011)
7	SDSA and FDO (slightly young)	90.3%	(Chang-Shing Lee & Mei-Hui Wang, 2011)
8	SDSA and FDO (slightly old)	91.2%	(Chang-Shing Lee & Mei-Hui Wang, 2011)
9	Fuzzy Expert System (Enhanced)	91.6%	(Prajapati et al., 2017)
10	Fuzzy Inference System	96%	(Niswati et al., 2018)
11	Fuzzy Logic Risk Assessment System	92.7%	(Korkmaz et al., 2019)
12	Fuzzy rule-based system	96.47%	(Aamir et al., 2021)
13	Fuzzy CNN	95%	(Deshmukh & Fadewar, 2018)
14	Fuzzy based expert system	94.55%	(Muhammad & Algehyne, 2021)
15	Fuzzy interference system	93.5%	(Ylenia et al., 2021)
16	Fuzzy C-means + Genetic Algorithm	95%	(Ghoushchi et al., 2021)

Integrative Biology Studies

Traditionally, research methods have made use of animal models and cell lines to understand the molecular basis of many biological processes. However, these do not tend to replicate their human counterparts very well, which creates a gap in our understanding. As a result, there is increasing demand for novel research methods that may reduce this gap and bring to light new biological insights and become the basis for novel treatment strategies. One such approach, known as Systems biology, has improved our understanding of the pathophysiology of diseases like diabetes. Systems biology is a field that forms the culmination of a variety of data, comprising -omics fields such as proteomics, transcriptomics, genomics, phenomics, amongst others. Further, the application of agnostic bioinformatics analysis techniques in systems biology has increased the discovery of significant insights into disease pathomechanisms (Pan et al., 2021).

Particularly for the case of Gestational Diabetes Mellitus (GDM), studies have tried to explore CpG signatures that could serve as potential biomarkers for GMD, as CpG methylation has been implicated in the development of the disease (Liu et al., 2021). For this, DNA methylation data was taken from GEO repository, and epigenome-wide association study (EWAS) was performed. Further, GO and KEGG pathway analyses was done along with construction of PPI network through use of STRING and cytoscape software. The selected CpG site -values were the predictor variable in the created SVM model, and the occurrence of GDM was taken into account as the outcome variable. Twelve hub genes connected to the PPI network's identified CpG sites were found using this study. AUC values of testing and training set were found to be 0.7576 and 0.8138. In a similar case for Diabetic Kidney Disease (DKD), a study used LASSO regression model and SVM feature elimination (SVM-RFE) for identifying potential biomarkers for the disease (Gao et al., 2022). About 110 differentially expressed (DEGs) were found from gene expression profile taken from GEO database. CXCL3 and LINC00282 were identified as diagnostic markers, with AUC 0.97 for CXCL3 and 1 for LINC00282.

In order to identify novel therapeutic targets (DT) that could provide aid for diabetic nephropathy (DN), a high performing machine learning system was developed in, known as the modified Group Method of Data Handling with Automatic Feature Selection (mGMDH-AFS) (Abedi et al., 2021). MiRNAs were found to be expressed differently in the kidney's cortex and medulla. Their enrichment studies and networks of miRNA-target interactions were developed. Proteins that had been utilised as targets of FDA-approved drugs were also identified. Afterwards, using the mGMDH-AFS method, these proteins were separated accordingly into DT and non-DT categories. The 88% accuracy of the ML framework allowed for the identification of notable DT candidates which were then targeted for DN.

From the above, it can be seen that combining both computational and experimental methods can be beneficial in developing a thorough understanding of biological processes and pathologies, which in turn would aid in introduction of new therapeutic strategies.

Discussion

Diabetes is one of the major health problems in the world that can cause many serious complications. The most important factor in treating diabetes and reducing other related complications is early detection. As a result, given the significance of diabetes, several computational methods for diabetes prediction and complications have been developed (R. & P., 2013). Figure III depicts how data mining and machine learning technique are used for diabetes prediction. There are a variety of diabetes databases available, each with a unique dataset and size. Computational methods could help predict diabetes at an early stage.

Figure 3. Graphical Representation of Diabetes Mellitus Prediction using Machine Learning Algorithms

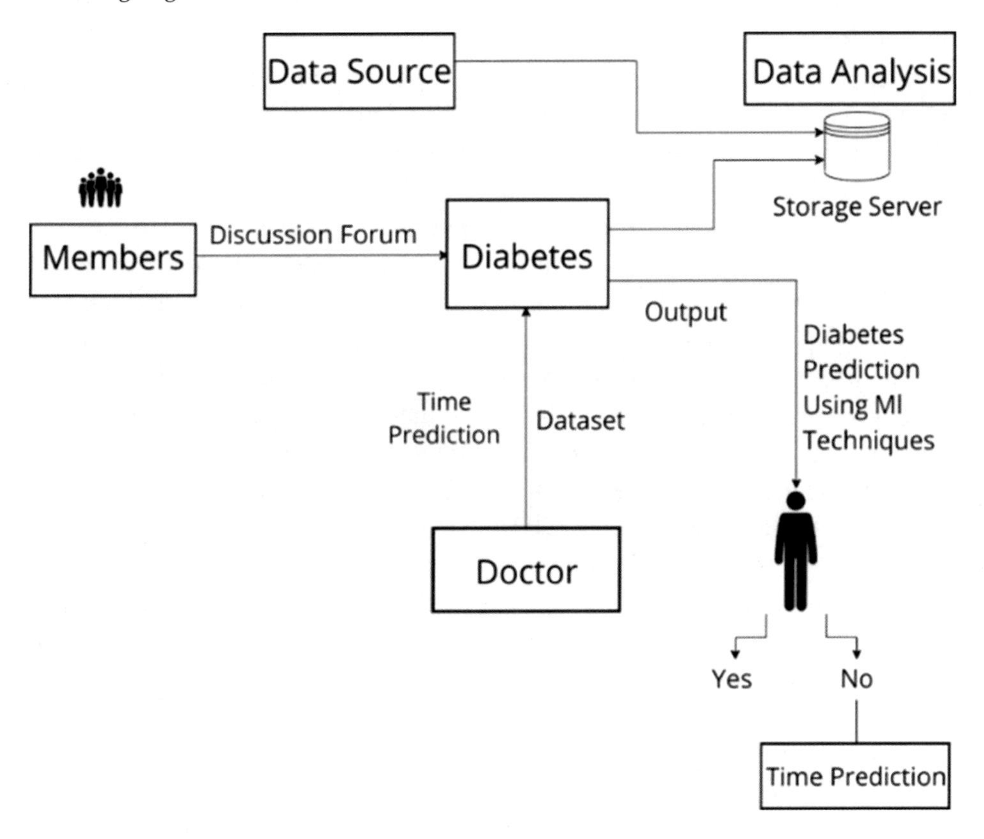

Various methods that use machine learning algorithms to help diagnose the disease quickly and efficiently have been developed in the past. Table III shows some of the methods that have been utilised in recent times for better prediction of

Diabetes. Previously, researchers have developed diabetes prediction methods that used algorithms such as Artificial Neural Networks (Abedi et al., 2021), Support Vector machine (Dewangan & Agrawal, 2015), Bayesian method (Dewangan & Agrawal, 2015), back propagation algorithm (Sridar & Shanthi, 2014), modified-PSO (Kohavi, 1995), Fuzzy Logic and Genetics Algorithm (Sanakal & Jayakumari, 2014), and others, and have achieved fairly good accuracy in experiments. In recent years, however, SVM Algorithm has emerged as one of the most widely used classifiers in the diagnosis and prediction of Diabetes Miletus, as seen from figure IV. It's also worth noting that, initially, only one machine learning algorithm was used for prediction at a time, but with time several ML algorithms were used to develop hybrid and collective models for higher accuracy (Table I).

Since PIDD has been used in the majority of studies, the need of data independent machine learning algorithm to decrease the requirement of datasets in diabetes prediction model is a must. Despite successful development and accuracy levels beyond 95%, no diabetes prediction model is being used in worldwide diabetes prediction. Diabetes is a major global issue, with lifestyle, race, and environment all having an impact on disease progression. The main difficulty in incorporating different diabetes datasets into ML models to establish prediction models is that the characteristic in each dataset is different (Negi & Jaiswal, 2016).

The majority of methods have only been tested and trained on one dataset, thus creating low reliability of the diabetes prediction model. Given the worldwide prevalence of diabetes, these methods must be trained, confirmed, and tested on varieties of populations. For fusing different datasets to build models, various data fusion methods are available. The best ML methods must be tested and trained on variety of representative populations around the world. ML methods can be more consistent, according to the current review, if they are trained, confirmed, and tested on a comprehensive population or at least a signified dataset from all datasets of diabetes obtainable (Jaiswal et al., 2021).

The unique aspect of various datasets presents a struggle when combining them, necessitating data fusion prior to model building (Soliman & AboElhamd, 2014). Finally, cutting-edge ML algorithms like Support Vector machine, Decision tree, and Logistic Regression can be used to develop prediction models for comparing the functioning of each algorithm individually and in grouping to determine the best diabetes detection method.

Figure 4. Differential use of several classifiers

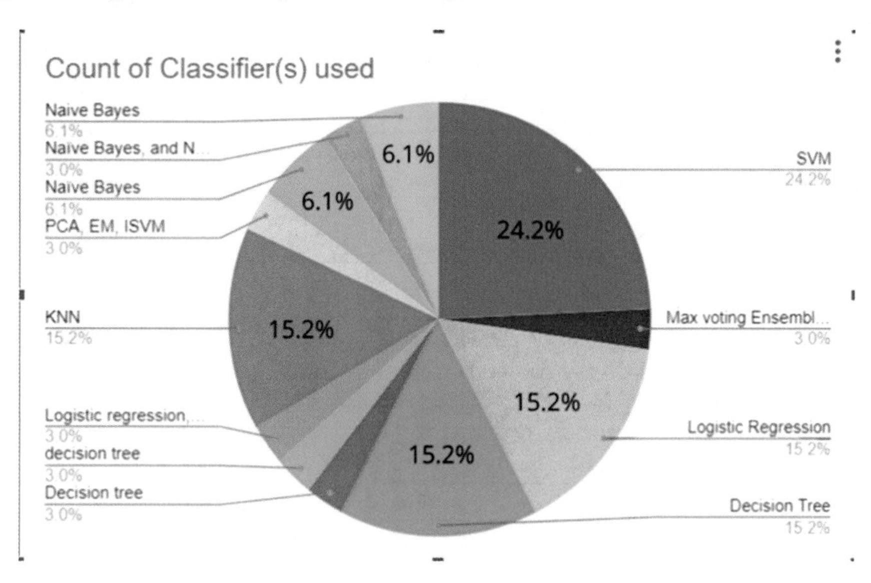

Table 3. Important Machine Learning based prediction methods and reported accuracy values

Sr. No.	Year	Methods	Dataset used	Accuracy	Reference
1	2016	Support Vector Machine	PIDD + Diabetes 130- US dataset	72%	(Negi & Jaiswal, 2016)
2	2017	Perceptron	NHANES0506, NHANES0708, and NHANES0090	75%	(Mirshahvalad & Zanjani, 2017)
4	2012	C4.5	Pima Indians Diabetes Database	91%	(Rajesh, 2012)
5	2013	Support Vector Machine	Pima Indians Diabetes Database	78%	(Kumari & Chitra, 2013)
6	2014	Artificial neural network	Pima Indians Diabetes Database	82%	(Dewangan & Agrawal, 2015)
7	2015	Decision Tree j48	Pima Indians Diabetes Database	73%	(Kandhasamy & Balamurali, 2015)
8	2018	Native Bayes Algorithm	Pima Indians Diabetes Database	76%	(Sisodia & Sisodia, 2018)
9	2016	Probabilistic neural network	Pima Indians Diabetes Database	81%	(Sisodia & Sisodia, 2018)
10	2017	Two-Class neural network	Pima Indians Diabetes Database	83%	(Kahn et al., 2006)

Continued on following page

Table 3. Continued

Sr. No.	Year	Methods	Dataset used	Accuracy	Reference
12	2014	LS-SVM-MPSO	Pima Indians Diabetes Database	97%	(Kohavi, 1995)
13	2015	Multi- Layer PNN+ Bayes Net	Pima Indians Diabetes Database	81%	(Mittal & Gill, 2016)
14	2016	SVM-ANN	Pima Indians Diabetes Database	96%	(Durairaj, 2015)
15	2014	Apriori + black propagation	Pima Indians Diabetes Database	91%	(Sridar & Shanthi, 2014)
16	2013	K-Means +Amalgam KN	Pima Indians Diabetes Database	97%	(Nirmaladevi et al., 2013)
17	2017	SVM	MESSIDOR Database	99%	(Murugeswari & Sukanesh, 2017)
18	2021	KNN	Pima Indians Diabetes Database	78.5%	(Saxena et al., 2021)
19	2020	Logistic Regression	Self-made dataset	74%	(Ye et al., 2020)
20	2018	PCA + EM + ISVM	Pima Indians Diabetes Database	97.95%	(Nilashi et al., 2016)

Future Scope and Challenges

Despite the various approaches and algorithms proposed in the areas of machine learning and deep learning, still many barriers remain, which yet to be researched upon. For the development of an efficient model, data comes first in the mind. One of the most arduous hurdles encountered while identifying the suitable research articles or studies in the Indian context is the absence of real-time data, owing to the inadequacy and compactness of datasets involved. Small datasets overfit the model and are more accurate, but cannot handle new test data. This means that the model cannot be implemented in real-time. In general, 80% of researchers' time is spent in cleaning and arranging data for model training. As data intricacy grows, so do costs and maintenance. The next step is the selection of features for model training. Some authors overlook certain features, while others group them for educational purposes. A previous study found that different test and training datasets reduced accuracy (Sharma & Shah, 2021). To create a diabetes prediction method based on multiple diabetes datasets, the data fusion technique that is fused with different diabetes datasets before training the model is required. However, it is very difficult to merge diabetic datasets to improve performance. In the future, hybrid ML / composite technology should be used to improve the performance of difficult and complex large datasets (Ashisha et al., 2022).

In healthcare, a ML model can only be helpful if it can help patients. The model's implementation in real-world applications is crucial in this scenario. In this continuous process, frequently forecasts or the number of applications essential should be considered for prediction model (Sharma & Shah, 2021).

Even with all of the foregoing obstacles, scholars and physicians will continue to develop larger and more accurate datasets, as well as more effective models and algorithms for improved organization and accuracy. In general, human resources are sparse in rural locations, notably in medicine. As a result, in the context of telemedicine, artificial intelligence plays a vital part in breaking down this barrier. Diabetes will be diagnosed utilising DL, AI, and cloud computing in the future (Chaki et al., 2020). Figure V displays graphically year-wise differential counts of publications in the last 7 years for several ML techniques usage. As research on early detection and diagnosis of Diabetes Mellitus is increasing drastically day by day, cutting-edge efficient models using machine learning for early diabetes detection and aiding people in making lifestyle changes can be developed. Because deep learning outperforms other algorithms on the great majority of datasets, it should be employed alongside it to improve accuracy and performance. This study demonstrates that future researchers can employ effective ML models to polish and refine them, as well as develop a pipeline or a collection of accurate and resourceful models to increase the possibilities of accurately anticipating the disease. These models can be improved further to systematize the system and enable it to handle novel data with ease (Sharma & Shah, 2021). One of the most significant areas for AI applications is biomedicine and healthcare systems, and medical imaging is perhaps the most promising domain (Castiglioni et al., 2021). First, the system computes image attributes that are thought to be crucial for producing the desired prediction or diagnosis. The machine learning algorithm system then decides which combination of these image attributes is most effective for categorising the image or calculating some metric for the specified image region (Erickson et al., 2017).

Figure 5. Represents year wise differential counts of publications for several machine-learning methods usage

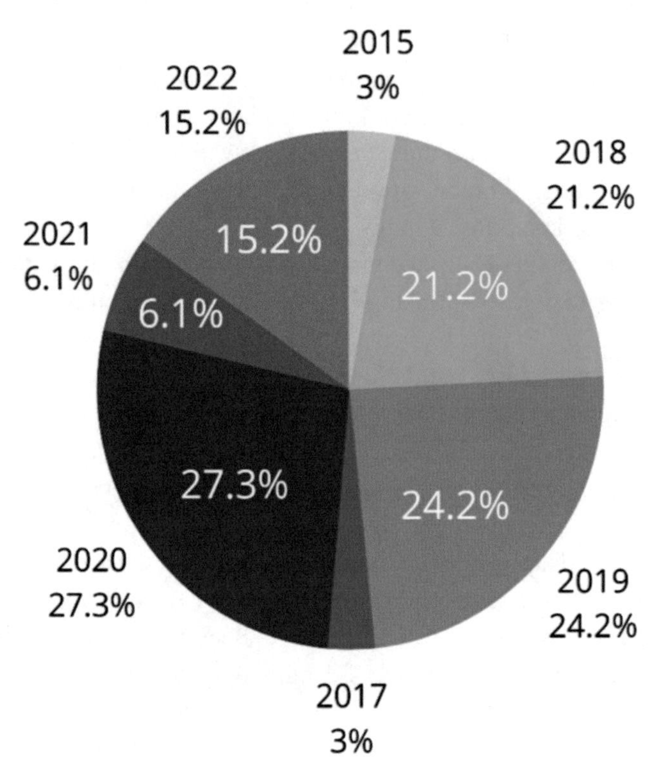

CONCLUSION

This study provides a comprehensive view of the machine learning techniques used to predict and diagnose diabetes through literature mining. Several machine classification and data mining techniques have emerged in the recent years. This paper outlines the use of such techniques for the prediction and diagnosis of diabetes in an effective way with recent updates.

For usage in the world's population, the goal of developing a prediction model for diabetes has changed from high prediction accuracy to high reliability. Very few developed methods exist that were tested and trained on variety of datasets (Dewangan & Agrawal, 2015; Jaiswal et al., 2021). Diabetes being a worldwide problem requires methods that are ready to be applied to the global population predicting diabetes from this particular dataset. The current algorithms frameworks and understanding helps researchers to develop algorithms/models that can be useful for early prognosis and diagnosis and open the new dimensions in the ensemble model development along with newer complex omics dataset for early prediction of diabetes.

ACKNOWLEDGMENT

We are thankful for Department of Biotechnology Jaypee Institute of Information Technology, NOIDA, INDIA for proving the necessary support

Conflict of Interest: On behalf of all authors, the corresponding author states that there is no conflict of interest

No funding

REFERENCES

Aamir, K. M., Sarfraz, L., Ramzan, M., Bilal, M., Shafi, J., & Attique, M. (2021). A Fuzzy Rule-Based System for Classification of Diabetes. *Sensors (Basel)*, *21*(23), 8095. https://doi.org/10.3390/s21238095

Abbas, H. T., Alic, L., Erraguntla, M., Ji, J. X., Abdul-Ghani, M., Abbasi, Q. H., & Qaraqe, M. K. (2019). Predicting long-term type 2 diabetes with support vector machine using oral glucose tolerance test. *PLoS One*, *14*(12), e0219636. https://doi.org/10.1371/journal.pone.0219636

Abedi, M., Marateb, H. R., Mohebian, M. R., Aghaee-Bakhtiari, S. H., Nassiri, S. M., & Gheisari, Y. (2021). Systems biology and machine learning approaches identify drug targets in diabetic nephropathy. *Scientific Reports*, *11*(1). https://doi.org/10.1038/s41598-021-02282-3

Agarwal, P., & Mehta, S. (2014). Nature-Inspired Algorithms: State-of-Art, Problems and Prospects. *International Journal of Computers and Applications*, *100*(14), 14–21. doi:10.5120/17593-8331

Ali, A., Alrubei, M. A. T., Hassan, L. F. M., Al-Ja'afari, M. A. M., & Abdulwahed, S. H. (2020). Diabetes diagnosis based on KNN. *IIUM Engineering Journal, 21*(1), 175–181. doi:10.31436/iiumej.v21i1.1206

Ashisha, G. R., George, S. T., Mary, X. A., Sagayam, K. M., & Pramanik, S. (2022). Analysis of Diabetes disease using Machine Learning Techniques: A Review. *Research Square*. https://doi.org/10.21203/rs.3.rs-1572946/v1

Azad, C., Bhushan, B., Sharma, R., Shankar, A., Singh, K. K., & Khamparia, A. (2021). Prediction model using SMOTE, genetic algorithm and decision tree (PMSGD) for classification of diabetes mellitus. *Multimedia Systems*. doi:10.1007/s00530-021-00817-2

Bukhari, M. M., Alkhamees, B. F., Hussain, S., Gumaei, A., Assiri, A., & Ullah, S. S. (2021). An Improved Artificial Neural Network Model for Effective Diabetes Prediction. *Complexity, 2021*, 1–10. doi:10.1155/2021/5525271

Castiglioni, I., Rundo, L., Codari, M., Di Leo, G., Salvatore, C., Interlenghi, M., Gallivanone, F., Cozzi, A., D'Amico, N. C., & Sardanelli, F. (2021). AI applications to medical images: From machine learning to deep learning. *Physica Medica*, *83*, 9–24. https://doi.org/10.1016/j.ejmp.2021.02.006

Chaki, J., Thillai Ganesh, S., Cidham, S. K., & Ananda Theertan, S. (2020). Machine learning and artificial intelligence based Diabetes Mellitus detection and self-management: A systematic review. *Journal of King Saud University - Computer and Information Sciences.* doi:10.1016/j.jksuci.2020.06.013

Choubey, D. K., Kumar, P., Tripathi, S., & Kumar, S. (2019). Performance evaluation of classification methods with PCA and PSO for diabetes. *Network Modeling and Analysis in Health Informatics and Bioinformatics*, *9*(1). https://doi.org/10.1007/s13721-019-0210-8

Choubey, D. K., Paul, S., & Dhandhania, V. K. (2018). GA_NN: An Intelligent Classification System for Diabetes. *Advances in Intelligent Systems and Computing*, 11–23. doi:10.1007/978-981-13-1595-4_2

Chuang, H.-Y., Hofree, M., & Ideker, T. (2010). A Decade of Systems Biology. *Annual Review of Cell and Developmental Biology*, *26*, 721–744. https://doi.org/10.1146/annurev-cellbio-100109-104122

Cui, C., Cui, Y., Fu, Y., Ma, S., & Zhang, S. (2017). Microarray analysis reveals gene and microRNA signatures in diabetic kidney disease. *Molecular Medicine Reports*. doi:10.3892/mmr.2017.8177 PMID:29207157

Das, H., Naik, B., & Behera, H. S. (2018). Classification of Diabetes Mellitus Disease (DMD): *Progress in Computing, Analytics and Networking*. Springer Singapore.

Derevitskii, I. V., & Kovalchuk, S. V. (2020). Machine Learning-Based Predictive Modeling of Complications of Chronic Diabetes. *Procedia Computer Science*, *178*, 274–283. doi:10.1016/j.procs.2020.11.029

Deshmukh, T., & Fadewar, H. S. (2018). Fuzzy Deep Learning for Diabetes Detection. *Advances in Intelligent Systems and Computing*, 875–882. doi:10.1007/978-981-13-1513-8_89

Dewangan, A. kumar, & Agrawal, P. (2015). Classification of Diabetes Mellitus Using Machine Learning Techniques. *International Journal of Engineering and Applied Sciences, 2*(5), 257905. https://www.neliti.com/publications/257905/classification-of-diabetes-mellitus-using-machine-learning-techniques

Ding, L., Fan, L., Xu, X., Fu, J., & Xue, Y. (2019). Identification of core genes and pathways in type 2 diabetes mellitus by bioinformatics analysis. *Molecular Medicine Reports*. doi:10.3892/mmr.2019.10522 PMID:31524257

Durairaj, M. (2015). Prediction Of Diabetes Using Back Propagation Algorithm.

Ephzibah, E. P. (2011). Cost Effective Approach on Feature Selection Using Genetic Algorithms and Fuzzy logic for Diabetes Diagnosis. *International Journal on Soft Computing*, *2*(1), 1–10. https://doi.org/10.5121/ijsc.2011.2101

Erickson, B. J., Korfiatis, P., Akkus, Z., & Kline, T. L. (2017). Machine Learning for Medical Imaging. *Radiographics*, *37*(2), 505–515. https://doi.org/10.1148/rg.2017160130

Gao, Q., Wang, Y., Xu, W., & Jin, H. (2022). Predicting diagnostic gene biomarkers in patients with diabetic kidney disease based on weighted gene co-expression network analysis and machine-learning algorithms. *Research Square*. https://doi.org/10.21203/rs.3.rs-1696152/v1

geo. (2019). *Home*. GEO - NCBI. Nih.gov. https://www.ncbi.nlm.nih.gov/geo/

Ghoushchi, S. J., Ranjbarzadeh, R., Dadkhah, A. H., Pourasad, Y., & Bendechache, M. (2021). An Extended Approach to Predict Retinopathy in Diabetic Patients Using the Genetic Algorithm and Fuzzy C-Means. *BioMed Research International,* 5597222. doi:10.1155/2021/5597222

Habibi, S., Ahmadi, M., & Alizadeh, S. (2015). Type 2 Diabetes Mellitus Screening and Risk Factors Using Decision Tree: Results of Data Mining. *Global Journal of Health Science*, *7*(5). https://doi.org/10.5539/gjhs.v7n5p304

Horgan, R. P., & Kenny, L. C. (2011). "Omic" technologies: genomics, transcriptomics, proteomics and metabolomics. *The Obstetrician & Gynaecologist, 13*(3), 189–195. doi:10.1576/toag.13.3.189.27672

Jaiswal, V., Negi, A., & Pal, T. (2021). A review on current advances in machine learning based diabetes prediction. *Primary Care Diabetes*, *15*(3), 435–443. https://doi.org/10.1016/j.pcd.2021.02.005

Jakkula, V. (n.d.). *Tutorial on Support Vector Machine (SVM)*. CCS. https://course.ccs.neu.edu/cs5100f11/resources/jakkula.pdf

Joshi, R. D., & Dhakal, C. K. (2021). Predicting Type 2 Diabetes Using Logistic Regression and Machine Learning Approaches. *International Journal of Environmental Research and Public Health, 18*(14), 7346. https://doi.org/10.3390/ijerph18147346

Kahn, S. E., Hull, R. L., & Utzschneider, K. M. (2006). Mechanisms linking obesity to insulin resistance and type 2 diabetes. *Nature, 444*(7121), 840–846. https://doi.org/10.1038/nature05482

Kandhasamy, J. Pradeep., & Balamurali, S. (2015, May). Performance Analysis of Classifier Models to Predict Diabetes Mellitus [Review of Performance Analysis of Classifier Models to Predict Diabetes Mellitus]. *Procedia Computer Science, 47*. doi:10.1016/j.procs.2015.03.182

Karahalil, B. (2016). Overview of Systems Biology and Omics Technologies. *Current Medicinal Chemistry, 23*(37), 4221–4230. https://doi.org/10.2174/0929867323666160926150617

Kaul, K., Tarr, J. M., Ahmad, S. I., Kohner, E. M., & Chibber, R. (2012). Introduction to Diabetes Mellitus. *Advances in Experimental Medicine and Biology, 771*, 1–11. doi:10.1007/978-1-4614-5441-0_1 PMID:23393665

Kohavi, R. (1995, August). A study of cross-validation and bootstrap for accuracy estimation and model selection [Review of A study of cross-validation and bootstrap for accuracy estimation and model selection]. *IJCAI'95: Proceedings of the 14th international joint conference on Artificial intelligence* – (Volume 2). IEEE.

Korkmaz, H., Canayaz, E., Birtane Akar, S., & Altikardes, Z. A. (2019). Fuzzy logic based risk assessment system giving individualized advice for metabolic syndrome and fatal cardiovascular diseases. *Technology and Health Care, 27*, 59–66. https://doi.org/10.3233/thc-199007

Kumari, V. A., & Chitra, R. (2013). Classification of Diabetes Disease Using Support Vector Machine. [IJERA]. *International Journal of Engineering Research and Applications, 3*, 1797–1801.

Kumari, S., Kumar, D., & Mittal, M. (2021, May). An ensemble approach for classification and prediction of diabetes mellitus using soft voting classifier [Review of An ensemble approach for classification and prediction of diabetes mellitus using soft voting classifier]. *International Journal of Cognitive Computing in Engineering, 2*, 40-46. doi:10.1016/j.ijcce.2021.01.001

Lee, C.-S., & Wang, M.-H. (2011). A Fuzzy Expert System for Diabetes Decision Support Application. *IEEE Transactions on Systems, Man, and Cybernetics. Part B, Cybernetics*, *41*(1), 139–153. https://doi.org/10.1109/tsmcb.2010.2048899

Liaw, A., & Wiener, M. (2002). Classification and Regression by randomForest. *R News*, *2*(3). https://cogns.northwestern.edu/cbmg/LiawAndWiener2002.pdf. doi:10.1057/9780230509993

Liu, Y., Geng, H., Duan, B., Yang, X., Ma, A., & Ding, X. (2021). Identification of Diagnostic CpG Signatures in Patients with Gestational Diabetes Mellitus via Epigenome-Wide Association Study Integrated with Machine Learning. *BioMed Research International*, *2021*, 1–10. https://doi.org/10.1155/2021/1984690

Lukmanto, R. B. Suharjito, N. A., & Akbar, H. (2019). Early Detection of Diabetes Mellitus using Feature Selection and Fuzzy Support Vector Machine. *Procedia Computer Science, 157*, 46–54. doi:10.1016/j.procs.2019.08.140

Marie-Sainte, L., Almohaini, A. & Saba. (2019). Current Techniques for Diabetes Prediction: Review and Case Study. *Applied Sciences, 9*(21), 4604. doi:10.3390/app9214604

Marselli, L., Thorne, J., Dahiya, S., Sgroi, D. C., Sharma, A., Bonner-Weir, S., Marchetti, P., & Weir, G. C. (2010). Gene Expression Profiles of Beta-Cell Enriched Tissue Obtained by Laser Capture Microdissection from Subjects with Type 2 Diabetes. *PLoS One*, *5*(7), e11499. https://doi.org/10.1371/journal.pone.0011499

Maulana, Y. I. R., Badriyah, T., & Syarif, I. (2018). Influence of Logistic Regression Models For Prediction and Analysis of Diabetes Risk Factors. *EMITTER International Journal of Engineering Technology*, *6*(1), 151–167. doi:10.24003/emitter.v6i1.258

Mirshahvalad, R., & Zanjani, N. A. (2017). Diabetes prediction using ensemble perceptron algorithm. In *2017 9th International Conference on Computational Intelligence and Communication Networks (CICN),* pp. 190–194. IEEE.

Mirza, S., Mittal, S., & Zaman, M. (2018). Decision Support Predictive model for prognosis of diabetes using SMOTE and Decision tree. *International Journal of Applied Engineering Research: IJAER*, *13*, 9277–9282. http://www.ripublication.com/ijaer18/ijaerv13n11_73.pdf

Mittal, P., & Gill, N. (2016, May). A computational hybrid model with two level classification using SVM and neural network for predicting the diabetes disease [Review of A computational hybrid model with two level classification using SVM and neural network for predicting the diabetes disease]. *Journal of Theoretical and Applied Information Technology.*

Mohammedhasan, M., & Uğuz, H. (2020). A New Early Stage Diabetic Retinopathy Diagnosis Model Using Deep Convolutional Neural Networks and Principal Component Analysis. *Traitement Du Signal, 37*(5), 711–722. doi:10.18280/ts.370503

Muhammad, L. J., & Algehyne, E. A. (2021). Fuzzy based expert system for diagnosis of coronary artery disease in nigeria. *Health and Technology, 11*(2), 319–329. https://doi.org/10.1007/s12553-021-00531-z

Murat Kirisci, M. Ubeydullah, S., & Yilmaz, H. (2019). An ANFIS perspective for the diagnosis of type II diabetes. *ANNALS of FUZZY MATHEMATICS and INFORMATICS, 17*(2), 101–113. doi:10.30948/afmi.2019.17.2.101

Murugeswari, S., & Sukanesh, R. (2017). Investigations of severity level measurements for diabetic macular oedema using machine learning algorithms. *Irish Journal of Medical Science (1971 -), 186*(4), 929–938. doi:10.1007/s11845-017-1598-8

National Institute of Diabetes and Digestive and Kidney Diseases. (2016, December). *What is Diabetes?* National Institute of Diabetes and Digestive and Kidney Diseases. https://www.niddk.nih.gov/health-information/diabetes/overview/what-is-diabetes

Negi, A., & Jaiswal, V. (2016, December 1). A first attempt to develop a diabetes prediction method based on different global datasets. *IEEE Xplore*. doi:10.1109/PDGC.2016.7913152

Nilashi, M., Bin Ibrahim, O., Mardani, A., Ahani, A., & Jusoh, A. (2016). A soft computing approach for diabetes disease classification. *Health Informatics Journal, 24*(4), 379–393. https://doi.org/10.1177/1460458216675500

Nirmaladevi, M., Appavu, S., & Swathi, U. V. (2013). An amalgam KNN to predict diabetes mellitus. *2013 IEEE International Conference ON Emerging Trends in Computing, Communication and Nanotechnology (ICECCN),* (pp. 691-695). IEEE.

Niswati, Z., Mustika, F. A., & Paramita, A. (2018). Fuzzy logic implementation for diagnosis ofDiabetes Mellitusdisease at Puskesmas in East Jakarta. *Journal of Physics: Conference Series, 1114*, 012107. https://doi.org/10.1088/1742-6596/1114/1/012107

Pan, W. W., Gardner, T. W., & Harder, J. L. (2021). Integrative Biology of Diabetic Retinal Disease: Lessons from Diabetic Kidney Disease. *Journal of Clinical Medicine, 10*(6), 1254. https://doi.org/10.3390/jcm10061254

Pei, D., Yang, T., & Zhang, C. (2020). Estimation of Diabetes in a High-Risk Adult Chinese Population Using J48 Decision Tree Model. *Diabetes, Metabolic Syndrome and Obesity, 13*, 4621–4630. https://doi.org/10.2147/dmso.s279329

Permana, B. A. C., Ahmad, R., Bahtiar, H., Sudianto, A., & Gunawan, I. (2021). Classification of diabetes disease using decision tree algorithm (C4.5). *Journal of Physics: Conference Series, 1869*(1), 012082. doi:10.1088/1742-6596/1869/1/012082

Posonia, A. M., Vigneshwari, S., & Rani, D. J. (2020, December 1). Machine Learning based Diabetes Prediction using Decision Tree J48. *IEEE Xplore*. doi:10.1109/ICISS49785.2020.9316001

Prajapati H, Jain A, Pal SK (2017). An enhance expert system for diagnosis of diabetes using fuzzy rules over PIMA dataset. *4*(9), 225-230.

Quinlan, J. R. (1986). Induction of decision trees. *Machine Learning, 1*(1), 81–106. https://doi.org/10.1007/bf00116251

R., P., & P., A. (2013). Diagnosis of diabetic retinopathy using machine learning techniques. Ictact *Journal on Soft Computing, 03*(04), 563–575. doi:10.21917/ijsc.2013.0083

Rahman, R. M., & Afroz, F. (2013). Comparison of Various Classification Techniques Using Different Data Mining Tools for Diabetes Diagnosis. *Journal of Software Engineering and Applications, 06*(03), 85–97. https://doi.org/10.4236/jsea.2013.63013

Rajendra, P., & Latifi, S. (2021). Prediction of diabetes using logistic regression and ensemble techniques. *Computer Methods and Programs in Biomedicine Update, 1,* 100032. doi:10.1016/j.cmpbup.2021.100032

Rajesh, K. (2012, September). Application of Data Mining Methods and Techniques for Diabetes Diagnosis (V. Sangeetha, Ed.) [Review of Application of Data Mining Methods and Techniques for Diabetes Diagnosis]. International Journal of Engineering and Innovative Technology (IJEIT), 2,(3).

Rajeswari, K., & Vaithiyanathan, V. (2011). Fuzzy based modeling for diabetic diagnostic decision support using Artificial Neural Network. *IJCSNS International Journal of Computer Science and Network Security, 11*(4), 126. http://paper.ijcsns.org/07_book/201104/20110419.pdf

Rakshit, S., Manna, S., & Biswas, S. (2017). *Prediction of Diabetes Type-II Using a Two-Class Neural Network* [Review of Prediction of Diabetes Type-II Using a Two-Class Neural Network]. Computational Intelligence, Communications, and Business Analytics, Springer Singapore.

Robertson, G., Lehmann, E. D., Sandham, W., & Hamilton, D. (2011). Blood Glucose Prediction Using Artificial Neural Networks Trained with the AIDA Diabetes Simulator: A Proof-of-Concept Pilot Study. *Journal of Electrical and Computer Engineering*, *2011*, 1–11. doi:10.1155/2011/681786

Sahebi, H. R., & Ebrahimi, S. (2015). A Fuzzy Classifier Based on Modified Particle Swarm Optimization for Diabetes Disease Diagnosis. *Advances in Computer Science: An International Journal*, *4*(3), 11–17. http://www.acsij.org/acsij/article/view/90/86

Sanakal, R., & Jayakumari, Smt. T. (2014). Prognosis of Diabetes Using Data mining Approach-Fuzzy C Means Clustering and Support Vector Machine. *International Journal of Computer Trends and Technology*, *11*(2), 94–98. doi:10.14445/22312803/ijctt-v11p120

Saxena, R. (2021). Role of K-nearest neighbour in detection of Diabetes Mellitus. [TURCOMAT]. *Turkish Journal of Computer and Mathematics Education*, *12*(10), 373–376. https://doi.org/10.17762/turcomat.v12i10.4182

Saxena, R., Sharma, S. K., & Gupta, M. (2021, April). Role of K-nearest neighbour in detection of Diabetes Mellitus [Review of Role of K-nearest neighbour in detection of Diabetes Mellitus]. *Turkish Journal of Computer and Mathematics Education*, *12*(10).

Sharma, T., & Shah, M. (2021). A comprehensive review of machine learning techniques on diabetes detection. *Visual Computing for Industry, Biomedicine, and Art*, *4*(1). doi:10.1186/s42492-021-00097-7

Sheik Abdullah, A., & Selvakumar, S. (2018). Assessment of the risk factors for type II diabetes using an improved combination of particle swarm optimization and decision trees by evaluation with Fisher's linear discriminant analysis. *Soft Computing*, *23*(20), 9995–10017. https://doi.org/10.1007/s00500-018-3555-5

Sisodia, D., & Sisodia, D. S. (2018). Prediction of Diabetes using Classification Algorithms. *Procedia Computer Science*, *132*, 1578–1585. https://doi.org/10.1016/j.procs.2018.05.122

Soliman, O. S., & AboElhamd, E. (2014). *Classification of Diabetes Mellitus using Modified Particle Swarm Optimization and Least Squares Support Vector Machine*. ArXiv:1405.0549 https://arxiv.org/abs/1405.0549

Sridar, K., & Shanthi, D. (2014, October). Medical diagnosis system for the diabetes mellitus by using back propagation-apriori algorithms [Review of Medical diagnosis system for the diabetes mellitus by using back propagation-apriori algorithms]. *Journal of Theoretical and Applied Information Technology*, *68*(1), 36–43.

Sun, Y., & Zhang, D. (2019, June). Machine Learning Techniques for Screening and Diagnosis of Diabetes: a Survey [Review of Machine Learning Techniques for Screening and Diagnosis of Diabetes: a Survey]. *Tehnicki vjesnik - Technical Gazette, 26*(3). https://hrcak.srce.hr/221017

Taser, P. Y. (2021). Application of Bagging and Boosting Approaches Using Decision Tree-Based Algorithms in Diabetes Risk Prediction. *Proceedings*, *74*(1), 6. https://doi.org/10.3390/proceedings2021074006

Thakkar, H., Shah, V., Yagnik, H., & Shah, M. (2021). Comparative anatomization of data mining and fuzzy logic techniques used in diabetes prognosis. *Clinical EHealth*, *4*, 12–23. doi:10.1016/j.ceh.2020.11.001

Wang, X., Zhai, M., Ren, Z., Ren, H., Li, M., Quan, D., Chen, L., & Qiu, L. (2021). Exploratory study on classification of diabetes mellitus through a combined Random Forest Classifier. *BMC Medical Informatics and Decision Making*, *21*(1), 105. doi:10.118612911-021-01471-4 PMID:33743696

Wang, Z., Wang, Z., Zhou, Z., & Ren, Y. (2016). Crucial genes associated with diabetic nephropathy explored by microarray analysis. *BMC Nephrology*, *17*(1), 128. doi:10.118612882-016-0343-2 PMID:27613243

World Health Organization. (2022). *Diabetes*. World Health Organization. https://www.who.int/health-topics/diabetes#tab=tab_1

Ye, Y., Xiong, Y., Zhou, Q., Wu, J., Li, X., & Xiao, X. (2020). Comparison of Machine Learning Methods and Conventional Logistic Regressions for Predicting Gestational Diabetes Using Routine Clinical Data: A Retrospective Cohort Study. *Journal of Diabetes Research*, *2020*, 1–10. https://doi.org/10.1155/2020/4168340

Ylenia, C., Chiara, D. L., Giovanni, I., Lucia, R., Donatella, V., Tiziana, S., Vincenzo, G., Ciro, V., & Stefania, S. (2021). A Clinical Decision Support System based on fuzzy rules and classification algorithms for monitoring the physiological parameters of type-2 diabetic patients. *Mathematical Biosciences and Engineering*, *18*(3), 2654–2674. https://doi.org/10.3934/mbe.2021135

Zadeh, L. A. (1965). Fuzzy sets. *Information and Control*, *8*(3), 338–353. https://doi.org/10.1016/s0019-9958(65)90241-x

Zadeh, L. A. (1969) Biological Applications of the Theory of Fuzzy Set and Systems, In: Proctor, L.D., Ed., *The Proceedings of an International Symposium on Biocybernetics of the Central Nervous System, Little,* 199-206. Brown and Company.

Zhang, J., Xu, J., Hu, X., Chen, Q., Tu, L., Huang, J., & Cui, J. (2017). Diagnostic Method of Diabetes Based on Support Vector Machine and Tongue Images. *BioMed Research International*, *2017*, 1–9. https://doi.org/10.1155/2017/7961494

Zhang, M., Luo, H., Xi, Z., & Rogaeva, E. (2015). Drug Repositioning for Diabetes Based on "Omics" Data Mining. *PLoS One*, *10*(5), e0126082. https://doi.org/10.1371/journal.pone.0126082

Zou, Q., Qu, K., Luo, Y., Yin, D., Ju, Y., & Tang, H. (2018). Predicting Diabetes Mellitus With Machine Learning Techniques. *Frontiers in Genetics, 9*. doi:10.3389/fgene.2018.00515

Chapter 9
Applications of Watermarking in Different Emerging Areas:
A Survey

Lalan Kumar
Independent Researcher, India

Ayush Kumar
G.L. Bajaj Institute of Technology and Management, India

Shravan Kumar
G.L. Bajaj Institute of Technology and Management, India

Indrajeet Kumar
https://orcid.org/0000-0003-2814-2900
Graphic Era Hill University, Dehradun, India

ABSTRACT

These days enormous amounts of information is at almost everyone's disposal with a single click of a button, and that too on a hand held device. Data can be present in various forms like still images, and slides of pictures like a video of GIF, over various websites present on the Internet. Because of the excessive use of this data, it also becomes important to secure it as it can be duplicated, transformed, stolen, tampered, or misused pretty easily. Recently, there has been a spike increase in the use of medical images in various E-health applications. In order to counter these potential threats, a number of watermarking techniques are being developed. A watermark is embedded in an image or document in the form of an image or pattern that can be used to authenticate the integrity of the image in question. As time goes by, the complexity of the problems that we are dealing with also keeps on increasing.

DOI: 10.4018/978-1-6684-6957-6.ch009

INTRODUCTION

Large amounts of data may now be stored on a page organiser and transferred to any system with the click of a mouse. Data may be found in a number of formats includes photographs, pictures image slideshows, video, and GIFs, (graphics interchange format), over various websites present on the Web. Because this data is so widely used, it is critical to keep it safe because it can easily be duplicated, transferred, stolen, hacked, or misused. The utilization of medical images in various E-health applications has increased recently. A variety of watermark approaches are being developed to counteract these potential threats. An image or pattern that serves as a watermark is added to an image or document so that its authenticity may be confirmed. As time progressed, the severity of the issues we face also continued to rise. The vast array of algorithms and strategies that have been created, advocated for, and applied in recent years to address the extremely difficult issues that have arisen when attempting to protect medical images from various threats are discussed in this survey study. Along with the methodologies survey, we also cover the idea of watermarking, its characteristics, new real-world applications, various difficulties encountered when watermarking medical photos, and a summary of the numerous watermarking approaches.

FURTHER INTRODUCTION

With the introduction of electronic, handheld devices, as well as advancements in Digital content creation is now easier than ever thanks to modern communication and technology. Then, this information is disseminated over the Internet to different communities. This content, which is essentially intellectual property, has been protected online using a variety of techniques, including steganography, encryption, and watermarking (Riaz, 2013), where anybody may read your data. To ensure security, steganography employs disguised communications without the end-or user's approval, whereas watermarking does not. Nonetheless, certain watermarking techniques are invisible by users (Imaduddin, 2014). Digital watermarking can be shared across several copies or unique to each copy (Mehta, 2014). Watermarking is a method of adding information (a watermark) to a digital image. The data is contained in the image here. The spatial domain of a watermarked image differs from that of the original work. When information is added to an image, the original work becomes deformed. It might be suggested as (Żurawski, 2013):

$$C_w = C_o + C_w \tag{1}$$

Where: Co= Original work, w = watermark, Cw = Watermarked work.

To read Digital watermarks, you are required to employ the appropriate software systems. Digitals watermarks help to secure the content while not leaving a perceivable mark on the work and the appearance of the work is not affected by the watermarking process either. For watermarking the content, a unique algorithm is used by the user to encrypt a specific pattern that can only be decrypted by the original created which is then embedded into the work.

In study (Miyazaki, 2005) Watermarking is preferred over comparable encrypting/ data concealment techniques. In contrast, the watermarking on medical images is more robust. The user's information and the hospital's logo may, if necessary, be added to the medical image using this technology. In the event of particularly sensitive data, these additional strategies can be utilised in addition to watermarking methods to increase effectiveness.

For any organisation, the patient's/client's info is highly confidential data leaking which can lead to millions of dollars lost in law-suits as well as data recovery or the impact of redoing various operations. The watermarking techniques are employed on various levels for the safety of intellectual property of the clients as well as the organisation. In the event of an illicit redistribution (Imaduddin, 2014), Watermarking can be used to detect this. Previously widespread, copyright infringement was largely limited because to the expense of duplicating and physically spreading them, but it is now simpler than ever to make their own high-quality copies utilizing contemporary technology like the Internet and portable devices, come with cameras. Because of this, watermarking is now more crucial than ever in preventing copyright violations.

Taking Perceptivity Into the Account, Watermarking is of the Following Two Types

Visible Watermarking

When the watermarking is evident on the content, the process is known as visible watermarking, such as when the original creator's name is inscribed on a piece of work or when a logo is embedded that the user can see. For example, television networks like CW, ABC, and NETFLIX (Kumar, 2018) affix their emblems on images and videos that belong to the network in the corner.

Invisible Watermarking

With the use of the required software, the creator can incorporate patterns or information into their work that cannot be seen but can be decoded. While using this method won't stop actual picture theft, It can aid in proving that the image was created by its original owner.

Watermarking in Frequency Domain

Taking frequency domain into the consideration, several types of watermarking techniques are categorized, Some of them are:

Discrete Cosine Transform (DCT):

The discrete Fourier transform separates a signal into its fundamental frequency components, such as the discrete cosine transform (Wu, 2000). When compared to other popular watermarking techniques, DCT is a strong watermarking technique. Reduced frequency insertion of the watermark into the component strengthens the watermarking process and results. The watermark, though, is more difficult to cover up. On the other hand, an image is less powerful but much easier to hide when a watermark is added to the higher frequency component (Hernandez, 2000).

Discrete Wavelet Transform (DWT):

For a discrete wavelet transform, wavelets are discretely sampled. In contrast to the Fourier transform, it records both frequency and location data. The four bands that make up the picture are LL, LH, HL, and HH. Although the LL band is stronger, it is also easier to see with the naked eye (Singh, A. K., 2017). The HH band is less durable but offers good imperceptibility.

Singular Value Decomposition (SVD)

In singular value decomposition, a matrix must be divided or split based on the following standards: (i) It is a diagonal of a matrix of the Eigenvalues of A and T, indicating matrix transposition (Singh, 2013). U and v are orthogonal matrices of dimensions M x M and N x N, respectively.

It has been demonstrated that the singular value decomposition technique produces robust images. Watermarking (Britanak, 2001, Hsieh, 2002) because of the following facts:

1. Even when we add distortions to the image, it's singular value remains intact.
2. We can perform SVD on both square and rectangular matrices.
3. Unlike DCT and DFT, Singular values can preserve one way as well as non-symmetric properties.

4. It helps us in representing the intrinsic algebraic properties of an audio signal/ digital image.

Watermarking in Spatial Domain

Initially, the watermark is added to the webpage utilizing spatial domain techniques, changing the pixels and other attributes of the image (Kamble, 2016). The host signal is combined with pixels using simple procedures in the pixel domain. This image is still blurry. The predicted data can be used as a key to identify the watermark image that was produced from the received signals. The real image and the original are contrasted. The Least Significant Bit (LSB) method is the most often utilized formula or technique in the spatial domain.

Least Significant Bit Algorithm

The least significant bit algorithm determines each picture bit's importance and uses that information to discriminate between various image regions. While certain portions of the image are busier and draw more user attention, others are less cluttered and draw the same amount of attention from users.

Spread Spectrum

Using this technique, a given stream of information can be encrypted by spreading it to as much of the frequency spectrum as possible (Sinha, 2014).

Correlation-based Techniques

We calculate the resemblance between the watermarked picture after transformation and the pseudorandom code used in correlation-based watermarking approaches to check for a watermark. The accuracy of this technique is determined by the host image's properties. a. Miyazaki showed in his paper (Miyazaki, 2005) that a fixed image can cause errors during watermark detection. They have implemented embedding process for watermarks to prevent such scenarios from happening.

Patchwork Methods

Patchwork can be described as a pseudo-random process in which a watermark is inserted into the real photo by employing redundant pattern encoding by implementing a Gaussian distribution (Begum, 2020). We randomly pick two patches i.e. Patch A and Patch B. The information from image A is faded while the information from image B is darkened. The patchwork method is quite robust against the non-geometric modifications that can be done to the original image. While the method is suitable for rand textures encompassing vast areas, it isn't suitable for images that comprise text mostly.

STANDARD WATERMARKING TECHNIQUES

DCT (Discrete Cosine Transform)

DCT is helpful in splitting images into different parts based upon their frequencies and then can discard frequencies that are less important which can also turn into a compression method for reducing the largeness of the image. Depending upon the requirement the watermarking can be embedded into the parts with higher or lower frequencies. DCT splits the image into M*M blocks, usually, m is equal to eight (Solanki, A. C., 2018).

DCT has the following advantages.

1. It can be used with a single integrated circuit.
2. It can reduce the blocks or jaggies (Blocking artefacts) that can appear when the sub-image boundaries can be perceived.
3. The most amount of information can be fit into the smallest number of frequency coefficients with the help of DC.

DCT can convert any signal into basic frequencies (Al-Naqeeb, 2017). DCT can also be used to switch the domain of a signal for time to frequency (Priyanka, 2014, Gahalod, 2018). DCT is of two types:

i) One dimensional DCT
ii) Two-dimensional DCT

Watermarking done by DCT is immune to any kind of attack (Pandya, 2018). DCT is found to be more robust for performing digital operations (When greater number of times are used to introduce the watermark into the zone). DCT can also leave a negative impact on the original image by having a negative effect on certain components with a higher frequency. DCT may also result in the destruction of the invariance property of the system (Rader, 1976). When it comes to an image the higher frequencies are in general of less importance than the lower frequencies as they are less perceivable to the human eye. Therefore, hiding the image in that part is more robust (Sinha, 2014) but in turn, it will make the watermark itself less visible which in turn will only help in detecting the piracy but won't remove the piracy in the first place which in turn lead to the same result. The 2-D DFT can be said to be similar to the 1-D DCT. DCT has a way higher time complexity compared to the other techniques. Also, it is easier to remove DCT watermark if it is visible using various loopholes like cropping, rotation and scaling of the image.

Steps involved in DCT:

1. Split the image into m*m blocks.
2. Use DCT individually every block as per the requirement.
3. Implement an algorithm for selection of blocks (Usually high-frequency ones).
4. Implement an algorithm for the selection of coefficients.
5. Insert the watermark into the selected blocks.
6. Apply inverse DCT individually to each of these blocks per the requirement.

The important properties of DCT that are taken into consideration when we are inserting a watermark are High compression of signal and high decorrelation in the coefficients (Rahman, 2014).

Discrete Fourier Transform (DFT)

DFT works by converting nonstop functions into frequency components. DFT is immune to various different kinds of attacks. As the watermarks are inserted in the magnitudes of the normal vectors it is almost impossible to transform the image in a track like scaling, cropping or rotating as doing so will cause data loss, in turn causing the image to become blurrier (Yadav, 2016, Robert, 2009). Like DCT, SFT is also complex and is harder to implement but unlike DFT it is less prone to attacks directly. The main limitation of using DFT is that it has significantly lower efficiency in terms of time complexity compared to DCT and DWT (Robert, 2009). In the mid-60s, highly advanced algorithms for getting an approximate value of the DFT were developed, known as *FAST FOURIER TRANSFORMS* (Rader, 1976). DFT has the capability to show the invariance in translation. An attack can change the image in terms of its phase representation, but the magnitude representation of the image is immune to any kind of attack (Rashid, 2016). One major advantage of DFT over DCT and DWT is that it is able to recover from attacks and modifications later on.

FFT algorithms convert the DFT matrices into their small products that are usually zero. Normally, the Discrete Fourier Transform having time complexity of $O(N^2)$ but employing Fast Fourier Transforms can reduce the time complexity to $O(N \log N)$.

Discrete Wavelet Transform (DWT)

DWT partitions a given signal into two portions, a low-frequency one and a higher-frequency one. Then, a low pass filter and a high pass filter are applied to these signals. This process is repeated in a number of iterations on each level (Mahajan, 2014) until a desired level of division is reached (Razak, 2018). The outputs from these filters are then included in the image (Inverse Discrete Wavelet transform), in other words, we can also say that the reconstruction of the image is known as IDWT. DWT can be used in image watermarking as well as compression and processing. DWT splits the image into three directions viz. Diagonal, horizontal and vertical. While DWT can not represent an image productively, it can still provide a multilevel time-frequency localization. DWT splits the image into four different parts/ wavelets i.e LL (Approximate), LH(vertical), HH (diagonal), HL (Horizontal).The LL or approximation is the one that is most visible to the human sense while the different three are the high-frequency ones that aren't largely perceptible to the human sense.

The letter L means low pass filter while the letter H means high pass filter (Mokhnache, S., 2018). Some commonly used filters are Daubechies Orthogonal filter, Haar Wavelet filter, and Daubechies bi- orthogonal Filter. First DWT is applied to tuples(rows) and after that all the attributes(columns) (Chaitanya, 2014). Changes made in LL, therefore, are more visible while the changes made in HH, HL, LH are less visible. The quality of the image produced by DWT is higher compared to other options available on an average. Due to all these advantages, it makes DWT almost perfect to find the right spot for embedding a watermark. In most of the cases, the watermark is inserted between HL and LH bands so a balance between robustness and accuracy (better hiding) is achieved. This problem of choosing the right balance between robustness and transparency can be categorized as an optimization problem and we can reach an optimal solution by the help of a genetic algorithm (Sood, 2014). A possible advantage for choosing DWT over DFT can be the fact that it could capture both the frequency and location information. DWT is better for signals that vary with time as the wavelets have their energy concentrated in time. In other words, DWT is better for signals that aren't stationary.

Singular Value Decomposition (SVD)

SVD employs linear algebra for watermarking (Gosavi, C. S., 2017). For a given picture x of size m*n, where m>=n. SVD can be defined by the equation:

$$X : \sum U_i * S_i * V_i \tag{2}$$

U: m*m orthogonal matrix
V: n*n transpose of orthogonal matrix
S_{ii}: Positive real number and X's singular value(Diagonal matrix)

Here U comprise of eigenvector AA^t termed as left singular vector while V comprises orthogonal vectors A^TA termed as the right singular vector.

Known properties of SVD are as:

1) SVD is decently stable.
2) SVD can also process matrices where m is not equal to n.
3) Svd can be used to represent image properties.
4) SVD is prone to little truncate error.

Combining SVD with DWT can have more efficiency compared to traditional DWT (Takore, 2016). SVD is a robust technique for image watermarking, which can be backed by the following facts:

1) Singular values are immune to any kind of disturbances in the image.
2) SVD has the capability to retaining booths one way as well as a non-symmetrical value which is impossible for DFT or DCT
3) By using SVD in the equation, one may additionally reflect the inherent algebraic qualities of any picture.
4) Regardless of the matrix being square or not (that is the comparison between m and n), SVD can be successfully applied on the image.

The visual details of the photo as far as human perceptibility goes can't be affected by SVD (Singh, 2013). One may also say that SVD converts images from a collection of related data/coefficients to a collection of unrelated coefficients/data.

While Svd is immune to a variety of different attacks, it is still not immune to attacks which may include rotation of images by ninety degrees in multiple iterations (Ali, 2016). This can be avoided by redistributing the various pixels and performing normalization in several iterations. In SVD, each singular value relates to a corresponding luminance value of the image while their corresponding singular vectors represent the geometric data on the image layer (Ahmed, 2018). When small values of the image are changed/ transformed due to various attacks, as a consequence large values for SVD will change. Hence SVD can be helpful in detecting even minute alterations in the original image. The basic concept behind the Singular value decomposition is that we can convert an image with a higher number of dimensions to an image of a smaller number of dimensions which in turn will be easier to understand to modify while also being able to detect any kind of changes more easily.

Least Significant bit Algorithm

LSB is the simple and the easiest to understand algorithm as far as the spatial domain is considered (Kavitha, 2012). The basic concept behind the least significant bit method is that not all the activity is going in all the regions in an image. Hence some parts of the image have most of the activity, that is they are mostly perceived by the human vision but there are not so busy parts in which any changes made won't be noticed. Such parts are known as least significant parts or least significant bits. Let's have a look at a typical grayscale image where each pixel is represented by one byte. Here the last two bits for any value will be the least significant bits, depending on the pixel and the watermark bit that has to be inserted the change made to the single-pixel will be so small that it won't be perceptible. Moreover, as the normal image will possibly have a large number of pixels, slight changes to a few original pixels will not alter the way humans perceive the image.

A watermark can be merged into an image using the least significant bit method as follows:

1) Convert the original image that will act as a host for the watermark from coloured to black and white i.e from RGB to grayscale.
2) Increase the precision of the image to double.
3) For the watermark image, shift it's most significant bits to the right.
4) The host image set the least significant bits to zero.
5) Add the results of step 3 and step 4.

While this method boasts losslessness it is also immune to spatial attacks to a large extent but it can still be affected by the signal processing attacks.

Spread Spectrum

Spread spectrum can be on the parts of the image which are perceivable to the human eye despite the potential risk of altering the original image to a larger than expected/needed extent (Pickholtz, 1982) Basically, spread spectrum spreads the overall watermark over the bandwidth of the host image. Spread spectrum is able to resist any kind of interference. Spread spectrum being highly sensitive to any kind of noise in the image might be one of its main disadvantages. Another disadvantage can be that spread spectrum ends up taking more bandwidth than required.

The following are some of the key benefits of employing spread spectrum technology:

1) Spread spectrum has high performance
2) Spread spectrum offers a moderate data rate
3) Spread spectrum is a highly robust method of robustness

Patchwork Method

In patchwork methods, we split the host image into two subsets and then apply opposite operations to each subset. In order to find if the image is watermarked or not, we take the variance between the two created subsets. If the variance is non-zero then the image is watermarked, otherwise, the image is not watermarked (Brown, 1993). A combination of DCT and patchwork can be implemented to make the watermarking process more robust. We take the image taken from the DCT domain and then the patchwork method is applied over it. Applying this method makes the final result more resistant to various filtering attacks and other signal based attacks like down-sampling, equalization etc. This technique was developed by a research group (Cho, 2006). In other words, we can also put the watermark into a statistic applied to the host picture using a Gaussian distribution. The two subsets are then transformed by lightning one and darkening the other. One drawback of the patchwork method is its inability to hide huge amounts of data.

PERFORMANCE METRICS FOR WATERMARKING TECHNIQUES

No matter what algorithm we apply for watermarking our image, we are concerned with the quality of the result or in other words, how effective a technique is. This efficiency can be measured by the help of different metrics so of which are as:

Mean Square Error (MSE)

The performance of an image can be computed by calculating the average value of the square of errors between the original picture and the end result (Kumar, 2022).

$$MSE = 1 / M*N \Sigma_i^M \Sigma_i^N (W_{ij} - H_{ij})^2$$

Here,

M, N: Pixel values from the host picture

W_{ij}: Pixel values extracted from the host picture
H_{ij}: Pixel values extracted from the host picture

Peak Signal to Noise Ratio (PSNR)

PSNR checks the performance of the technique by taking into account the value of noise in the final result. The PSNR value and visual quality are inversely correlated (Singh, 2023). PSNR may also be defined as the magnitude of the ratio of maximul likely power of the picture and noise that's altering that image. It's basically being used to calculate the imperceptibility. PSNR can be expressed using the given formula:

$$PSNR = 10 * \log_{10}(P^2/MSE)$$

Where p= maximum value in the host image.

Signal to Noise Ratio (SNR)

SNR is employed to calculate the level of sensitivity in any given image is (Singh, 2023). It can be represented by the given equation:

$$SNR = 10 * \log_{10}(P_{signal}/P_{noise})$$

Bit Error Rate (BER)

The ratio of error-prone bits to total bits is known as the bit error rate.

BER can be represented by the given equation:

BER = Error prone Bits / Actual number of Bits

Normalized Correlation

The peak value of NC is1 i.e for NC=1, the given two images are equal otherwise the given two images are not equal. It is employed to fetch the degree to which the watermark in the target image and the original, undisturbed watermark resemble each other (Pant, 2021). In the same way it can be used with the host picture and the final result. It can be represented by the given equation.

$$NC = \Sigma_i \Sigma_j [I(a,b) - Iw(a,b)]$$

$$\Sigma_i \Sigma_j [I(a,b)+Iw(a,b)]$$

LITERATURE SURVEY OF ALL THE STANDARD WATERMARKING TECHNIQUES

Table 1 shows the literature study of standard watermarking techniques.

Table 1. Tabular survey of all the popular watermarking techniques

Technique	Methodology	Advantages	Limitations
DCT (Discrete Cosine Transform)	Splitting the image into m*m blocks, and applying DCT to every single individual block that divides the image different sub-parts depending upon frequencies and discarding the less important ones.	1) Can reduce the blocks or jaggies that can appear when the sub-image boundaries are perceived 2)The most amount of information can be fit into the smallest number of frequency coefficient 3)It can be used with a single integrated circuit	1) Higher complexity compared to the other techniques 2)Easier to remove with the help of various spatial attacks.
DFT (Discrete Fourier Transform)	Converting continuous functions into frequency components	1)Almost immune to spatial attacks as the image becomes too distorted 2)shows invariance in translation	1) Higher complexity compared to other techniques
DWT (Discrete Wavelet Transform)	Splitting the image into lower and higher frequency parts and then inserting the watermark into them depending upon the requirement, This process is continious recursively till the want level is given .	It is better for signals that vary with time	1)It isn't good for stationary signals 2)It is slower than DCT
SVD (Singular Value decomposition)	For a given picture x of size m*n, with m>=n. SVD can be defined by the equation: $X = \Sigma U_i * S_i * V_i$ U: m*m orthogonal matrix V: n*n transpose of orthogonal matrix S_{ii}: Non negative real number and X's singular value(Diagonal matrix).	1)SVD can be said to be quite stable. 2)SVD can also process matrices where m is not equal to n. 3)SVD can be used to represent image properties.	1)Takes a lot of time for 3d volumes 2)Not flexible enough to include geometric penalty function
Least Significant Bit Algorithm	Inserting pixel bits from the watermark (By shifting important data to least significant bits) in the least significant bits of the pixels present in the host picture.	1)Slight changes to a few original pixels will not affect the way humans perceive any given image 2) It is also immune to spatial attacks to a large extent	1) It can still be affected by the signal processing attacks
Spread Spectrum	Spread spectrum spreads the overall watermark over the bandwidth of the host image	1)Spread spectrum has high performance 2)Spread spectrum offers a moderate data rate 3)Spread spectrum is a highly robust method of robustness.	1)Spread spectrum is highly sensitive to any kind of noise in the image. 2)Spread spectrum ends up taking more bandwidth than required
Approaches based on correlation	When using correlation-based watermarking methods, we determine how closely the final product resembles the pseudorandom code that must be verified in order to establish the watermark's presence.	1) Watermarks are clearly detectable.	1) A certain image may result in mistakes while identifying watermarks. 2) The properties of the host picture will determine how accurate this approach.
Patchwork method	We split the host image into two subsets and then apply opposite operations to each subset.	1)This method makes the final result more resistant to various filtering attacks and other signal based attacks like down-sampling, equalization etc.	1) One drawback of the patchwork method is the inability to hide vast amounts of data.

WATERMARKING TECHNIQUES WITH MEDICAL DATA

Medical data can be watermarked using a DICOM image security approach that uses the reversible watermarking technique (Kumar, 2020). In this method, the RS vector is first identified and a hash value based on the image's MD5 checksum is retrieved. Next, the R-S vector is compressed using Huffman's algorithm to get the watermark value. This approach has a BER of zero, an SNR of 53 dB, an MSE of 0.12, and a standard deviation of 0.02. As a consequence, we may infer that the host picture is not significantly impacted by the injected watermark.

This technique makes use of a key that is only known to the creator for choosing the coefficients hence no one besides the owner can modify or remove the watermark from the original image. A dynamic block-based watermark algorithm (Wolfgang, 1999) has also been developed to watermark medical data. The algorithm examines the properties of the coefficients after decomposing the wavelet. While the watermark is being added to the original host image, mean and variance are taken into consideration to dynamically alter the intensity at which the watermark is being added. This creates a range where the watermark may be effectively extracted. The intensity of the inserting is discovered to be inversely proportional to the image quality, as determined by the PSNR value. This watermark can then be inserted into the original host picture by using linear interpolation. The extraction process for the approach can also detect any kind of alterations. Table 2 shows a literature survey of recent watermarking techniques proposed.

Table 2. Literature survey of recent watermarking techniques proposed.

Authors	Objective	Methodology	Advantages	Limitations
Mohamed M. Abd-Eldayem. (Abd-Eldayem, 2013)	Suggested security method for digital communications and images in medicine that uses watermarking and encryption	First, the image's R-S vector is retrieved using an MD5 checksum-based hash value. The R-S vector is then compressed using Huffman's algorithm, which is then combined with the hash value and the patient credentials to produce a watermark value that can be injected using the AES encryption method.	This method has a BER of 0, SNR of 53 dB, MSE of 0, standard deviation of 0, and a BER of 0. The encoded watermark does not significantly alter the original image, we may infer from this. Because of the high PSNR value (57 dB), the watermark is almost impossible to detect.	It is not robust against the modification attacks but can detect the modifications
Lu-Ting Ko, Jwu-E. Chen, Yaw-Shih Shieh, Hsi-Chin Hsin, and Tze-Yun Sung (Ko, L. T., 2012)	Nested Quantization Index Modulation for Reversible Watermarking and Its Application to Healthcare Information Management Systems	The nested structure of the embedded watermark allows this technique to increase its capacity.	It also has the ability to precisely recreate the original image, making it ideal for watermarking medical data.	More complex compared the normal QIM
Abhilasha Sharma, Amit Kumar Singh, and S.P. Ghrera. (Sharma, A., 2015)	"Medical Image Watermarking Method that is Secure and Robust"	In this strategy, the EPR data is placed in the ROI zone while the somewhat less sensitive data, such as the logo, is placed in the NROI region.	1)It boasts robustness while facing signal processing attacks 2)It has high imperceptibility	Encypted algorithms like RSA that are used have high time complexity
Kuo-Kun Tseng, Xialong He, Woon-Man Kung, Shuo-Tsung Chen, Minghong Liao, and Huang-Nan Huang. (Tseng, K. K., 2014)	Wavelet-Based Watermarking and Compression for ECG Signals with Verification Evaluation	The watermark in the ECG data can be embedded into the low-frequency coefficients	This method has better robustness as well as SNR value	DWT used has high complexity and is slower than DCT
Aleš Roček, Karel Slavíček, Otto Dostál, and Michal Javorník (Roček, A., 2016)	Fully reversible watermarking in medical images using novel visibility parameters	Medical data may also be watermarked using a hybrid of zero and reversible watermarking.	This approach yields an average PSNR value of between 81 and 105.	10% of image still gets distorted in the RONI

Continued on following page

Table 2. Continued

Authors	Objective	Methodology	Advantages	Limitations
R. Eswaraiah, and E. Sreenivasa Reddy (Eswaraiah, R., 2014)	Medical Image Watermarking Technique for Exact ROI Recovery and Accurate Tamper Detection	Additionally, a block-based fragile watermarking method that can assist in both the recovery of the original picture and the identification of image manipulation has been presented.	This technique allows us to locate the changed blocks in the ROI and restore them to their initial states.	This method is efficient only when the border if the final image are unmodified from the intruders
Lu-Ting Ko, Jwu-E Chen, Yaw-Shih Shieh, Massimo Scalia, and Tze-Yun Sung (Ko, L. T., 2012)	A New Reversible Watermarking Method Based on Fractional Discrete Cosine Transform for Healthcare Information Management Systems	An algorithm that may be used to improve the transparency of the finished image is FDCT-based reversible watermarking.	It has the capability to fully recover the original image	DCT used inside has higher complexity compared to the normal techniques for watermarking
Anthony T. S. Ho, Xunzhan Zhu, and Yong Liang Guan. (Ho, A. T., 2004)	Using the Pinned Sine Transform, image content authentication	Pinned sine transform PST can be used to selectively authenticate the content of the digital images	1) This technique may be used to find even the tiniest changes in a picture's texture. 2) This technique is shown to be quite resilient while having a 98% detection rate for the alterations.	With more compression, there is a lower chance of detecting tampering.
Shrinivas Khandare, and Urmila Shrawankar. (Khandare, S., 2016)	Watermarking in the Image Bit Depth Plane for Secure Transmission of Classified Images	*IBDPDI* watermarking is another technique that can be helpful in increasing data security	As long as the image is on the internet, this technique can keep the image's authenticity.	The value of correlation between the original watermark before to insertion and recovered watermark is taken into consideration when the watermark quality degrades.
N. Aherrahrou, and H. Tairi. (Aherrahrou, 2015)	PDE-based method for watermarking multimodal medical images	Watermarking RONI with a DWT-SVD hybrid transform while watermarking ROI in the spatial domain	1)Increase in robustness against attacks 2)Authenticity of the product is increased	The quality of ROI pictures alongside RONI pictures has to be increased.
K. Kuppusamy, and K. Thamodaran (Kuppusamy, 2012)	Optimized Image Watermarking Scheme Based On PSO	A combination of Daubechies and PSO based transformation can be employed on the original picture.Later we can make use of DCT on the watermark that is to be inserted in the original image.	This technique makes use of a key that is only known to the creator for choosing the coefficients hence no one besides the owner can modify or remove the watermark from the original image	Performing DCT on watermark increases the complexity of the Algorithm

Continued on following page

Table 2. Continued

Authors	Objective	Methodology	Advantages	Limitations
Guoyan Liu, Hongjun Liu, and Abdurahman Kadir. (Guoyan Liu, 2012)	Watermarking a Color Pathological Image Using Wavelets by Dynamically Modulating Embedding Intensity	After the decomposition of the wavelet, the algorithm analyzes the characteristics of the coefficients. While the watermark is being inserted into the original image, we take into account mean as well as the variance to dynamically adjust the intensity at which we are inserting the watermark	1)There is an effective range to extract the watermark as well 2)Additionally, it has been discovered that this technique is resistant to spatial data changes.	According to the PSNR value, the intensity of the signal is discovered to be inversely related to the quality of the picture.
Lamri Laouamer, Muath Alshaikh, Laurent Nana, and Anca Chrisitine Pascu (Laouamer, 2015)	Tamper detection using a strong watermarking system and a threshold versus intensity approach	The produced watermark to be inserted can be informed of its construction location using an approach based on the Weber Excitation Deferential descriptor.. This watermark can then be inserted in the original host picture while employing linear interpolation.	During the recovering this method can also detect any kind of alterations	Watermark is imperceptible, so it can be detected but won't prevent piracy in the first place
Chaiwoot Seetha, Suthida Goollawattanaporn, and Chularat Tanprasert. (Seetha, 2013)	Transparent Digital Watermark on Drug's Images	Applying a transparent digital watermark with alpha blending and alpha channels on drug pictures		It can't prevent piracy in the first place.
Dominik Heider, Martin Pyka, and Angelika Barnekow (Heider, 2009)	DNA watermarks in non-coding regulatory sequences	Using DNA watermarks to detect illegal use of genetically modified organisms		Can't recommend integrating watermark alongside the regulatory regions
Atheer Bassel Al-Naqeeb and Md Jan Nordin, (Naqeeb, 2017)	Robustness Watermarking Authentication Using Hybridisation DWT-DCTand DWT-SVD,	Using a hybrid DWT-DCT and DWt-SVD technique		Correlation value of degradation attack high degradation although not due to algorithm itself
Sharbani Bhattacharya (Bhattacharya, 2014)	Utilizing the Neighborhood Set and the Fuzzy Matrix Rule, you can watermark digital images.	Using a neighbourhood set of fuzzy matrices to insert the watermark.	It reduces the chances of the watermark getting detected or tampered	In some case the PSNR value is 0

In most of the watermarking techniques, It is difficult to strike a balance between imperceptibility and resilience. That is, either the technique is effective at detecting changes or it is effective at discouraging tampering by drastically distorting the image when tampered with. Many methods rely on time-consuming encryption and decryption algorithms such as RSA and MD5 checksums. It becomes difficult to manage #d photos while keeping security and compression in mind. Some techniques make use of hybrid technologies.

RESEARCH GAP

There is still a need for a technique that can demote alteration as well as detect alteration. Higher the quality of the images and results, higher is the complexity of the techniques. There is a need for a technique which can achieve the goal at low complexity. There is always some kind of distortion with the watermarking and if there is no distortion then it can be altered too easily. Using encryption or key to recover the original image back easily also increases the over complexity Most techniques lose their efficiency as the compression is increased.

CONCLUSION

A great deal of private information is at risk with medical imaging. With the increase of access to the internet, Stealing private patient information or medical photographs has gotten a lot simpler as well. In this study, we cover numerous methods that can be used to watermark medical photos as well as different performance indicators that we can use to evaluate the effectiveness of the method that we have used. We also then take into consideration various recent techniques that have been used to incorporate watermarks in the medical images and their advantages as well as disadvantages in a tabular format. We have also mentioned various research gaps that still need to be met to make watermarking more efficient and robust in the medical field. Researchers who want to accomplish their study objectives can use this poll to assist them choose the best technological combinations to use.

REFERENCES

Abd-Eldayem, M. M. (2013). A proposed security technique based on watermarking and encryption for digital imaging and communications in medicine. *Egyptian Informatics Journal*, *14*(1), 1–13. doi:10.1016/j.eij.2012.11.002

Aherrahrou, N., & Tairi, H. (2015). PDE based scheme for multi-modal medical image watermarking. *Biomedical Engineering Online*, *14*(1), 1–19. doi:10.118612938-015-0101-x PMID:26608730

Ahmed, R., Riaz, M. M., & Ghafoor, A. (2018). Attack resistant watermarking technique based on fast curvelet transform and Robust Principal Component Analysis. *Multimedia Tools and Applications*, *77*(8), 9443–9453. doi:10.100711042-017-5128-5

Al-Naqeeb, A. B., & Nordin, M. J. (2017). Robustness Watermarking Authentication Using Hybridisation DWT-DCTand DWT-SVD. *Pertanika Science & Technology, 25*(0128-7680*)*, 73-86.

Ali, M., Ahn, C. W., & Pant, M. (2016). Intelligent Watermarking Scheme Employing the Concepts of Block Based Singular Value Decomposition and Firefly Algorithm. *GCSR*, *5*, 37–57.

Begum, M., & Uddin, M. S. (2020). Digital image watermarking techniques: A review. *Information (Basel)*, *11*(2), 110. doi:10.3390/info11020110

Bhattacharya, S. (2014). *Watermarking Digital Images Using Fuzzy Matrix Rules and Neighborhood Set. International Journal of Advanced Computing, Recent Science Publications*. ISSN.

Britanak, V., & Rao, K. R. (2001). An efficient implementation of the forward and inverse MDCT in MPEG audio coding. *IEEE Signal Processing Letters*, *8*(2), 48–51. doi:10.1109/97.895372

Brown, C. A., Charles, P. D., Johnsen, W. A., & Chesters, S. (1993). Fractal analysis of topographic data by the patchwork method. *Wear*, *161*(1-2), 61–67. doi:10.1016/0043-1648(93)90453-S

Chaitanya, K., Reddy, S., & Rao, G. (2014). Digital Color Image Watermarking In RGB Planes Using DWT-DCT-SVD Coefficients. *International Journal of Computer Science and Information Technologies*, *5*(2), 2413–2417.

Cho, J. W., Chung, H. Y., & Jung, H. Y. (2006, September). A robust blind audio watermarking using distribution of sub-band signals. In *International Workshop on Multimedia Content Representation, Classification and Security* (pp. 106-113). Springer. 10.1007/11848035_16

Eswaraiah, R., & Sreenivasa Reddy, E. (2014). Medical image watermarking technique for accurate tamper detection in ROI and exact recovery of ROI. *International Journal of Telemedicine and Applications*, *2014*, 2014. doi:10.1155/2014/984646 PMID:25328515

Gahalod, L., & Gupta, S. K. (2018). A Review on Digital Image Watermarking using 3-Level Discrete Wavelet Transform. *IJSRSET, 4099 Themed Section. Engineering and Technology*, *4*(1), 2395–1990.

Gosavi, C. S., & Mali, S. N. (2017). Watermarking for Video using single channel block based schur decomposition. *Global Journal of Pure and Applied Mathematics*, *12*(2), 1575–1585.

Heider, D., Pyka, M., & Barnekow, A. (2009). DNA watermarks in non-coding regulatory sequences. *BMC Research Notes*, *2*(1), 1–6. doi:10.1186/1756-0500-2-125 PMID:19583865

Hernandez, J. R., Amado, M., & Perez-Gonzalez, F. (2000). DCT-domain watermarking techniques for still images: Detector performance analysis and a new structure. *IEEE Transactions on Image Processing*, *9*(1), 55–68. doi:10.1109/83.817598 PMID:18255372

Ho, A. T., Zhu, X., & Guan, Y. L. (2004). Image content authentication using pinned sine transform. *EURASIP Journal on Advances in Signal Processing*, *2004*(14), 1–11. doi:10.1155/S111086570440506X

Hsieh, C. T., & Sou, P. Y. (2002, July). Blind cepstrum domain audio watermarking based on time energy features. In *2002 14th International Conference on Digital Signal Processing Proceedings. DSP 2002 (Cat. No. 02TH8628)* (*Vol. 2,* pp. 705-708). IEEE.

Imaduddin, M. D., & Pullarao, G. (2014). Real Time Simulation Based on Image Protection Using Digital Watermarking Techniques. *International Journal of New Trends in Electronics and Communication (Vol. 2).*

Kamble, M. V. A Review of Different Techniques on Digital Image Watermarking Scheme. *International Journal of Innovative Science, Engineering & Technology, 3*(2).

Kavitha, K. K., Koshti, A., & Dunghav, P. (2012). Steganography using least significant bit algorithm. *International Journal of Engineering Research and Applications (IJERA).*

Khandare, S., & Shrawankar, U. (2016). Image bit depth plane digital watermarking for secured classified image data transmission. *Procedia Computer Science*, *78*, 698–705. doi:10.1016/j.procs.2016.02.119

Ko, L. T., Chen, J. E., Shieh, Y. S., Hsin, H. C., & Sung, T. Y. (2012). Nested quantization index modulation for reversible watermarking and its application to healthcare information management systems. *Computational and Mathematical Methods in Medicine*, *2012*, 2012. doi:10.1155/2012/839161 PMID:22194776

Ko, L. T., Chen, J. E., Shieh, Y. S., & Sung, T. Y. (2012, June). A novel fractional discrete cosine transform based reversible watermarking for biomedical image applications. In *2012 International Symposium on Computer, Consumer and Control* (pp. 36-39). IEEE. 10.1109/IS3C.2012.19

Kumar, I., Bhatt, C., Vimal, V., & Qamar, S. (2022). Automated white corpuscles nucleus segmentation using deep neural network from microscopic blood smear. *Journal of Intelligent & Fuzzy Systems*, (Preprint), 1-14.

Kumar, L., & Singh, K. U. (2020). An analysis of different watermarking schemes for medical image authentication. *European Journal of Molecular & Clinical Medicine*, *7*(4), 2250–2259.

Kumar Jaiswal, R., & Ravi, S. (2018). Robust Imperceptible Digital Image Watermarking based on Discrete Wavelet & Cosine Transforms. *International Journal of Advanced Research in Computer Engineering & Technology (IJARCET), 7*(2).

Kuppusamy, K., & Thamodaran, K. (2012). Optimized image watermarking scheme based on PSO. *Procedia Engineering*, *38*, 493–503. doi:10.1016/j.proeng.2012.06.061

Laouamer, L., AlShaikh, M., Nana, L., & Pascu, A. C. (2015). Robust watermarking scheme and tamper detection based on threshold versus intensity. *Journal of Innovation in Digital Ecosystems*, *2*(1-2), 1–12. doi:10.1016/j.jides.2015.10.001

Liu, G., Liu, H., & Kadir, A. (2012). Wavelet-based color pathological image watermark through dynamically adjusting the embedding intensity. *Computational and Mathematical Methods in Medicine*, *2012*, 2012. doi:10.1155/2012/406349 PMID:23243463

Mahajan, P. H., & Bhalerao, P. B. (2014). A Review of Digital Watermarking Strategies. *International Journal of Advanced Research in Computer Science And Management Studies, 7*.

Mehta, B., & Rani, S. (2014). Segmentation of broken characters of handwritten Gurmukhi script. *International Journal of Engineering Science*, *3*, 95–105.

Miyazaki, A. (2005). An improved correlation-based watermarking method for images using a nonlinear programming algorithm. NSIP 2005. Abstracts. IEEE-Nonlinear Signal and Image Processing. IEEE.

Miyazaki, A. (2005, May). An improved correlation-based watermarking method for images using a nonlinear programming algorithm. In NSIP 2005. Abstracts. IEEE-Eurasip Nonlinear Signal and Image Processing, 2005. (p. 5). IEEE. doi:10.1109/NSIP.2005.1502212

Mokhnache, S., Bekkouche, T., & Chikouche, D. (2018). A Robust Watermarking Scheme Based on DWT and DCT Using Image Gradient. *International Journal of Applied Engineering Research*, *13*(4). Research India Publications.

Pandya, J. B., & Gupta, R. V. (2018). A Study of ROI based Image Watermarking Techniques. *International Journal of Scientific Research in Computer Science. Engineering and Information Technology*, *3*(1), 1213–1217.

Pant, B., Bordoloi, D., & Gangodkar, D. (2021). A neural network classifier for payload-based online worms detection. *Webology*, *18*(5), 3235–3240.

Pickholtz, R., Schilling, D., & Milstein, L. (1982). Theory of spread-spectrum communications-a tutorial. *IEEE Transactions on Communications*, *30*(5), 855–884. doi:10.1109/TCOM.1982.1095533

Priyanka, B., Krishna, D. P., & Purushottam, E. (2014). Attestation Performance on Digital Watermarking. [IJCSNS]. *International Journal of Computer Science and Network Security*, *14*(1), 94.

Rader, C., & Brenner, N. (1976). A new principle for fast Fourier transformation. *IEEE Transactions on Acoustics, Speech, and Signal Processing*, *24*(3), 264–266. doi:10.1109/TASSP.1976.1162805

Rahman, F., & Mandaogade, N. N. (2014). Digital audio watermarking techniques with musical audio feature classification. *Int. J. Curr. Eng. Technol*, *4*(5).

Rashid, A. (2016). Digital watermarking applications and techniques: A brief review. *International Journal of Computer Applications Technology and Research*, *5*(3), 147–150. doi:10.7753/IJCATR0503.1006

Razak, N. A. (2018). Digital Image watermarking base on DWT and SVD techniques. [JNCET]. *J Netw Commun Emerging Technol*, *8*(02).

Riaz, S., & Lee, S. W. (2013, January). Image authentication and restoration by multiple watermarking techniques with advance encryption standard in digital photography. In *2013 15th International Conference on Advanced Communications Technology (ICACT)* (pp. 24-28). IEEE.

Robert, L., & Shanmugapriya, T. (2009). A study on digital watermarking techniques. *International journal of Recent trends in Engineering, 1*(2), 223.

Roček, A., Slavíček, K., Dostál, O., & Javorník, M. (2016). A new approach to fully-reversible watermarking in medical imaging with breakthrough visibility parameters. *Biomedical Signal Processing and Control*, *29*, 44–52. doi:10.1016/j.bspc.2016.05.005

Seetha, C., Goollawattanaporn, S., & Tanprasert, C. (2013). Transparent digital watermark on Drug's images. *Procedia Computer Science*, *21*, 302–309. doi:10.1016/j.procs.2013.09.040

Sharma, A., Singh, A. K., & Ghrera, S. P. (2015). Secure hybrid robust watermarking technique for medical images. *Procedia Computer Science*, *70*, 778–784. doi:10.1016/j.procs.2015.10.117

Singh, A. K., Kumar, B., Singh, G., & Mohan, A. (2017). BMedical image watermarking: techniques and applications. *Book series on Multimedia Systems and Applications*.

Singh, D. P., Bordoloi, D., & Shukla, S. (2021). Utilizing Steganography and Cryptography to Conceal Information Within BMP Images. *Webology*, *18*(5), 3005–3009.

Singh, Y. S., Devi, B. P., & Singh, K. M. (2013). A review of different techniques on digital image watermarking scheme. *International Journal of Engine Research*, *2*(3), 194–200.

Sinha, M. K., Rai, R., & Kumar, G. (2014). Literature survey on digital watermarking. *International Journal of Computer Science and Information Technologies*, *5*(5), 6538–6542.

Solanki, A. C., & Bakaraniya, P. V. (2018). Different video watermarking techniques-a review. *International Journal of Scientific Research in Computer Science. Engineering and Information Technology*, *3*(1), 1890–1894.

Sood, S. (2014). Digital Watermarking Using Hybridization of Optimization Techniques: A Review. *International Journal of Computer Science and Information Technologies*, *5*(4), 5249–5251.

Takore, T. T., Kumar, P. R., & Devi, G. L. (2016, March). A modified blind image watermarking scheme based on DWT, DCT and SVD domain using GA to optimize robustness. In 2016 international conference on electrical, electronics, and optimization techniques (ICEEOT) (pp. 2725-2729). IEEE.

Tseng, K. K., He, X., Kung, W. M., Chen, S. T., Liao, M., & Huang, H. N. (2014). Wavelet-based watermarking and compression for ECG signals with verification evaluation. *Sensors (Basel)*, *14*(2), 3721–3736. doi:10.3390140203721 PMID:24566636

Wolfgang, R. B., Podilchuk, C. I., & Delp, E. J. (1999). Perceptual watermarks for digital images and video. *Proceedings of the IEEE*, *87*(7), 1108–1126. doi:10.1109/5.771067

Wu, C. F., & Hsieh, W. S. (2000). Digital watermarking using zerotree of DCT. *IEEE Transactions on Consumer Electronics*, *46*(1), 87–94. doi:10.1109/30.826385

Yadav, V., & Verma, N. (2016). Secure Multimedia Data using Digital Watermarking: A Review. *International Journal of Engineering Research and General Science*, *4*(1), 181–187.

Żurawski, C., & Skłodowski, P. (2013). Standard Deviation-Based Image Fidelity Measure for Digital Watermarking. In XIV International Conference-System Modelling and Control. Łódź.

Chapter 10
Application of Deep Learning Techniques for Pneumonia Detection Using Chest X-Ray Images

Deepak Vishwakarma
DIT University, India

Hritik Bhandari
DIT University, India

Nikhil Agrawal
DIT University, India

Kriti
DIT University, India

Jyoti Rawat
DIT University, India

ABSTRACT

Pneumonia is one of the major diseases affecting the large proportion of the population. The detection of pneumonia can be done by an X-ray scan of the patient which is observed by a radiologist to look for abnormalities indicative of pneumonia. This observation is highly subjective and depends on the experience of the radiologist, leading to ambiguity in appropriate diagnosis, and thus producing some false negatives. To overcome these issues, it is imperative that radiologists be provided with a tool that acts as second set of eyes for them and helps them gain confidence in their diagnosis. Keeping in view the aforementioned objectives, many researchers have proposed various computer-assisted classification (CAC) systems based on machine learning and deep learning methods. The present work compared the performance of MobileNetv2, VGG16, and XceptionNet for classifying chest X-ray images into normal and pneumonia classes, reporting the highest accuracy of 96.0% using VGG16.

DOI: 10.4018/978-1-6684-6957-6.ch010

INTRODUCTION

Pneumonia is a dangerous disease that affects our body in a severe manner. It is a harmful illness in which the air sacs present in the lungs are filled with different liquids which causes difficulty in breathing (Chu et al., 2020). These microbes causing pneumonia to go into the lungs and then to alveoli. Alveoli functions like an exchange-point where there is continuous exchange of blood and air from the outside world. When pathogens enter the lungs, the immune system start releasing white blood cells (WBCs) for alveoli to help and as these WBC cells fight the pathogens, it leads to inflammation. As the level of carbon-di-oxide keeps on rising the body breathes more quickly to clear out and get more oxygen in. Thus, common symptoms of pneumonia include heavy breathing. Pneumonia is found predominantly in young adults, with a high mortality rate of 5% of inpatients (Mayo Clinic, 2022). The germs that cause pneumonia in children and adults are the same, and many respiratory viruses are successfully transmitted from one generation to another between families. In growing countries, in which diagnosis and treatment are behind schedule because of a scarcity of experienced radiologists, pediatric pneumonia is related to alarming mortality charges. The large gap between the quantity of physicians and the population of a specific vicinity also hinders well timed diagnosis. 800,000 children who are less than 5 every year old are killed or affected by pneumonia in their life. This includes over 153,000 newborns (WHO, 2021). Timely diagnosis and appropriate treatment of the disease leads to increased survival rates. Different methods are available for lung imaging to diagnose pneumonia in patients; however, chest X-rays (CXRs) are widely used. The study of the X-ray scan for accurate diagnosis may be a difficult problem even for knowledgeable radiologists due to the presence of noise and artifacts (Sousa et al., 2018). Therefore, to overcome these challenges and assist radiologists in their diagnosis, researchers have used a variety of computer-assisted classification (CAC) systems to identify chest X-ray images into various stages of common pneumonia. We are able to distinguish normal and pneumonia cases of patients by observing the opacities present in the chest X-ray. In pneumonia cases we get the darker elements near the spine which shows the presence of the disease (UNICEF, 2021). Sample chest X-ray images indicating healthy lungs and lungs affected by viral and bacterial pneumonia are shown in Figure. 1.

Figure 1. Sample chest X-ray images indicating healthy lungs and lungs affected by viral and bacterial pneumonia

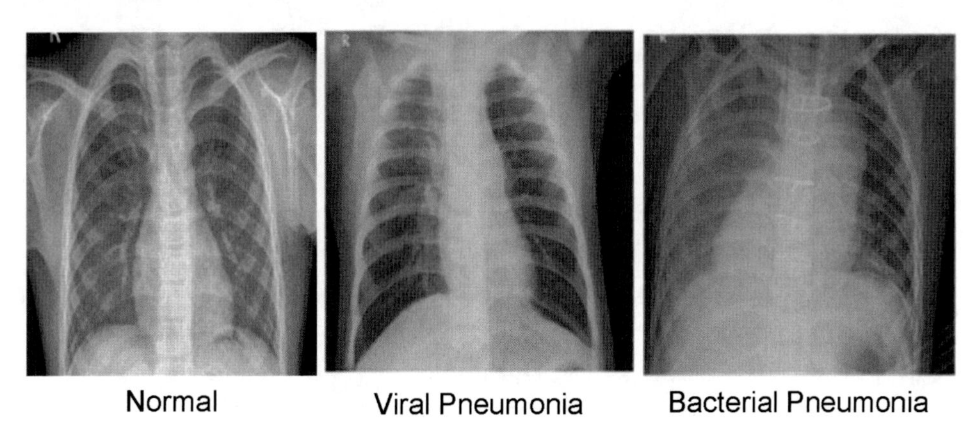

Normal   Viral Pneumonia   Bacterial Pneumonia

In Figure 1, normal chest X-rays indicate the blood vessels and the movement of the hemidiaphragm which shows the healthy and proper functioning of lungs. For viral pneumonia chest X-ray it is observed that virus affects both side of the lungs which causes to increase in cellular debris and mucus where previously open lung pockets were present. In the case of bacterial pneumonia chest X-ray we it is observed that a white condensed area or opacity is present on one side of lung. The reason for this is that bacteria attack on one side of the lung that causes inflammation which take over the cells that are filled with air.

RELATED WORK

Many researchers have attempted to build unique CAC systems for the identification of results. We have given a detailed study of the papers we studied in the field of pneumonia detection using deep learning in Table 1.

Table 1. Brief description of related studies carried out for detection of pneumonia using chest X-ray images

Author (Year)	Dataset Description	Methodology
Xianghong et al. (2018)	4513 (Bacterial/Viral)	Segmentation: AlexNet FCN Features: Deep features + Handcrafted features Classifier: SVM (Ac.: 80.4%)
Rajaraman et al. (2018)	5856 (Normal/Pneumonia)	Classifier: Customized VGG16 (Ac.: 96.2%)
Ayan et al. (2019)	5856 (Normal/Viral/ Bacterial pneumonia)	Classifier: VGG16 (Ac.: 87.0%)
Jain et al. (2019)	5840 (Normal/Pneumonia)	Classifier: VGG19 (Ac.: 88.7%)
Sousa et al. (2019)	3883 (Viral/ Bacterial pneumonia)	Classifier: Self-designed CNN (Ac.: 83.1%)
Varshni et al. (2019)	2862 (Normal/Pneumonia)	Features: Deep features using DenseNet169 Classifier: SVM (Ac.: 80.02%)
Stephen et al. (2019)	5856 (Normal/Pneumonia)	Classifier: Self-designed CNN (Ac.: 93.73%)
Chouhan et al. (2020)	5856 (Normal/Pneumonia)	Classifier: Ensemble model of DL networks (Ac.: 96.4%)
Togacar et al. (2020)	5849 (Normal/Pneumonia)	Features: Deep features from AlexNet, VGG16, VGG19 Feature selection: mRMR Classifier: LDA (Ac.: 99.41%)
Rahman et al. (2020)	5247 (Normal/Pneumonia)	Classifier: DenseNet201 (Ac.: 98.0%)
Irfan et al. (2020)	25596 (Normal/Pneumonia)	Classifier: DenseNet121 (Ac.: 71.0%)
	203 (Normal/Pneumonia)	Classifier: DenseNet121 (Ac.: 76.0%)
Sharma et al. (2020)	5863 (Normal/Pneumonia)	Classifier: Self-designed CNN (Ac.: 90.68%)
Yue et al. (2020)	5840 (Normal/Pneumonia)	Classifier: MobileNet (Ac.: 92.98%)
Al Mamlook et al. (2020)	5856 (Normal/Pneumonia)	Classifier: Self-designed CNN (Ac.: 98.46%)
Hashmi et al. (2020)	5836 (Normal/Pneumonia)	Classifier: DL models based weighted classifier (Ac.: 98.43%)
Liang et al. (2020)	5856 (Normal/Pneumonia)	Classifier: Self-designed CNN (Ac.: 90.5%)

Continued on following page

Table 1. Continued

Author (Year)	Dataset Description	Methodology
Ebiele et al. (2020)	17050 (Normal/Pneumonia)	Features: PCA Classifier: SVM (Ac.: 90.0%)
Habib et al. (2020)	5856 (Normal/Pneumonia)	Pre-processing: HE Classifier: CheXNet (Ac.: 92.6%)
		Pre-processing: HE Features: Deep features using ChexNet Feature selection: PCA Classifier: LR (Ac.: 96.1%)
Elshennawy et al. (2020)	5856 (Normal/Pneumonia)	Classifier: ResNet152v2 (Ac.: 99.2%)
Wu et al. (2020)	5863 (Normal/Pneumonia)	Pre-processing: Adaptive median filter Features: Deep features from self-designed CNN Classifier: RF (Ac.: 96.85%)
Ferreira et al. (2020)	5856 (Normal/Pneumonia)	Pre-processing: CLAHE Segmentation: U-Net Features: VGG16 based deep features Classifier: MLP (Ac.: 97.4%)
Dey et al. (2021)	7150 (Normal/Pneumonia)	Features: Deep features using VGG19 + handcrafted features Feature selection: PCA Classifier: RF (Ac.: 97.94%)
Chowdhary (2021)	5863 (Normal/Pneumonia)	Features: Deep features using VGG16 Classifier: SVM (Ac.: 96.61%)
Naveen et al. (2021)	5216 (Normal/Pneumonia)	Classifier: VGG16 (Ac.: 95.67%)
GM et al. (2021)	5863 (Normal/Pneumonia)	Classifier: Self-designed CNN (AUC: 0.9582)
Ieracitano et al. (2022)	121 (COVID-19 pneumonia/ non-COVID-19 pneumonia)	Pre-processing: Fuzzy enhancement Deep features: CovNNet Classifier: MLP (Ac.: 80.9%)
Ayan et al. (2022)	5856 (Normal/Pneumonia)	Classifier: Ensemble of deep learning models (ResNet50, MobileNet, XceptoinNet) (Ac.: 95.8%)
Mujahid et al. (2022)	7750 (Normal/Pneumonia)	Classifier: Ensemble of deep learning models (Ac.: 99.29%)
Alharbi et al. (2022)	800 (Normal/Pneumonia)	Classifier: Improved BoxENet (Ac.: 95.4%)

Continued on following page

Table 1. Continued

Author (Year)	Dataset Description	Methodology
Guail et al. (2022)	5856 (Normal/Pneumonia)	Deep features: PNA-GCN Classifier: MLP (Ac.: 97.7%)

Recent improvements in deep learning models and the availability of large datasets have made algorithms perform better in detecting pneumonia. As can be seen from the recent studies carried out for classification of chest X-ray images (2018-2022), most of the studies have been carried out using deep learning based techniques (Al Mamlook et al., 2020; Ayan & Unver, 2019; Chouhan et al., 2020; Elshennawy & Ibrahim, 2020; GM et al., 2021; Hashmi et al., 2020; Irfan et al., 2020; Jain et al., 2020; Liang & Zheng, 2020; Naveen & Diwan, 2021; Rahaman et al., 2020; Rajaraman et al., 2018; Sharma et al., 2020; Sousa et al., 2019; Stephen et al., 2019; Yue et al., 2020). It can also be observed that very few studies have made use of hybrid classification methods, wherein the features from the images have been computed using deep networks while classification has been done using conventional machine learning classifiers (Alharbi et al., 2022; Ayan et al., 2022; Chowdary 2021; Dey et al., 2021; Ebiele et al. 2020; Ferreira et al., 2020; Gu et al., 2018; Guail et al. 2022; Habib et al., 2020; Ieracitano et al., 2022; Mujahid et al., 2022; Togacar et al., 2020; Varshni et al., 2019; Wu et al., 2020). It has been observed that highest accuracy of 99.4% has been obtained by Togacar et al. (2020) using a combined deep feature set obtained from AlexNet, VGG16 and VGG19 networks. The obtained feature set was then subjected to minimal redundancy maximal relevance (mRMR) for selection of optimal features which were further fed to linear discriminant analysis (LDA) classifier. Habib et al. (2020) in their study compared the performance of deep learning method and hybrid classification method using images pre-processed by histogram equalization (HE) technique. In the deep learning technique pre-trained CheXNet network has been used for classification of normal and pneumonia chest X-ray images achieving an accuracy of 92.6%. In case of hybrid branch, the deep features computed from CheXNet were reduced using principal component analysis (PCA) and fed to logistic regression (LR) classifier achieving an accuracy of 96.1%.

As observed from Table 1, most of the studies have been carried out for classifying chest X-rays into normal and pneumonia classes therefore, in the present work performance of different deep learning models has been compared to classify chest X-rays into normal and pneumonia classes.

METHODOLOGY

The present work aims to propose a technique for classifying chest X-ray images into normal and pneumonia classes based on state-of-the-art deep learning networks. The workflow of the proposed methodology is shown in Figure. 2.

Figure 2. Workflow of the proposed methodology for classification of chest X-ray images

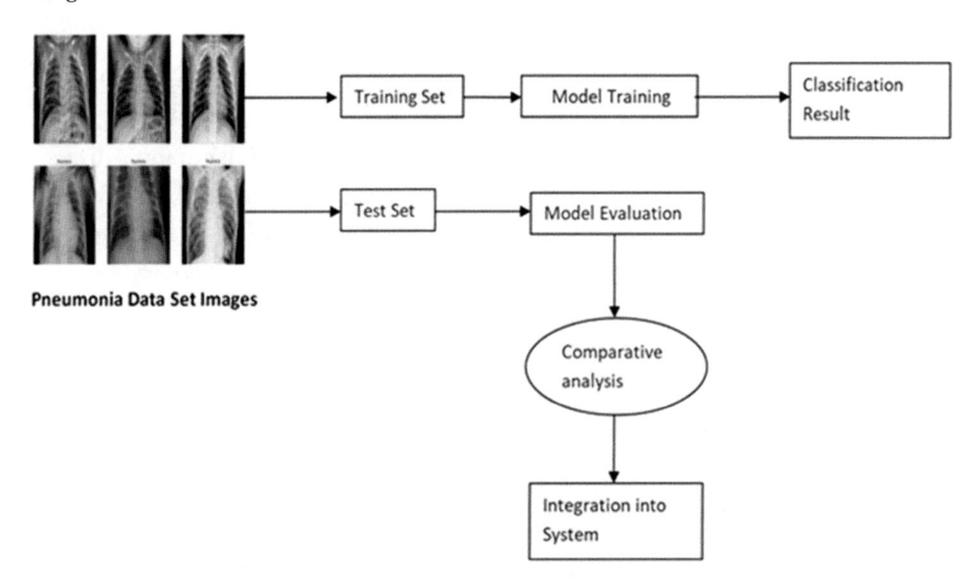

Dataset Description

The labelled dataset of chest X-rays has been taken from an online available source provided on the Kaggle website (Kermany et al., 2018) This dataset contains a total of 5856 chest X-rays images where 1583 chest X-ray images are of normal patients and 4273 files are of patients with pneumonia.

Data Pre-Processing

In the present work, different deep learning models have been trained which have many trainable parameters and need large amounts of data to train efficiently otherwise the problem of overfitting occurs. Basic pre-processing of data in order to avoid this problem is.

Data Compression and Resizing

In the present work, the data has been compressed to reduce irrelevance and redundancy of the images to store or transmit data in an efficient form. We need to understand that image resizing is one of the most important steps for preprocessing. The data has been resized to 512 × 512 pixels for our models to train faster in comparison to the data without resizing.

Data Balancing

Balancing training data is an important part of data preprocessing. Data imbalance can lead to potential risks in training a model. We have total of 5856 images of chest X-rays out of which 1583 are normal and 4273 images of pneumonia affected patients. After resizing we have balanced the data of both classes by using 1583 normal images and 1598 pneumonia images. In the next step we have split the training set, validation set and testing set in the ratio of 7:1:2 respectively.

Convolutional Neural Networks

The CNNs are said to be multi-layer perceptrons which will readily identify the important distinctions from the input image. One of the most important features of CNN is that when we take any image as input, we are able to assign the weights and also differentiate objects from other (Yamashita et al., 2018). The convolutional layer and the pooling layer are two additional layers that distinguish the CNN. There is also a completely linked layer and a RELU (rectified linear unit) layer. As data passes through each layer of the network, the RELU layer acts as an activation function, maintaining non linearity. The dataset will be classified with the help of a fully connected layer. The most crucial layer is the convolution layer, which applies a filter to an array of image pixels, resulting in a convoluted feature map. The pooling layer minimizes the sample size of a given road map and speeds up processing by minimizing the number of parameters that the network must process. The filters are what actually detect the pattern. Pattern could be of any type so it may be called edge detector. Earlier these filters were able to only detect specific objects like eyes, nose, and ear but later on they were able to detect the sophisticated images like cat, dog etc. While adding convolutional layer to the model it should also be specified that how many filters and layers to have in the network. There are many layers comprising of filters which have their own parameters, and we get a deep insight of inside volume but it also comprises of small receptive field. The activation layer comes in handy because it can be used to approximate practically any nonlinear function. The activation layer receives the feature map from the convolutional layer as input (Yamashita et al., 2018). The basic flow of a deep CNN network for image classification is shown in Figure. 3.

Figure 3. The basic flow of a deep CNN network for image classification

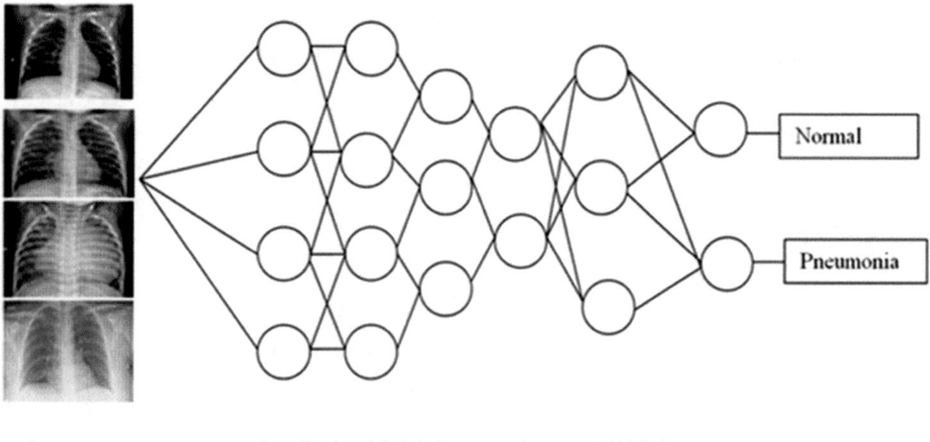

Pre-Trained Neural Networks and Transfer Learning

Pre-trained neural networks are the deep learning networks that have already been trained on a large dataset for the identification and extraction of important underlying features in images useful for the differentiation between objects of distinct classes. These networks serve as a starting point for making a network learn a new task. This is the main idea behind the process of transfer learning.

We are successful in the determination of the classification performance of three pre-trained networks namely VGG16, XceptionNet and MobileNet that are able to differentiate between pneumonia and normal classes.

(a) VGG16: VGGNet may be a classical convolutional neural specification designed as an improvement over the preliminary deep network AlexNet. The VGGNet model, employs 3×3 convolutional filters instead of big filter sizes. This leads to the reduced number of parameters required which successively leads to faster convergence and reduced overfitting. For detailed architecture, readers are directed to Simonyan & Zisserman, (2014).

(b) XceptionNet: François Chollet created Xception in 2017, drawing inspiration from the architecture of Inception V3 [34]. The Xception model's main contribution is that it employs a slightly modified depthwise separable convolution process. Depth wise separable convolution is reversed in the Xception architecture. There are 14 modules in each of the convolutional layers, which has linear residual connections. For detailed architecture, readers are directed to Chollet, (2017).

(c) Mobile Net V2 - A CNN that can be said as mobile friendly is MobileNetv2. The MobileNet model is a network model in which the basic unit is a light-weight depthwise convolution. It also helps in reducing the network size and the number of parameters. For detailed architecture, the readers are directed to Sandler et al., (2018).

RESULTS

The performance of pre-trained networks namely VGG16, XceptionNet and MobileNetv2 has been compared in the present work. The classification results of each of these networks are shown in Figure. 4.

Figure 4. Classification performance of pre-trained networks

Classification Report

	precision	recall	f1-score	support
NORMAL	0.97	0.95	0.96	300
PNEUMONIA	0.95	0.97	0.96	300
accuracy			0.96	600
macro avg	0.96	0.96	0.96	600
weighted avg	0.96	0.96	0.96	600

Classification report of VGG16

Classification Report

	precision	recall	f1-score	support
NORMAL	0.94	0.95	0.95	300
PNEUMONIA	0.95	0.94	0.95	300
accuracy			0.95	600
macro avg	0.95	0.95	0.95	600
weighted avg	0.95	0.95	0.95	600

Classification report of XceptionNet

Classification Report

	precision	recall	f1-score	support
NORMAL	0.92	0.92	0.92	300
PNEUMONIA	0.92	0.92	0.92	300
accuracy			0.92	600
macro avg	0.92	0.92	0.92	600
weighted avg	0.92	0.92	0.92	600

Classification report of MobileNetv2

As seen from classification reports presented in Figure. 4, it is noted that deep network VGG16 achieves maximum accuracy of 96.0% for classification of chest X-rays into normal and pneumonia classes. Out of the total of 600 testing instances, a total of 23 instances were misclassified out of which 15 normal instances were misclassified while 8 misclassified cases belonged to pneumonia class.

The accuracy and loss values for VGG16 are shown in Figure. 5 during training and validation phases, indicating the performance of the pre-trained network.

Figure 5. Performance of pre-trained network VGG16, indication accuracy and loss values for training and validation datasets

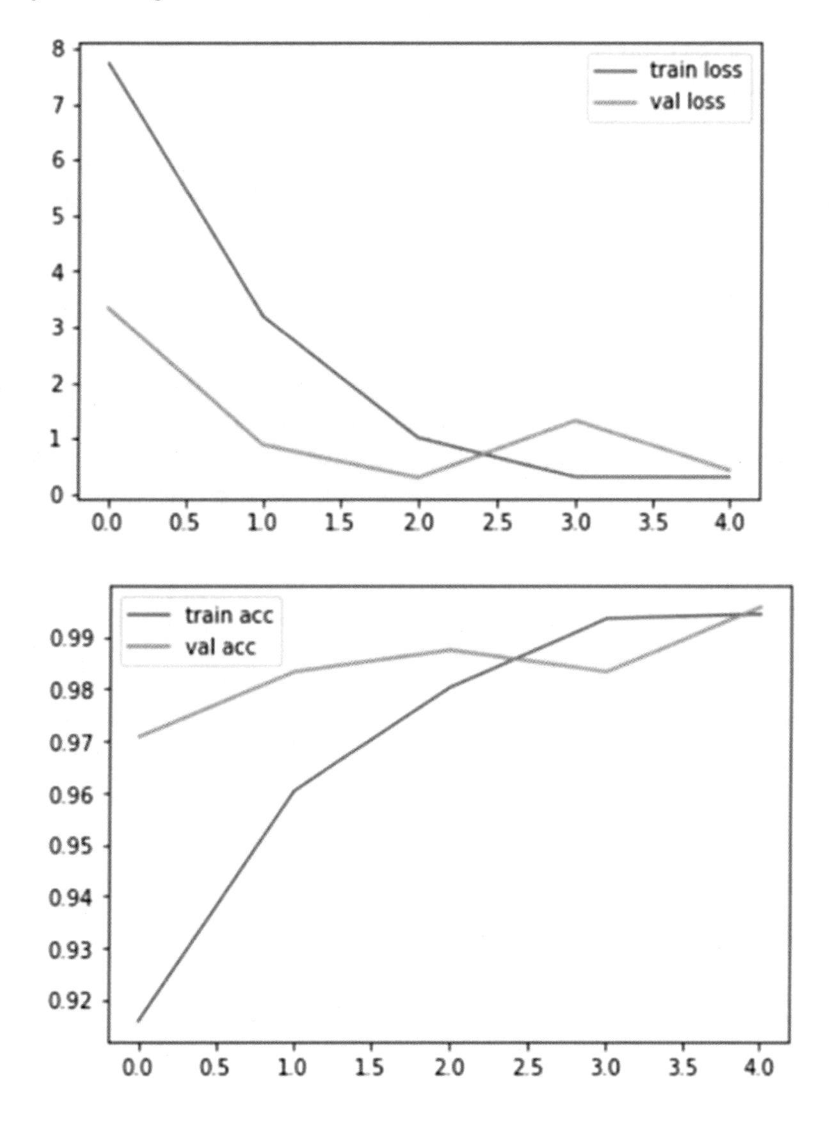

CONCLUSION AND FUTURE SCOPE

Pneumonia is one of the dangerous diseases and we should detect it by observing any symptoms and plan for a medication in order to improve the likelihood of survival. However, the visual analysis of the chest X-rays is a subjective task and highly operator dependent which might sometimes result in misdiagnosis. To overcome these issues, researchers have tried to develop various CAC system designs useful in diagnosis of abnormalities through X-ray images. The present work also tries to portray a simple and effective algorithm for the identification of chest X-rays into normal and pneumonia classes. The authors compare the classification performance of three pre-trained networks, and it was observed that the best accuracy of 96.0% has been achieved using VGG16. The results obtained in the present work indicate the usefulness of proposed classification system in routine medical practice by radiologists for validating their diagnosis as the system is fully automated after the data entry stage.

One of the future directions for extending the present work and increasing the utility of the proposed system is to integrate the CAC system as an algorithm into the X-ray imaging machines used in routine medical practice by radiologists. In that case, the radiologist can input the captured image into the system wherein the underlying algorithm runs the trained model on the captured image and outputs the probable predicted class as normal or pneumonia based on the captured features. The work can also be further extended by using the deep features extracted from the VGG16 and feeding them to classical machine learning classifiers for differentiation between normal and pneumonia chest X-rays, thus forming a hybrid CAC system design.

REFERENCES

Al Mamlook, R. E., Chen, S., & Bzizi, H. F. (2020, July). Investigation of the performance of machine learning classifiers for pneumonia detection in chest x-ray images. In *2020 IEEE International Conference on Electro Information Technology (EIT)* (pp. 098-104). IEEE. 10.1109/EIT48999.2020.9208232

Alharbi, A. H., & Hosni Mahmoud, H. A. (2022, May). Pneumonia transfer learning deep learning model from segmented X-rays. []. MDPI.]. *Health Care*, *10*(6), 987. PMID:35742039

Ayan, E., Karabulut, B., & Ünver, H. M. (2022). Diagnosis of pediatric pneumonia with ensemble of deep convolutional neural networks in chest x-ray images. *Arabian Journal for Science and Engineering*, *47*(2), 2123–2139. doi:10.100713369-021-06127-z PMID:34540526

Ayan, E., & Ünver, H. M. (2019, April). Diagnosis of pneumonia from chest X-ray images using deep learning. In 2019 Scientific Meeting on Electrical-Electronics & Biomedical Engineering and Computer Science (EBBT) (pp. 1-5). IEEE. doi:10.1109/EBBT.2019.8741582

Chollet, F. (2017). Xception: Deep learning with depthwise separable convolutions. In *Proceedings of the IEEE conference on computer vision and pattern recognition* (pp. 1251-1258). 10.1109/CVPR.2017.195

Chouhan, V., Singh, S. K., Khamparia, A., Gupta, D., Tiwari, P., Moreira, C., Damaševičius, R., & De Albuquerque, V. H. C. (2020). A novel transfer learning based approach for pneumonia detection in chest X-ray images. *Applied Sciences (Basel, Switzerland)*, *10*(2), 559. doi:10.3390/app10020559

Chowdary, G. J. (2021). Impact of machine learning models in pneumonia diagnosis with features extracted from chest x-rays using VGG16. [TURCOMAT]. *Turkish Journal of Computer and Mathematics Education*, *12*(5), 1521–1530.

Chu, D. K., Pan, Y., Cheng, S. M., Hui, K. P., Krishnan, P., Liu, Y., Ng, D. Y. M., Wan, C. K. C., Yang, P., Wang, Q., Peiris, M., & Poon, L. L. (2020). Molecular diagnosis of a novel coronavirus (2019-nCoV) causing an outbreak of pneumonia. *Clinical Chemistry*, *66*(4), 549–555. doi:10.1093/clinchem/hvaa029 PMID:32031583

Dey, N., Zhang, Y. D., Rajinikanth, V., Pugalenthi, R., & Raja, N. S. M. (2021). Customized VGG19 architecture for pneumonia detection in chest X-rays. *Pattern Recognition Letters*, *143*, 67–74. doi:10.1016/j.patrec.2020.12.010

Ebiele, J., Ansah-Narh, T., Djiokap, S., Proven-Adzri, E., & Atemkeng, M. (2020, September). Conventional machine learning based on feature engineering for detecting pneumonia from chest X-rays. In Conference of the South African Institute of Computer Scientists and Information Technologists 2020 (pp. 149-155). doi:10.1145/3410886.3410898

Elshennawy, N. M., & Ibrahim, D. M. (2020). Deep-pneumonia framework using deep learning models based on chest x-ray images. *Diagnostics (Basel)*, *10*(9), 649. doi:10.3390/diagnostics10090649 PMID:32872384

Ferreira, J. R., Cardenas, D. A. C., Moreno, R. A., de Sá Rebelo, M. D. F., Krieger, J. E., & Gutierrez, M. A. (2020, July). Multi-view ensemble convolutional neural network to improve classification of pneumonia in low contrast chest x-ray images. In *2020 42nd Annual International Conference of the IEEE Engineering in Medicine & Biology Society (EMBC)* (pp. 1238-1241). IEEE. 10.1109/EMBC44109.2020.9176517

GM, H., Gourisaria, M. K., Rautaray, S. S., & Pandey, M. (2021). Pneumonia detection using CNN through chest X-ray. [JESTEC]. *Journal of Engineering Science and Technology*, *16*(1), 861–876.

Gu, X., Pan, L., Liang, H., & Yang, R. (2018, March). Classification of bacterial and viral childhood pneumonia using deep learning in chest radiography. In *Proceedings of the 3rd International Conference on Multimedia and Image Processing* (pp. 88-93). 10.1145/3195588.3195597

Guail, A. A. A., Jinsong, G., Oloulade, B. M., & Al-Sabri, R. (2022). A principal neighborhood aggregation-based graph convolutional network for pneumonia detection. *Sensors (Basel)*, *22*(8), 3049. doi:10.339022083049 PMID:35459035

Habib, N., Hasan, M. M., & Rahman, M. M. (2020). Fusion of deep convolutional neural network with PCA and logistic regression for diagnosis of pediatric pneumonia on chest X-rays. *The New Biologist*, *10*(3), 62–76.

Hashmi, M. F., Katiyar, S., Keskar, A. G., Bokde, N. D., & Geem, Z. W. (2020). Efficient pneumonia detection in chest xray images using deep transfer learning. *Diagnostics (Basel)*, *10*(6), 417. doi:10.3390/diagnostics10060417 PMID:32575475

Ieracitano, C., Mammone, N., Versaci, M., Varone, G., Ali, A. R., Armentano, A., Calabrese, G., Ferrarelli, A., Turano, L., Tebala, C., Hussain, Z., Sheikh, Z., Sheikh, A., Sceni, G., Hussain, A., & Morabito, F. C. (2022). A fuzzy-enhanced deep learning approach for early detection of Covid-19 pneumonia from portable chest X-ray images. *Neurocomputing*, *481*, 202–215. doi:10.1016/j.neucom.2022.01.055 PMID:35079203

Irfan, A., Adivishnu, A. L., Sze-To, A., Dehkharghanian, T., Rahnamayan, S., & Tizhoosh, H. R. (2020, July). Classifying pneumonia among chest x-rays using transfer learning. In *2020 42nd Annual International Conference of the IEEE Engineering in Medicine & Biology Society (EMBC)* (pp. 2186-2189). IEEE. 10.1109/EMBC44109.2020.9175594

Jain, R., Nagrath, P., Kataria, G., Kaushik, V. S., & Hemanth, D. J. (2020). Pneumonia detection in chest X-ray images using convolutional neural networks and transfer learning. *Measurement*, *165*, 108046. doi:10.1016/j.measurement.2020.108046

Kermany, D., Zhang, K., & Goldbaum, M. (2018). Labeled optical coherence tomography (OCT) and chest x-ray images for classification. Mendeley Data. doi:10.17632/rscbjbr9sj.2

Liang, G., & Zheng, L. (2020). A transfer learning method with deep residual network for pediatric pneumonia diagnosis. *Computer Methods and Programs in Biomedicine*, *187*, 104964. doi:10.1016/j.cmpb.2019.06.023 PMID:31262537

Mayo clinic staff. (June 2022), *Pneumonia*. May Clinic. https://www.mayoclinic.org/diseases-conditions/pneumonia/symptoms-causes/syc-20354204

Mujahid, M., Rustam, F., Álvarez, R., Luis Vidal Mazón, J., Díez, I. D. L. T., & Ashraf, I. (2022). Pneumonia Classification from X-ray images with inception-v3 and convolutional neural network. *Diagnostics (Basel)*, *12*(5), 1280. doi:10.3390/diagnostics12051280 PMID:35626436

Naveen, P., & Diwan, B. (2021, March). Pre-trained VGG-16 with CNN Architecture to classify X-Rays images into Normal or Pneumonia. In *2021 International Conference on Emerging Smart Computing and Informatics (ESCI)* (pp. 102-105). IEEE 10.1109/ESCI50559.2021.9396997

Rahman, T., Chowdhury, M. E., Khandakar, A., Islam, K. R., Islam, K. F., Mahbub, Z. B., Kadir, M. A., & Kashem, S. (2020). Transfer learning with deep convolutional neural network (CNN) for pneumonia detection using chest X-ray. *Applied Sciences (Basel, Switzerland)*, *10*(9), 3233. doi:10.3390/app10093233

Rajaraman, S., Candemir, S., Kim, I., Thoma, G., & Antani, S. (2018). Visualization and interpretation of convolutional neural network predictions in detecting pneumonia in pediatric chest radiographs. *Applied Sciences (Basel, Switzerland)*, *8*(10), 1715. doi:10.3390/app8101715 PMID:32457819

Sandler, M., Howard, A., Zhu, M., Zhmoginov, A., & Chen, L. C. (2018). Mobilenetv2: Inverted residuals and linear bottlenecks. In *Proceedings of the IEEE Conference on Computer Vision and Pattern Recognition* (pp. 4510-4520).

Sharma, H., Jain, J. S., Bansal, P., & Gupta, S. (2020, January). Feature extraction and classification of chest x-ray images using CNN to detect pneumonia. In *2020 10th International Conference on Cloud Computing, Data Science & Engineering (Confluence)* (pp. 227-231). IEEE. 10.1109/Confluence47617.2020.9057809

Simonyan, K., & Zisserman, A. (2014). Very deep convolutional networks for large-scale image recognition. *arXiv preprint arXiv:1409.1556*.

Sousa, A. S., Ferrito, C., & Paiva, J. A. (2018). Intubation-associated pneumonia: An integrative review. *Intensive & Critical Care Nursing*, *44*, 45–52. doi:10.1016/j.iccn.2017.08.003 PMID:28869146

Sousa, G. G. B., Fernandes, V. R. M., & Paiva, A. C. D. (2019, August). Optimized deep learning architecture for the diagnosis of pneumonia through chest X-rays. In *International Conference on Image Analysis and Recognition* (pp. 353-361). Springer. 10.1007/978-3-030-27272-2_31

Stephen, O., Sain, M., Maduh, U. J., & Jeong, D. U. (2019). An efficient deep learning approach to pneumonia classification in healthcare. *Journal of Healthcare Engineering*, *2019*, 1–7. doi:10.1155/2019/4180949 PMID:31049186

Toğaçar, M., Ergen, B., Cömert, Z., & Özyurt, F. (2020). A deep feature learning model for pneumonia detection applying a combination of mRMR feature selection and machine learning models. *IRBM*, *41*(4), 212–222. doi:10.1016/j.irbm.2019.10.006

UNICEF. (2021). *Pneumonia*. UNICEF. https://data.unicef.org/topic/child-health/pneumonia/

Varshni, D., Thakral, K., Agarwal, L., Nijhawan, R., & Mittal, A. (2019, February). Pneumonia detection using CNN based feature extraction. In *2019 IEEE International Conference on Electrical, Computer and Communication Technologies (ICECCT)* (pp. 1-7). IEEE. 10.1109/ICECCT.2019.8869364

WHO. (2021). *Pneumonia* WHO. https://www.who.int/news-room/fact-sheets/detail/pneumonia

Wu, H., Xie, P., Zhang, H., Li, D., & Cheng, M. (2020). Predict pneumonia with chest X-ray images based on convolutional deep neural learning networks. *Journal of Intelligent & Fuzzy Systems*, *39*(3), 2893–2907. doi:10.3233/JIFS-191438

Yamashita, R., Nishio, M., Do, R. K. G., & Togashi, K. (2018). Convolutional neural networks: An overview and application in radiology. *Insights Into Imaging*, *9*(4), 611–629. doi:10.100713244-018-0639-9 PMID:29934920

Yue, Z., Ma, L., & Zhang, R. (2020). Comparison and validation of deep learning models for the diagnosis of pneumonia. *Computational Intelligence and Neuroscience*, *2020*, 1–8. doi:10.1155/2020/8876798 PMID:33014032

Chapter 11
Pneumonia Detection Through X-Ray Images Using Convolution Neural Network

Puneet Garg
ABES Engineering College, India

Akhilesh Kumar Srivastava
ABES Engineering College, India

Anas Anas
ABES Engineering College, India

Bhavye Gupta
ABES Engineering College, India

Chirag Mishra
ABES Engineering College, India

ABSTRACT

Pneumonia is a very contagious illness that spreads quickly among newborns. According to UNICEF, pneumonia was to blame for 16% of all baby deaths under the age of five. The main objective of this study is to determine whether a patient has pneumonia using a chest X-ray picture. CNN is used for this for this process, as it's great processing capability makes them the most effective choice for image processing and categorization. By the use of CNN, results will be obtained rapidly, and dependence on medical personnel will be reduced. Additionally, it will produce more precise findings than human vision, which could overlook a little X-Ray feature. More than17,000 chest X-ray pictures of pneumonic and healthy lungs are included in the collection. This model's total accuracy is 88.62%.

DOI: 10.4018/978-1-6684-6957-6.ch011

INTRODUCTION

Breathing becomes difficult when the air sacs in the lungs become infected. This condition is known as pneumonia, a lung infection generally brought on by viruses present in the environment (Kaushik, 2020). Due to the low cost of this method, it is frequently used to identify pneumonia. Due of Pneumonia's resemblance to other lung infections, its detection might be challenging (Szepesi & Szilágyi, 2022). The lungs with pneumonia are depicted in Figure 1. Radiologists performed the majority of the laborious and time-consuming analysis of the acquired images (Kundu & Das, 2021). Due to this issue, there is a lot of interest in this field to create software that solely analyses X-rays of the chest and determines whether or not an individual has pneumonia Regardless of whether they are male or female, everyone may utilize this effortlessly (Rajasenbagam & Jeyanthi 2021).

Figure 1. Pneumonia in Lungs (Source: Browsed on Web Page (Hacking, n.d.) Pneumonia)

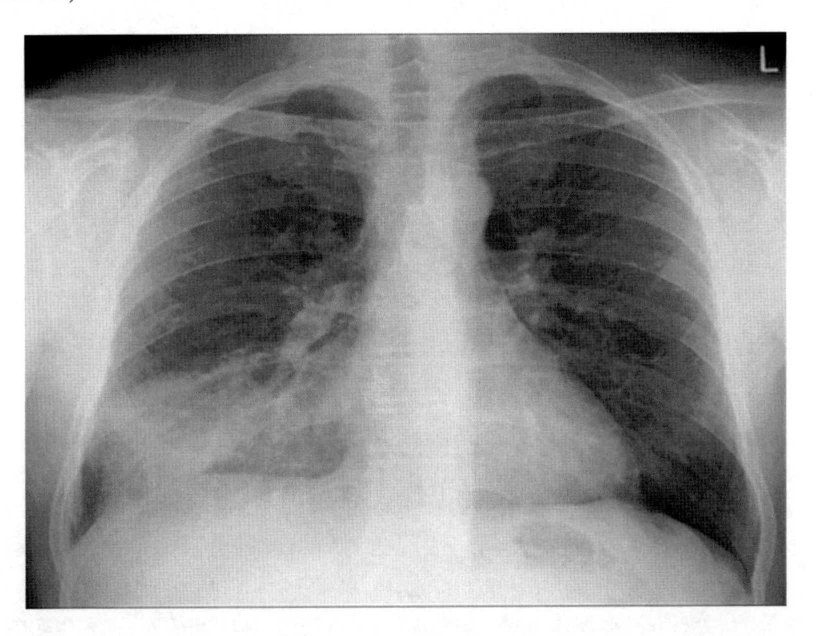

This project's main objective is to identify whether a patient has pneumonia by using images from a chest X-ray (Wang & Zhang, 2021). Due to its high accuracy and the fact that it is more effective than SVM image classification, the model that would be developed would be based on convolutional neural networks (Varshney & Lamba). Because it is readily available and less expensive than other detection methods, chest X-ray pictures are used to diagnose pneumonia in the majority of countries (Yadav & Khan, 2022). The implementation of the machine learning model will lessen reliance on the medical staff and make it simple to identify lung infections. In comparison to results examined by the human eye, this software will provide more accurate results (Pustokhina & Pustokhin 2021). The lung infection caused by pneumonia is seen in Figure 2. Computer-assisted methods.

Image classification, which first pre-processes photos before training a model based on what it learns from the images and then delivering the most accurate results, is the current demanding area of research as a result of advancements in the machine learning domain (Gabruseva & Poplavskiy, 2020). The identification of numerous disorders that are challenging to observe with the naked eye has been assisted by image categorization (Rajpurkar & Irvin, 2017). Because of its highly accurate and efficient outcomes that enable early disease identification and timely delivery of drugs, artificial intelligence is a discipline that is expanding every day (Garg & Dixit, 2022). The construction of models for the classification of medical pictures using machine learning (ML), a branch of artificial intelligence, has achieved notable success (Sharma & Gupta, 2022).

Figure 2. Person with Pneumonia(Source: Browsed on Web Page (Pneumonia Classification, 2009, November 5)).

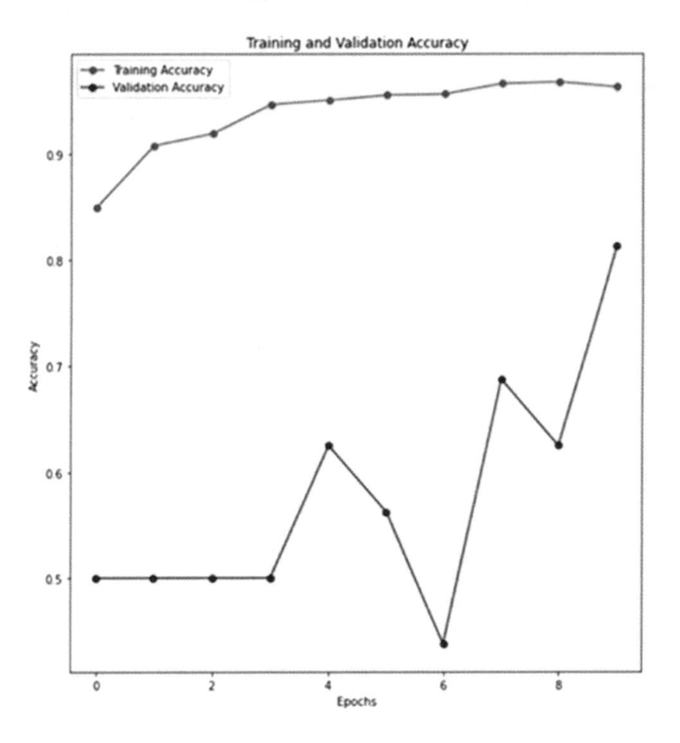

Medical personnel describe pneumonia as an infectious lung disease that destroys the lung's alveoli, making it harder for the organ to function (Sethi & Garg, 2020). According to medical professionals, the most frequent symptoms are chest pain, fever, a dry cough, and breathing difficulties. Individual differences will be seen in this infection's symptoms (Sharma & Garg 2022). Asthma, heart attacks, a compromised immune system, and other significant risk factors for pneumonia are listed below . X-rays of the chest are typically used to diagnose this infection, but blood samples can also be used to do so.

Convolutional Neural Networks will be used for this project because, because to their powerful processing capabilities, they are best suited for image processing and categorization (Khanna, Rani, & Garg (2021)). CNN is a popular and quick image processing and classification technology that many scientists and academics in this field employ (Saraswat & Mohanty (2022)). CNN is an application of artificial neural networks. This model can be used to determine whether or not a person has pneumonia (Beniwal, Saini, &bGarg(2021)). The Chest X-Ray image must be provided in this model in order to determine whether the patient has pneumonia or is healthy (Sonib& Nagpal (2022)). It will generate results rapidly and lessen the need for medical personnel. Additionally, it will provide more accurate results compared to human eyes, which could overlook a little feature in an X-Ray (Maggo & Garg (2022)). Figure 3 shows a woman with Pneumonia Infection. The Chest X-Ray Images were collected from Kaggle due to its enormous dataset and the fact that it is classified into two kinds, Pneumonia and Normal. More than 17,000 photos of pneumonic and healthy lungs from chest X-rays are included in the dataset (Chaudhary & Garg, 2014).

Figure 3. Pneumonia Infection(Source: Browsed on Web Page (C., n.d.) Aspiration Pneumonia).

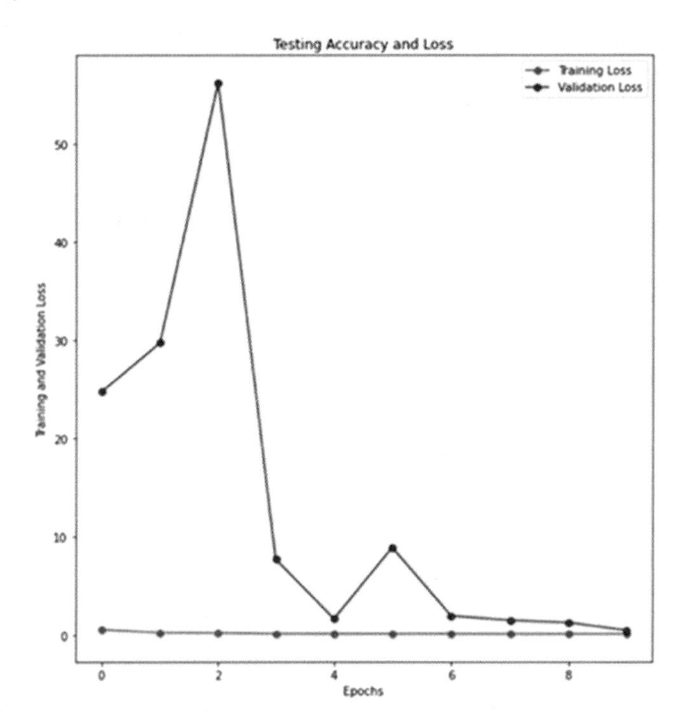

BACKGROUND

A type of acute respiratory infection that affects the lungs called pneumonia (Varshni & Thakra, 2019). A healthy person's lungs are made up of tiny sacs called alveoli that fill with air when they breathe. When someone gets pneumonia, their alveoli are stuffed with fluid and pus, which makes breathing difficult and reduces oxygen absorption. Infectious diseases account for the majority of pediatric fatalities worldwide (Varshney, Lamba, & Garg, 2022). 2019 had 740 180 pediatric deaths from pneumonia, which accounted for 14% of all pediatric deaths in that age group but 22% of all pediatric deaths in children from 1 to 5 years (Chouhan & Singh, 2020). Children and families are affected by pneumonia everywhere, although deaths are most common in southern Asia and sub-Saharan Africa. Pneumonia can be avoided in children, prevented with straightforward measures, and treated with affordable, low-tech medicine and care (Pustokhina & Pustokhin, 2021).

The signs and symptoms of pneumonia can range from mild, you hardly notice them, to severe, you need to be hospitalized. The type of bacteria that causes the infection, your age, and your general state of health all affect how your body reacts to pneumonia (Khanna & Rani, 2021).

Pneumonia may exhibit the following symptoms and signs:

1. Coughing up green, yellow, or even bloody mucous.
2. Coughing up green, yellow, or even bloody mucous.
3. Breathing difficulty
4. Chest pain that is piercing or stabbing and worsen when person cough or breathe deeply
5. Lack of hunger, lower energy levels, and exhaustion
6. Recurrent vomiting, infants mainly felt that problem.
7. Perplexity, particularly in the elderly

PROPOSED METHODOLOGY

The suggested methodology is demonstrated in the following ways:

I. Dataset: Kaggle was employed to get the images due to its sizable dataset and segmentation of the chest X-ray images into two categories, namely pneumonia and normal (Garg, Dixit (2020)). Three subfolders are included in the folder for the training, testing, and validation datasets that we utilize to develop our model. The training dataset contains about 5863 chest X-ray pictures, both normal and pneumonic (Garg & Sethi 2019).
II. Image Pre-Processing: Then, we pre-processed the dataset of X-ray pictures to make it consistent with our training model. Label encoding, data augmentation, and resizing are all included in the image pre-processing (Sethi & Singh, 2020).
III. Developing a Model: The chest x-ray image collection will be preprocessed before our model is trained using a convolutional neural network (CNN) machine learning technique.
IV. Testing: Next, the testing dataset in the test dataset folder will be used to make a prediction about whether the subject has pneumonia or not.
V. Output label: Based on chest X-ray images, the output label will either say Pneumonia or Normal. The proposed methodology is described in Figure 3.

The methodology is shown in depth in the following points:

Importing the Libraries

For building and running our machine-learning model, the relevant libraries must be imported. Convolutional network models are created using these significant libraries. The libraries used in this design model, such as NumPy, Matplotlib, Seaborn, Keras, OpenCV, open dataset, and Panda, offer great performance, accuracy, data structures, and algorithms. Python's NumPy library is used to perform logical and mathematical operations on one- and two-dimensional arrays. An API called Keras is utilized to depict quick neural network experimentation. The module to forecast the outcome is simpler to use and more user-friendly.

Data Loading, Training, Validation, and Testing

The Kaggle dataset is divided into three folders: Val (testing dataset), Train (training dataset), and (validation dataset). These subfolders house images from chest X-rays (greyscale). Images go into one of two categories: pneumonia or typical. These datasets were obtained from Kaggle and used to train the model. It eliminates all low-quality chest x-ray images after analyzing the photos. The artificial intelligence system is trained using the photos that have been diagnosed. The third expert could fix any errors in the system to increase accuracy if they arise.

Data Augmentation

Add more datasets to the existing data to increase accuracy while avoiding the overfitting issue. Adding datasets improves performance, accuracy, and variation generation. These modified processes—known as data augmentation strategies—modify the array representation while keeping the same label. These methods can be improved in a variety of ways, including with colour-based greyscales, translations, vertical flips, random colour, rotations, and colour jitters, among others. The model can enhance the number of trainings based on our training datasets and create a very robust model by applying these augmentations.

Points for data augmentation:

1. Some training photos are rotated by about 30 degrees at random, which is a point for data augmentation.
2. A 20% random zoom increment on some photographs
3. 10% of the width of each image is horizontally scaled.
4. Photos are reduced in height by 10% vertically.
5. Image flipping from vertical to horizontal. After the model is complete or prepared, work on the training dataset.

IMPLEMENTATION

The CNN technique, which is best suited for image processing and classification, is used in the implementation of this model to train machine learning. The following examples demonstrate how the CNN model is implemented in detail:

Train Model Based on Neural Network

The CNN model, which is based on a neural network, is trained during this stage of deployment to diagnose pneumonia accurately and effectively from chest X-ray images. For further processing at different levels, the best weights would be used during model training. The weights will then be further modified using the activation function to ensure that the model is produced with the best outcomes possible. The model's performance against a certain task will then be evaluated by calculating the Loss, which is used to measure the model's effectiveness.

This training's major goal is to reduce this loss function for more precise and efficient outputs. There are two different sorts of approaches, namely batch and epochs, for giving the pictures dataset to the images. Epochs are used by this model during model training. Instead of merely supplying batches of photographs for training the model, all the images folder is provided in epochs. For more accurate results, this model employs Epochs=10, which feeds it 10 times the whole picture dataset. The dataset had 17457 chest X-ray pictures, with an accuracy of 88.62% and a loss function value of 0.29. It took around an hour to complete 10 epochs. The model that has been developed is shown in Figure 4.

The summary of this model contains all pertinent information about it, such as the number of layers, the nature of the output layers, the parameters used, and the weights applied.

Figure 4. CNN Model Created

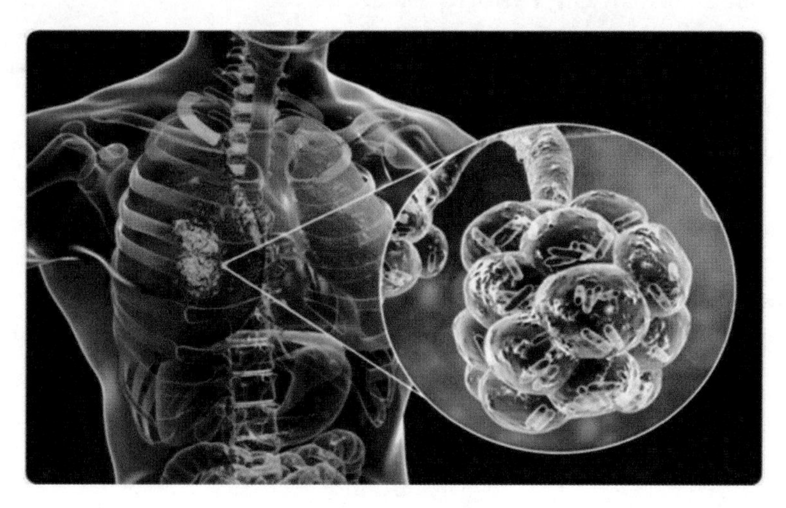

A string about the constructed model is returned by the summary() method, which may then be printed in the desired format. Summary of the model is shown in Figure 5.

Figure 5. Model Summary (Sequential Model)

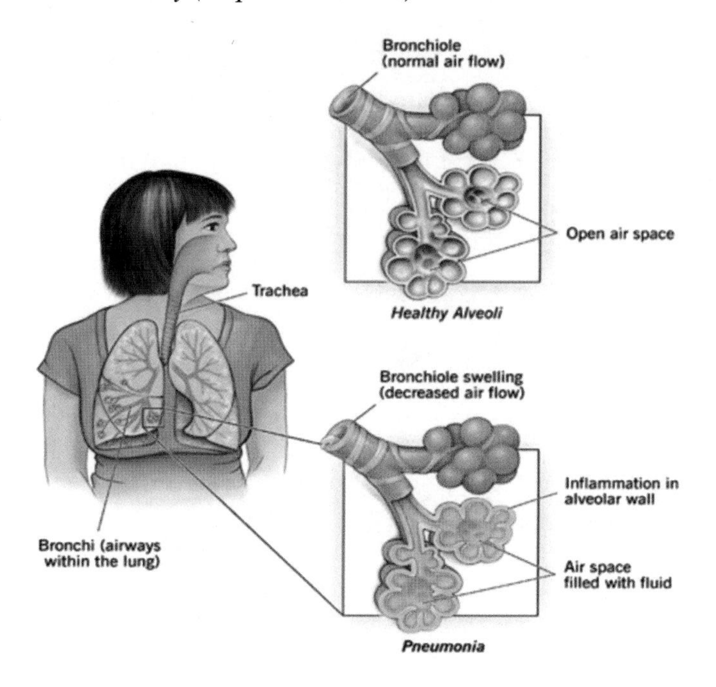

Model Evaluation on Testing Dataset

The metric for classification used in it contains various parameters like Precision, recall, F1 scores using which model easily provides support to the model for pneumonia and normal to find the different averages and weights of a model on this particular dataset. When the accuracy indicator for classification is not giving the expected correct results model makes the use of accuracy for classification to predict the result of model performance and its achievement in case the data given is variance. The Recall parameter is used to find the parts of the sample which is correctly anticipated by the model in the given dataset. The two parameters precision and recall are combined to get the result of F1 score as shown in Figure 6.

Figure 6. Table for Precision, Recall, f1-Score

```
model = Sequential()
model.add(Conv2D(32,(3,3),strides=1,padding='same',activation='relu',input_shape=(150,150,1)))
model.add(BatchNormalization())
model.add(MaxPool2D((2,2),strides=2,padding='same'))

model.add(Conv2D(64,(3,3),strides=1,padding='same',activation='relu'))
model.add(Dropout(0.1))
model.add(BatchNormalization())
model.add(MaxPool2D((2,2),strides=2,padding='same'))

model.add(Conv2D(64,(3,3),strides=1,padding='same',activation='relu'))
model.add(BatchNormalization())
model.add(MaxPool2D((2,2),strides=2,padding='same'))

model.add(Conv2D(128,(3,3),strides=1,padding='same',activation='relu'))
model.add(Dropout(0.2))
model.add(BatchNormalization())
model.add(MaxPool2D((2,2),strides=2,padding='same'))

model.add(Conv2D(256,(3,3),strides=1,padding='same',activation='relu'))
model.add(Dropout(0.2))
model.add(BatchNormalization())
model.add(MaxPool2D((2,2),strides=2,padding='same'))

model.add(Flatten())
model.add(Dense(units=128,activation='relu'))
model.add(Dropout(0.2))
model.add(Dense(units=1,activation='sigmoid'))
model.compile(optimizer="rmsprop",loss='binary_crossentropy',metrics=['accuracy'])
model.summary()
```

Generating Confusion Matrix

Accuracy is not only the parameter by which the model can predict the result of the whole model to make it more precise. Also, model can make use of another matrix known as the Confusion matrix as shown in Figure 7. A confusion matrix helps in the visualization of the model and the results of model in tabular form which also make it easy to understand the wholesome result of a model to some unknown person. Every individual row of the Confusion matrix provides the occurrence of a concluded class and on the other hand, each column helps in finding the occurrence of a class.

Figure 7. Confusion Matrix

```
Model: "sequential"
_________________________________________________________________
 Layer (type)                Output Shape              Param #
=================================================================
 conv2d (Conv2D)             (None, 150, 150, 32)      320

 batch_normalization (BatchN  (None, 150, 150, 32)     128
 ormalization)

 max_pooling2d (MaxPooling2D  (None, 75, 75, 32)       0
 )

 conv2d_1 (Conv2D)           (None, 75, 75, 64)        18496

 dropout (Dropout)           (None, 75, 75, 64)        0

 batch_normalization_1 (Batc  (None, 75, 75, 64)       256
 hNormalization)

 max_pooling2d_1 (MaxPooling  (None, 38, 38, 64)       0
 2D)

 conv2d_2 (Conv2D)           (None, 38, 38, 64)        36928

 batch_normalization_2 (Batc  (None, 38, 38, 64)       256
 hNormalization)

 max_pooling2d_2 (MaxPooling  (None, 19, 19, 64)       0
 2D)

 conv2d_3 (Conv2D)           (None, 19, 19, 128)       73856

 dropout_1 (Dropout)         (None, 19, 19, 128)       0

 batch_normalization_3 (Batc  (None, 19, 19, 128)      512
 hNormalization)

 max_pooling2d_3 (MaxPooling  (None, 10, 10, 128)      0
 2D)

 conv2d_4 (Conv2D)           (None, 10, 10, 256)       295168

 dropout_2 (Dropout)         (None, 10, 10, 256)       0

 batch_normalization_4 (Batc  (None, 10, 10, 256)      1024
 hNormalization)

 max_pooling2d_4 (MaxPooling  (None, 5, 5, 256)        0
 2D)

 flatten (Flatten)           (None, 6400)              0

 dense (Dense)               (None, 128)               819328

 dropout_3 (Dropout)         (None, 128)               0

 dense_1 (Dense)             (None, 1)                 129

=================================================================
Total params: 1,246,401
Trainable params: 1,245,313
Non-trainable params: 1,088
```

Testing Images on Model

The final step of training is to determine whether or not the trained model, which has undergone extensive training, accurately predicts the X-Ray pictures from the sample dataset. The images that were used as the model's input successfully predicted the result, as seen in Figures 10 and 11. Figure 8 displays an X-ray of lungs that are in good condition and devoid of pneumonia. In contrast, Figure 9 shows an X-Ray picture of lungs with pneumonia infection.

Result 1

Figure 8. Normal Class

	precision	recall	f1-score	support
Pneumonia (Class 0)	0.94	0.87	0.91	390
Normal (Class 1)	0.81	0.91	0.86	234
accuracy			0.89	624
macro avg	0.88	0.89	0.88	624
weighted avg	0.89	0.89	0.89	624

Result 2

Figure 9. Pneumonia Class

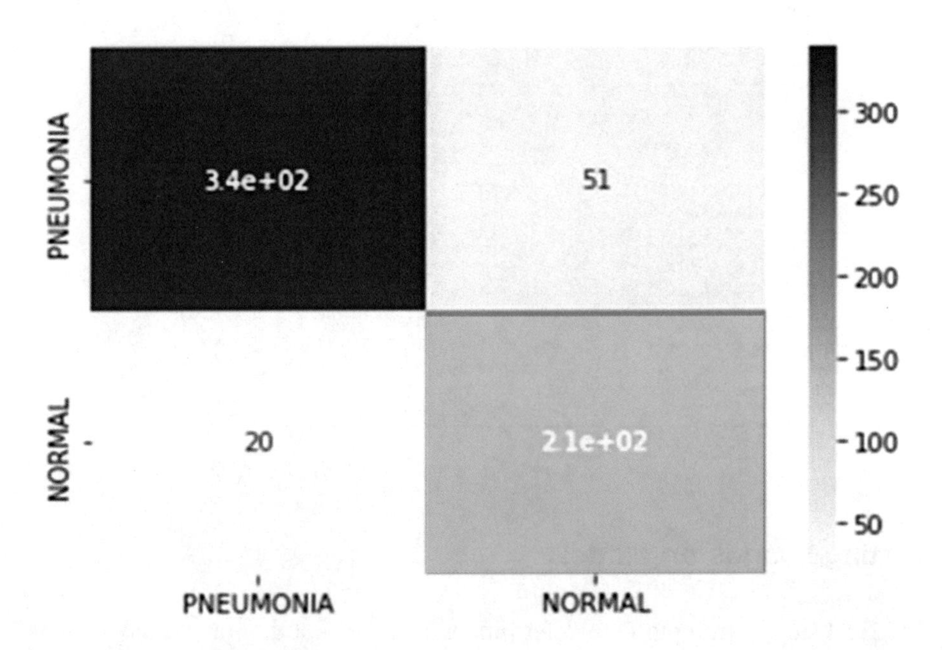

RESULT AND ANALYSIS

The findings and analyses of the above-mentioned CNN model are shown in the following point:

- With recall and F1 score as parameters for classification, the accuracy displayed by this CNN Model is 88.62%, which aids in anticipating the right outcome. The computed F1-Score is approximately 89%. The high percentage of recall value demonstrates that our CNN model predicts the False-Negative incidence is very low, which aids in properly forecasting the patient X-Ray result and facilitating prompt treatment.
- In this stage, the trained model's results are plotted to demonstrate its training and validation accuracy as well as the model's training loss, which is depicted in Figure 10. Loss Function is computed using epoch-based training. Then, in the dataset depicted in Figure 11, the curve was drawn for each iteration.

Figure 10. Accuracy Graph for Training and Validation

```
In [60]:  a='C:/Users/bhavye/Downloads/chest-xray-pneumonia/chest_xray/val/NORMAL/NORMAL2-IM-1442-0001.jpeg'
          predict = pneumoniaPrediction([prepare(a)])
          print(predict,"\n")
          IPython.display.Image(filename=a,width=250,height=250)

          1/1 [==============================] - 0s 37ms/step
          Normal

Out[60]:
```

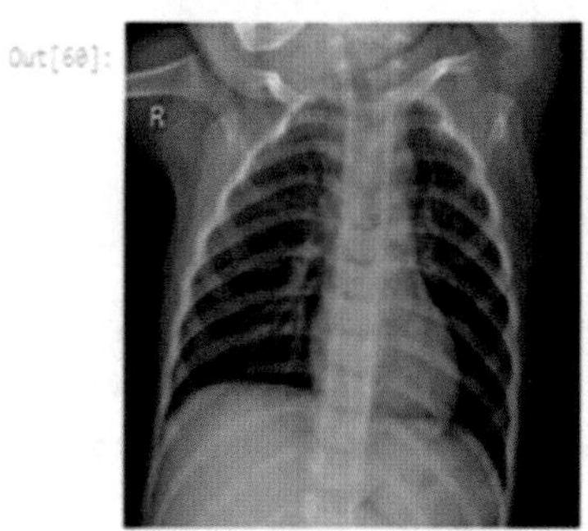

Figure 11. Losses from Training and Validation

```
In [55]:
a='C:/Users/bhavye/Downloads/chest-xray-pneumonia/chest_xray/val/PNEUMONIA/person1950_bacteria_4881.jpeg'
predict = pneumoniaPrediction([prepare(a)])
print(predict,"\n")
IPython.display.Image(filename=a,width=250,height=350)

1/1 [==============================] - 0s 36ms/step
Pneumonia

Out[55]:
```

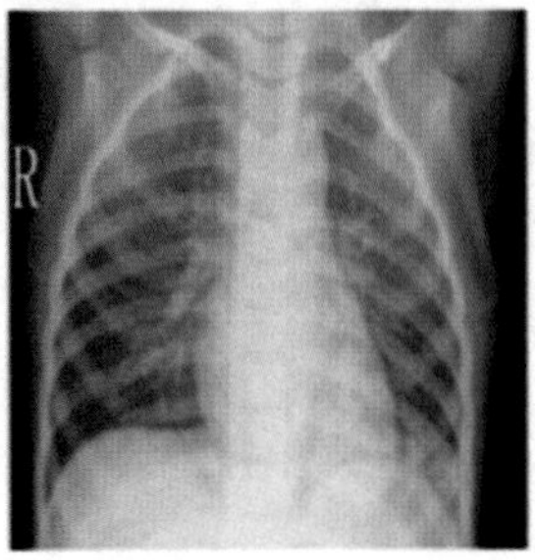

SUMMARY

- It is challenging to distinguish between different lung infections with the naked eye due to the similarity of these infections. Additionally, radiologists and other medical workers must through a laborious and time-consuming process in order to diagnose pneumonia.
- The main goal of this chapter is to more accurately and effectively diagnose pneumonia using chest X-ray pictures. Given that CNN's neural network topology makes it the most effective for classifying images, this model was created using CNN.
- In order to predict outcomes based on chest X-ray scans, this algorithm underwent extensive training on a huge dataset. It is also producing extremely good effects, according to the findings and observations. In order to save a patient's life, medical personnel can quickly determine by utilizing this CNN Model whether a patient is suffering from pneumonia by looking at their symptoms.
- The vast amount of X-ray pictures used as a dataset makes it possible to forecast outcomes quickly, lowering the number of pneumonia-related deaths worldwide and advancing societal causes by sparing a person's precious life.
- With the help of machine learning techniques and neural networks, it is anticipated that this trained model would deliver accurate results for several datasets on schedule.

- Additionally, it is projected that in the future, this three-layer CNN model will operate on a Generative Neural Network that is based on unsupervised learning and discover an effective method of outcome prediction.
- The CNN classifier model can, therefore, be employed efficiently by medical professionals for diagnostic purposes for the early diagnosis of pneumonia in both children and adults.
- It is possible to quickly process a huge number of X-ray images to get extremely accurate diagnostic results, assisting healthcare systems in providing effective patient care services and lowering death rates.
- By using a variety of parameter tuning techniques, such as adding dropout, altering learning rates, batch size, number of epochs, adding more sophisticated fully connected layers, and altering various stochastic gradient optimizers, these convolutional neural network models were effectively created.
- Our research helps with the early detection of pneumonia to avoid negative effects in such remote locations. There hasn't been much effort done to far precisely to identify Pneumonia from the aforementioned dataset. The creation of algorithms in this area could be very helpful for delivering improved healthcare services.

REFERENCES

Beniwal, S., Saini, U., Garg, P., & Joon, R. K. (2021). Improving performance during camera surveillance by integration of edge detection in IoT system. [IJEHMC]. *International Journal of E-Health and Medical Communications*, *12*(5), 84–96.

Chaudhary, A., & Garg, P. (2014). Detecting and diagnosing a disease by patient monitoring system. *International Journal of Mechanical Engineering And Information Technology*, *2*(6), 493–499.

Chouhan, V., Singh, S. K., Khamparia, A., Gupta, D., Tiwari, P., Moreira, C., & De Albuquerque, V. H. C. (2020). A novel transfer learning based approach for pneumonia detection in chest X-ray images. *Applied Sciences*, *10*(2), 559.

Chow, S. (2009, November 5). *Pneumonia Classification.* News-Medical.net. https://www.news-medical.net/health/Pneumonia-Classification.aspx

Cleaveland Clinic. (n.d.). *Aspiration Pneumonia: What It Is, Causes, Diagnosis, Treatment*. Cleveland Clinic. https://my.clevelandclinic.org/health/diseases/21954-aspirat
ion-pneumonia

Dixit, A., Garg, P., Sethi, P., & Singh, Y. (2020, April). TVCCCS: Television Viewer's Channel Cost Calculation System On Per Second Usage. [). IOP Publishing.]. *IOP Conference Series. Materials Science and Engineering*, *804*(1), 012046.

Gabruseva, T., Poplavskiy, D., & Kalinin, A. (2020). Deep learning for automatic pneumonia detection. In *Proceedings of the IEEE/CVF conference on computer vision and pattern recognition workshops (*pp. 350-351). IEEE.

Garg, P., Dixit, A., & Sethi, P. (2019). Wireless sensor networks: An insight review. *International Journal of Advanced Science and Technology*, *28*(15), 612–627.

Garg, P., Dixit, A., & Sethi, P. (2022). Ml-fresh: Novel routing protocol in opportunistic networks using machine learning. *Computer Systems Science and Engineering*, *40*(2), 703–717.

Garg, P., Dixit, A., Sethi, P., & Pinheiro, P. R. (2020). Impact of node density on the qos parameters of routing protocols in opportunistic networks for smart spaces. *Mobile Information Systems*.

Hacking, C. (n.d.). Pneumonia: Radiology Reference Article. *Radiopaedia.org*. https://radiopaedia.org/articles/pneumonia

Khanna, A., Rani, P., Garg, P., Singh, P. K., & Khamparia, A. (2021). An Enhanced Crow Search Inspired Feature Selection Technique for Intrusion Detection Based Wireless Network System. *Wireless Personal Communications*, 1–18.

Kundu, R., Das, R., Geem, Z. W., Han, G. T., & Sarkar, R. (2021). Pneumonia detection in chest X-ray images using an ensemble of deep learning models. *PLoS One*, *16*(9), e0256630.

Maggo, C., & Garg, P. (2022). From linguistic features to their extractions: Understanding the semantics of a concept. *2022 Fifth International Conference on Computational Intelligence and Communication Technologies (CCICT)*, (pp. 427-431). Research Gate. doi:10.1109/CCiCT56684.2022.00082

Pustokhina, I. V., Pustokhin, D. A., Lydia, E. L., Garg, P., Kadian, A., & Shankar, K. (2021). Hyperparameter search based Convolutionneural network with Bi-LSTM model for intrusion detection system in multimedia big data environment. *Multimedia Tools and Applications*, 1–18.

Pustokhina, I. V., Pustokhin, D. A., Lydia, E. L., Garg, P., Kadian, A., & Shankar, K. (2021). Hyperparameter search based Convolutionneural network with Bi-LSTM model for intrusion detection system in multimedia big data environment. *Multimedia Tools and Applications*, 1–18.

Rajasenbagam, T., Jeyanthi, S., & Pandian, J. A. (2021). Detection of pneumonia infection in lungs from chest X-ray images using deep Convolutionalal neural network and content-based image retrieval techniques. *Journal of Ambient Intelligence and Humanized Computing*, 1–8.

Rajpurkar, P., Irvin, J., Zhu, K., Yang, B., Mehta, H., Duan, T., & Ng, A. Y. (2017). *Chexnet: Radiologist-level pneumonia detection on chest x-rays with deep learning.* arXiv:1711.05225.

Saraswat, L., Mohanty, L., Garg, P., & Lamba, S. (2022). Plant Disease Identification Using Plant Images. *2022 Fifth International Conference on Computational Intelligence and Communication Technologies (CCICT)*, (pp. 79-82). Research Gate. doi:10.1109/CCiCT56684.2022.00026

Sethi, P., Garg, P., Dixit, A., & Singh, Y. (2020, April). Smart number cruncher–a voice based calculator. *IOP Conference Series. Materials Science and Engineering*, *804*(1), 012041.

Sharma, N., & Garg, P. (2022). Ant colony based optimization model for QoS-Based task scheduling in cloud computing environment. Measurement. *Sensors (Basel)*, 100531.

Sharma, R., Gupta, S., & Garg, P. (2022). Model for Predicting Cardiac Health using Deep Learning Classifier. *2022 Fifth International Conference on Computational Intelligence and Communication Technologies (CCICT)*, (pp. 25-30). Research Gate. doi:10.1109/CCiCT56684.2022.00017

Sirish Kaushik, V., Nayyar, A., Kataria, G., & Jain, R. (2020). Pneumonia detection using Convolutionalal neural networks (CNNs). In *Proceedings of First International Conference on Computing, Communications, and Cyber-Security (IC4S 2019)* (pp. 471-483). Springer, Singapore.

Soni, E., Nagpal, A., Garg, P., & Pinheiro, P. R. (2022). Assessment of Compressed and Decompressed ECG Databases for Telecardiology Applying a ConvolutionNeural Network. *Electronics (Basel)*, *11*(17), 2708.

Szepesi, P., & Szilágyi, L. (2022). Detection of pneumonia using Convolutionalal neural networks and deep learning. *Biocybernetics and Biomedical Engineering*, *42*(3), 1012–1022. doi:10.1016/j.bbe.2022.08.001

Varshney, S. L., & Garg, P. (2022). A Comprehensive Survey on Event Analysis Using Deep Learning. *2022 Fifth International Conference on Computational Intelligence and Communication Technologies (CCICT)*, (pp. 146-150). Research Gate. doi:10.1109/CCiCT56684.2022.00037

Varshney, S. L., & Garg, P. (2022). A Comprehensive Survey on Event Analysis Using Deep Learning. *2022 Fifth International Conference on Computational Intelligence and Communication Technologies (CCICT)*, pp. 146-150, doi: 10.1109/CCiCT56684.2022.00037

Varshni, D., Thakral, K., Agarwal, L., Nijhawan, R., & Mittal, A. (2019, February). Pneumonia detection using CNN based feature extraction. In *2019 IEEE international conference on electrical, computer and communication technologies (ICECCT)* (pp. 1-7). IEEE.

Yadav, P. S., Khan, S., Singh, Y. V., Garg, P., & Singh, R. S. (2022). A Lightweight Deep Learning-Based Approach for Jazz Music Generation in MIDI Format. *Computational Intelligence and Neuroscience*, 2022.

Yu, X., Wang, S. H., & Zhang, Y. D. (2021). CGNet: A graph-knowledge embedded Convolutionalal neural network for detection of pneumonia. *Information Processing & Management*, *58*(1), 102411.

Chapter 12
Investigating COVID-19 Vaccination Patterns in Europe:
Is the End of the Pandemic Still Foreseeable?

Frank Adusei-Mensah
https://orcid.org/0000-0001-8237-5305
University of Eastern Finland, Finland

Ivy E. Inkum
Mantyla Kotihoito, Finland

Kennedy J. Oduro
Cape Coast Teaching Hospital, Ghana

ABSTRACT

The present chapter aims to investigate the occurrence of COVID-19 vaccine administration patterns in Europe for effective vaccination and booster shot scheduling towards COVID-19 pandemic control. Method: Data were obtained from the ECDC on COVID-19 vaccination radar on 5th March 2021 and processed for statistical analysis with IBM's SPSS version 21. Statistically, a significant difference was considered at p less than 0.05. Results: The authors observed statistically significant lower vaccine uptake compared to delivered doses (average at 62.678 ± 3.928%). Uptake for Oxford-AstraZeneca vaccines (50.927 ± 4.626%) compared to Pfizer-Biontech vaccine (86.285 +/- 2.1052%) was observed compared to previous prospective study on the wiliness to receive COVID-19 vaccine in the region (75%). Conclusion: The early COVID-19 acceptance pattern based on vaccine type or manufacturer was observed. The findings will be useful for policymakers to introduce policies on educational campaigns to enhance vaccine and booster uptake for smooth and effective control of the pandemic.

DOI: 10.4018/978-1-6684-6957-6.ch012

INTRODUCTION

The coronavirus pandemic is a global challenge affecting the lives and livelihoods of billions globally. The unprecedented speed of the pandemic tested every ounce of science, and it led to the development of vaccines by different vaccine makers at an unprecedented pace than ever experienced before. Being one of the most important advances in modern medicine, vaccines have saved the lives of many from vaccine-preventable deaths. Credit to the success of vaccination, some of the world's devastating pandemics including smallpox has been controlled and/ or eradicated. Vaccination is undoubtedly one of the efficacious public health arsenals of modern medicine. However, it is important to note that having safe and efficacious vaccines alone does not save lives and control a pandemic; rather, vaccination plus other public health measures do! The scale of the pandemic, vaccination, and boosters are indispensable elements for controlling the COVID-19 outbreak. Although there still could be many unanswered questions about the degree of protection, the duration of the waning of the vaccine-triggered immunity to COVID-19, how often, the variants, and the efficacy against different variants (Paul et al., 2021). During the initial drafting, there were over 175.3 million vaccine doses administered between Early December 2020 to mid-March 2021 in the EU region, however the pattern of vaccine acceptance and the emergence of new COVID-19 variants and waves of the outbreaks have barely changed compared to the current 13 billion + of vaccine doses administered globally (as of 5th January 2023) (WHO, 2023). There is still much to be desired including attitudinal changes for effective control and eradication of the COVID-19 pandemic. To achieve an efficient vaccination campaign and future boosters, public health professionals and vaccination planners need to overcome many bottlenecks including miscommunication, perceptions of vaccine safety, side effects, and efficacy (Gerussi et al., 2021, Paul et al., 2021). The 'ever-existing' COVID-19 with ever-changing variants and epicenters including the most recent wave in China (December 2023 wave) calls for unparalleled concerted effort and speed. With as resource intensive as vaccine development is, and vaccine producers stretched, production and supply chains tested, for the populace to rely on a single producer alone will prolong the pandemic (Sauramäki, et al, 2022). Since most of the vaccines available on the market have impeccable results in averting severe covid-19 infection and mortality, it is advisable to say that 'the best vaccine to safe one's life is the one that reaches him/her in time'. Reports on vaccine hesitancy and COVID-19 vaccine acceptance bias have been document with multiple reasons, some preferring one vaccine to the other. Earlier reports suggested cancelling vaccination appointment times, preferring mRNA vaccine to AstraZeneca/Oxford University vaccines and close to 80% of the Oxford/AstraZeneca vaccine doses delivered to EU countries remained un-used for reasons of efficacy, safety and region of manufacturing (Boffey, 2021). With billions of lives at risk and tens of thousands of lives lost every day to COVID-19, it is important to evaluate the vaccines available today for their efficacy and safety from epidemiologic point of view and to promote vaccine uptake. The main aim of this paper is therefore to investigate the pattern of vaccination and vaccine acceptance retrospectively for effective control of the pandemic. This retrospective view is for future planning and for effective control of future outbreaks.

OVERVIEW OF SELECTED VACCINE-PREVENTABLE DISEASE AND MODEL PROPOSAL

Ebola Viral Disease

Zoonotic diseases are emerging and re-emerging at a faster rate than before. The Ebola Virus Disease (EVD) is one of the sporadic but severe and often fatal condition characterized with signs and symptoms including fever, sore throat, muscle and joint pain, extreme headache and, looseness of the bowels, and hemorrhaging from orifice, bruising and red eyes. First reported in 1976 near the Ebola River in Democratic Republic of Congo, the EVD has since then had about 22 periodic outbreaks in several African countries. The 2014 epidemic was more trans-national with close to 30,000 cases and CF ranging from 0 (0%) in the UK to 75% in the Dr Congo. It was one of the worse Ebola outbreaks in history. The outbreak of Ebola virus disease in and across countries including developing - developed countries and outside its endemic regions highlights the need for cross-border corporation for infection control. The widespread infection in 2014 also among developed countries like the UK, Spain and the USA attracted attention. Currently, there are 2 licensed vaccines; ERVEBO® (Ebola Zaire Vaccine, Live also known as V920, rVSVΔG-ZEBOV-GP or rVSV-ZEBOV) which are both endorsed by the United States Food and Drug Administration (FDA) against Ebola. The authorized EVD vaccines are acceptably safe and protective against the Zaire ebolavirus variant. The most recent November 2022 flare-up in Ugandan with 142 already confirmed cases of Sudan Ebola viral disease (SVD), case fatality rate of 39% (CFR: 39%) including seven health care workers (ECDC 2023).

Ebola Virus Disease (EVD) was reported to have its maiden outbreak in 1976 with two outbreaks in Sudan and Zaire; after that, there have been over 20 outbreaks in Central Africa. During the 2000 outbreak in Uganda, over 400 confirmed cases of Ebola within the first three months of the outbreak were reported (WHO, 2014). As high as 28 000+ confirmed cases of EVD with over 11000 deaths were reported in 3 African countries – Sierra Leone, Liberia and Guinea and during the

2014 outbreak alone. In 2014, the primary case of the EVD outbreak was reported in Guinea and spread to about 10 countries (CF: 40.01%) (WHO, 2014). Though national and international agencies supported the extensive mobilization of personnel, equipment and resources, there were still challenges with containment of the EVD. This is because, besides the virus, and health factors, social conditions such as poverty, inadequate health infrastructure and community opposition to the Ebola control campaigns were hugely impeding control effort and negatively accounted for the unprecedented rate of spread of the EVD. Other social conditions including infrastructure, logistics, lack of health practitioners; surveillance, governance, health knowledge, and management of health services were suboptimal. The 2014/2015 epidemic presented unique problems. However, the fragile pre-existing health systems also presented opportunities to learn towards the 2019 coronavirus pandemic globally. Many criticized the international response for being "too little and too late", an experience which the authors believe facilitated the quick development of the mRNA COVID-19 vaccines in 2020.

In West Africa, the scale of the emergency by the international response encompassed training teams, boosting Ebola treatment centres, and strengthening social mobilization capacities (WHO, 2014). Again, the engagement of communities, the capacities for case finding, contact tracing communication, surveillance, and laboratory testing and clinical trial management were strengthened. These measures were also translated unto the control of the ongoing COVID-19 pandemic. Other Ebola intervention programmes were focused on basic services and socio-economic revitalization, nutrition and water, governance, peace building and social cohesion, sanitation and hygiene, and infrastructure.

Although efforts have been made by various Government and other International Organizations to control EVD and mortality by developing new technologies, creating awareness of the virus, building more treatment facilities, and given appropriate orientations to health workers involved in the treatments and vaccine development would be helpful.

Democratic Republic of Congo (DRC) is a Central African country in the Sub-Saharan region. Among other countries, DRC has had the most episodes of the EVD in history. The socioeconomic, humanitarian, and geopolitical issues surrounding the region and the Ebola viral diseases presented a volatile but complex situation for the control strategy. There are, however, critical questions worth considering. What is the knowledge gap of the affected populace towards the Ebola viral disease and the possible treatments and vaccines? How to address issues regarding Ebola vaccines and therapeutic misconception? Is there any external interference for effective control campaign? Are there any fears, mistrust towards the healthcare providers, and any potential selection bias? Similarly, the willingness of populace to participate in Ebola vaccine trials and/ or inoculations has been strongly coupled with alleged risk of Ebola infection as was reported of HIV (Jenkins et al., 2000) and neuroticism (Johnson MO, 2000). Health promotion on the benefits of getting vaccinated and the potential risk of severe infection without vaccination is crucial; individuals who feel more vulnerable are more likely to be vaccinated than those who are not.

There is however the danger of potential of 'preventive misconception' after being vaccinated. It is worth noting that the two approved Ebola vaccines by the American FAD and the EMEA are effective against certain Ebola variants, and they do not give broad protection against ALL variants of the Ebola virus disease. "Preventive misconception" (PM) is a state whereby participants of an intervention overestimate the potential protection they will receive from the intervention and may indulge in risky behaviors (Simon et al., 2007). In shingles vaccine study, 32% of respondents demonstrated evidence of PM, 24% of participants overestimated the likelihood of personal effects of the vaccine, while under 15% underestimated the protection (Joffe., 2014).

These misconceptions of PM and increased risky behaviors may occur among certain participants thwarting control efforts amidst the availability of vaccines (Jenkins et al., 2000). Ebola, HIV, and hepatitis vaccines trials clearly differ due to the variableness of the received protection and the case fatalities of these conditions, but participants' view in each of these sets of trials may have some similarities. Therefore, the lack of trust and the misunderstandings of the risk compensation of the health condition could result in the exponential spread of the disease. This scenario is applicable in the ongoing COVID-19 pandemic despite the availability of effective vaccines (Adusei-Mensah et al., 2021). Ebola vaccine studies and treatment/ prevention interventions should thus seek to develop better ways of communicating with the affected communities. Miscommunication has been reported to be one of the banes against COVID-19 vaccine acceptance globally (Adusei-Mensah et al., 2022). Thus, better methods of public education including platforms like this book chapter are urgently needed to examine the extent to which such misconceptions, risk disinhibition, fear and beliefs leading to lack of trust for healthcare systems and providers. Modern technological tools poses another window for brighter and an 'all encompassing' opportunity to address these challenges and to deal with the attitudinal and behavioral factors to probe for instance, against communication barriers in the hard to reach areas of the endemic regions. Participants' potential misunderstandings of the Ebola vaccine efficacy and safety communication could also pose challenges in the acceptance of the various Ebola interventions in the region (Fink., 2015).

Care must also be taken on the best means to convey the complexities of the situation and the need for the preventive interventions in participants' own local languages. These can help to overcome miscommunication and miscomprehension. For instance, some participants in a malaria vaccine trial were reported of misunderstanding the basic concepts of the trial (Krosin et al., 2006). It is believed that most of the sub-Saharan African languages, may not have words for "experimental drug/ vaccine trial," (Fink., 2015) which, makes it more challenging for accurate communication of the same. Health promotion interventions aimed at improving health knowledge would promote confidence of affected communities in the health services, and it is a critical step in the case of the Ebola virus disease.

Technological Development and Impact

The development of new technologies including temperature sensors, the Agent-Based Simulations of Siettos et al (2015), and the Oppia mobile for learners and tutors, education, and treatment facilities to fight the Ebola disease have help to chalk some successes in the fight against the disease. However, the Ebola outbreak in the crisis faced DR. Congo and the ongoing 2023 outbreak in Uganda present a complex situation for public health professionals due to multiple factors. One of such is the non-existing variant specific vaccine for the Uganda ongoing outbreak which is impeding the progress in the control of the Ebola disease despite the availability of two brands of vaccines (ECDC 2023). In addition, lack of conformity to Ebola control strategies by Ebola patients has been identified as one of the obstacles against the control effort.

The major challenges faced by field health professionals in the DR Congo Ebola outbreak were outlined previously.

- lack of knowledge and understanding of the disease and the treatment options by the local community leading to mistrust of the health professionals and the information provided by the health professionals.
- Mobility and transportation of health professionals to some parts of the country was also affected by political instability
- Mistrust and miscommunication
- Lack of definitive treatment modalities
- Partly due to lack of effective vaccines for all Ebola disease virus' variants

Transmission and Pathogenesis of EVD

Ebola virus disease (EVD) is a zoonotic disease with animals like fruit bats, chimpanzees, monkeys, etc as reservoir (Fauci, 2014). Infection is through contact with the fluids from the reservoir or another infected person. EVD is endemic in the Central African region, the natural geographic distribution of fruit bats. Inter-human transmission occurs through direct contact with the bodily fluids of infected person, and secondary contact with contaminated environments with such fluids. Infectivity is less during the asymptomatic phase (first 1-3 days), and it increases with time as the disease progresses. Health care professionals are especially at risk with the EVD when they are not well protected; seven out of the confirmed 55 deaths (CF 39%) in the ongoing Uganda outbreak are health care workers (ECDC, 2023). Access to Personal protective equipment (PPE), and maintaining social distances helps curtail the transmission (WHO, 2014). Two approved vaccines for some variants of the virus but currently there are no definitive therapy for EVD treatment. Recovery has been hugely due to the immune system and supportive care; the supportive care's quality is crucial in informing the management outcome. During the 2014 outbreak, the case fatality was 0% in the UK and Spain, 25% in the USA compared to 39-100% in some developing countries in the West and Central Africa (CDC 2022). The gastrointestinal EVD begins as a feverish illness, often with myalgia and exhaustion and progress with vomiting and diarrhea which occurs in about 70% EVD cases (Fowler et al., 2014). Body fluid replacement, body electrolyte and acid management are essential components of the supportive care. Unexplained hemorrhaging from the gastrointestinal tract is experienced by some 20% of EVD cases in the late phase of the disease trajectory (Fowler et al., 2014).

Treatment Options

Responses to the past and recent Ebola outbreaks are met with several treatment options to the affected population; different kinds of viruses including Ebola virus (EBV), convalescent whole blood, and convalescent plasma are used to treat the affected individuals. In a 1995 outbreak of Ebola virus disease in the DRC, blood of convalescent patients was administered to affected patients resulting in a fatality rate less than 80% (Mupapa et al., 1999). Other potential management therapies like small antiviral molecules (Favipiravir), RNA based drugs, Ribavirin, and monoclonal antibodies exist (Fisher-Hoch et al., 1995). As the episodes of the EBV keeps emerging at an unprecedented rate, more vaccines and therapeutic interventions and inter-state collaborations are encouraged including the upscaling of the ZMapp by Defyrus, (Qiu, et al. 2014).

MODEL PROPOSAL

In a viral non-curable disease like Ebola, interventions aimed at prevention is key in achieving the ultimate health outcome, but most of the available models falls short in this regard especially reducing zoonotic host-human transmission. In addition, the political instability in some of the countries in the region also impedes information flow, reducing trust and thwarts the health outcomes of the available interventions.

A modified SEIHFR model is believed to give health returns with the intent of improving health outcomes in all the three interventions in the model while educating and promoting transmission reduction effort from the zoonotic host to humans. We propose a multidirectional strategy in tackling this complex situation and improve health outcomes-

The SEIHFR Model

Figure 1 is an illustration of a modified SEIHFR model. SEIHFR is an acronym for S (susceptible and at-risk persons), E (exposed population), I (infectious persons posing risk in the community), H (hospitalized patients), F (funerals of the dead from EVD) and R (persons removed from the model via recovery/ death). The green is the intervention aiming at reducing transmission in the target population. The orange represents the intervention aiming at enhancing hospitalization of the infected to lessening infectivity. The blue is aimed at plummeting spread at burials. The interventional transitions are represented with broken arrows (Seitos et al., 2014).

Figure 1. SEIHFR model

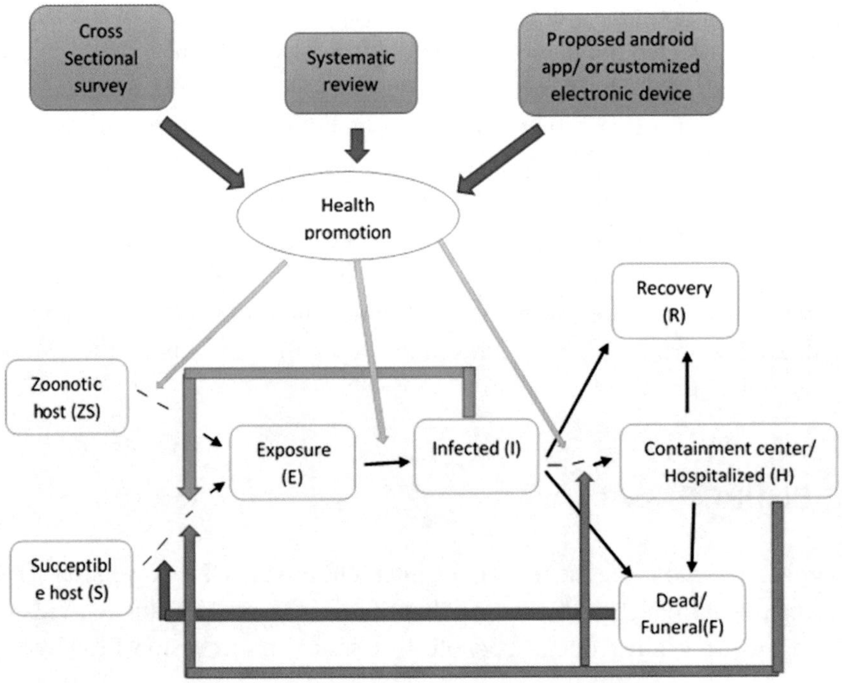

COVID-19 DISEASE

Attitude to get Vaccinated

As it is known that vaccines do not save lives; vaccination does. Nearly 2 decades after the approval of rotavirus vaccine by the FDA and the WHO, yet only about 60% of the world's children have received complete dose of the rotavirus vaccine (Kim et al., 2021). COVID-19 vaccine preferences, hesitancy and an 'access gap' would have dramatic consequences on lives (Kim et al., 2021). There are questions that are common to vaccines globally; access issues, logistics and supply chain management, and vaccine administration (Kim et al., 2021). The scale and urgency of the current pandemic makes it even more dicey, requiring continues research to promote acceptance rate. Briefly, some of these several factors that may thwart the use of COVID-19 vaccines include: The programmatic scale for different working and age groups, logistics with consideration on cold-chain facilities for mRNA vaccines of Moderna (−20 °C, lasting maximum 7-days) and Pfizer (−70 °C lasting maximum 3 days) which are exclusively thought-provoking issue for use in Low- and Middle-income countries (LMICs). Again, of particularly important in Europe is the acceptability of the various COVID-19 vaccine platforms under mass use. In a previous study, acceptance in the region was about 75% (Lazarus et al., 2021a). But this was a prospective study without the existence of various platforms with varying phase III efficacy and safety profiles.

Of great interest of vaccine acceptability is the public's attitude towards vaccine safety, their importance, and effectiveness. Distrust in the safety and effectiveness of vaccines have been consistently associated with vaccine uptake (de Figueiredo et al., 2020). Although the general population of Europe have previously indicated positive attitudes towards vaccines (Paul et al., 2021), they did not indicate which vaccines types or platforms they would like to be vaccinated with. Previous study suggests close to 26% of the adults population across seven European countries were uncertainty and unwilling to get a COVID-19 vaccine when available (Neumann-Böhme et al., 2020b), the real figures in practice are much higher favoring certain vaccine platforms (Boffey, 2021). In the same study, about 70-80% of Europeans were ready to receive the COVID-19 vaccine when available (Neumann-Böhme et al., 2020b). Specifically, 73.9% of the participants (n=7664) from Denmark, France, Germany, Italy, Portugal, the Netherlands, and the UK were willing to get vaccinated against COVID-19. Though, Neumann-Böhme and colleagues identified fear of possible side effects of the future COVID-19 vaccines as a major reason for not wanting to be vaccinated against COVID-19, it has become clear that most of the riot in Europe towards COVID-19 vaccine preferences are related to efficacy.

The above poses significant challenge in achieving the high vaccination coverage required to control the pandemic and return to near normal life.

With the global supply and production chain stretched to the limit and scarcity of raw materials to meet high vaccine demand, it is important to evaluate the available vaccines to see if it is worth being choosy and picky or accepting whichever vaccine made available to you to help control the pandemic.

Characteristics of the COVID-19 Vaccines in Mass Administration in Europe

The Pfizer/BioNTech and Modena are mRNA vaccines expressing the COVID-19 spike glycoprotein. In principle, these vaccines use the body's DNA to translate the genetic message from the COVID-19's viral mRNA into the spike glycoprotein's De novo synthesis. The translated spike glycoprotein then induces the body's immune response against future viral infection. However, the vaccines from Gamaleya and AstraZeneca-Oxford University express the spike protein from adenovirus vector platforms. In principle, the AstraZeneca vaccine uses a spike protein expressed from chimpanzee's adenovirus (Kim et al., 2021). It is worth noting that, effective vaccination is a part of active, all-inclusive control of a pandemic (Kim et al., 2021). Data from the AstraZeneca's vaccine phase III trial suggest that, the overall vaccine efficacy 14 days after the second dose was 66·7% (ChAdOx1 nCoV-19), (Table 1), and no hospital admissions was observed after the initial 21-day (Voysey et al., 2021). Less than 1% of the 12,282 participants had serious adverse events but no vaccine related death observed (Voysey et al., 2021). They had a tentatively efficacy of 76·0% with a single standard dose between 22 to day 90 days after vaccination (Voysey et al., 2021). The Pfizer BionTech vaccine reported 94% - 95% efficacy in their phase three trials after their second dose administered weeks apart whiles Modena reported similar efficacies with similar dose variations (Pfizer Inc., n.d.). The Modena's mRNA-1273 vaccine against COVID-19 encrypting for a prefusion stabilized form of the Spike (S) protein(Moderna, 2020). According to the WHO report, the Modena vaccine has efficacy of approximately 92% in protecting against COVID-19, 14 days after the first dose (*The Moderna COVID-19 (MRNA-1273) Vaccine*, n.d.), (Table 1).

Table 1. Basic information on the COVID-19 vaccines in mass use

Vaccine	Trial type	Trial centers	Adverse effect	Total participants	Prev. of infection	Prev. severe and hospitalized COVID-19	Prev. mortality to COVID-19
Oxford-AstraZeneca (ChAdOx1 nCoV-19)	Phase III double blind PCT	The UK, South Africa, and Brazil	0·9% transverse myelitis and headache	32,459	66·7 - 76·0% after 22 days of single dose.	Over 86%	100%
Pfizer-Biontech BNT162b2	Phase III double blind PCT	US, Brazil, Argentina, Turkey, South Africa, and Germany	3.8% fatigue and headache at 2.0%	43,000	94%-95%	Close to 100%.	100%
Modena (mRNA-1273)	Phase III double blind PCT	US and multiple countries	Fatigue, myalgia, arthralgia, headache, and erythema	30,000	94.1%	Nearly 100	100%

Key: PCB = placebo control trial, prev. = Preventing,
Sources: (Voysey et al., 2021; Pfizer Inc., n.d.; WHO, 2021; Pfizer Inc, 2020; AstraZeneca, 2021).

Study Design

A correlational research design was chosen in the present study to measures a association or the impact of the SARS-COV-2 vaccine types and its preferential uptake in the EU region. The researchers did not alter the effect or the outcome in the present study.

Methods

Vaccination data in the European region on the EU member states was obtained from EU center for disease control's vaccine tracker (EUCDC) (EUCDC, 2021) on the 5th March 2021. The data is publicly available for academic and non-for-profit use. However, the authorities were informed through email communication on the intent to use the data. As a result, all ethical or legal requirements for the use of the data was met. The extracted data was organized for analysis using Microsoft's Excel 2010. Descriptive and statistical analysis were performed using IBM's SPSS version 21 and analysis at 95% confidence interval and statistically significant difference was considered at $p < 0.05$.

Results

Data was obtained from European Centre for Disease Prevention and Control, COVID-19 vaccine tracker (EUCDC, 2021). The difference between the total vaccines distributed to the member states (n=47,319,245) and the vaccines administered by the members (n=34,827,459) as of by 5th March 2021 was significantly low ($p < 0.05$) at 95%CI (p=0.00) (EUCDC, 2021). Though there have been production challenges by vaccine producers in meeting the huge demand, the figure 2 presents a clear difference in the doses received compared to the doses administered in the EU region. The received-administered differences vary between countries but very conspicuous in countries like France, Germany for AstraZeneca vaccines for AstraZeneca vaccines (Figure 2). The overall administered by platform was observed to be low as 50.927 +/- 4.6258 SE for AstraZeneca, 50.822 +/- 5.0502 SE for Modena and as high as 86.285 +/- 2.1052 SE for Pfizer/Biontech vaccines (Table 2 figure 3).

Figure 2. COVID-19 vaccine doses received and administer in Europe as at 05th March 2021
Note: AZ = AstraZeneca, PB = Pfizer-Biotech and M = Modena.

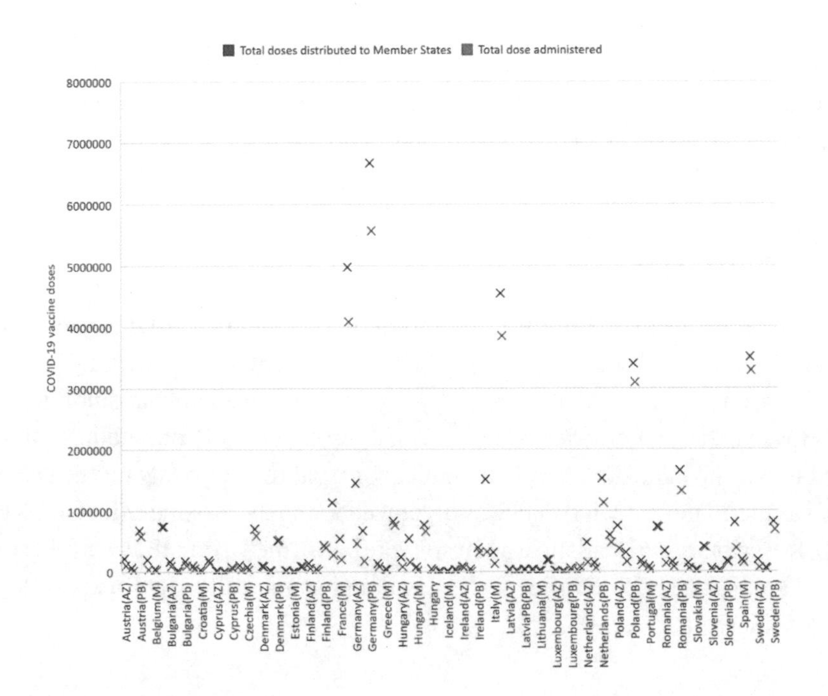

In univariate automatic modeling analysis, there observed a model effect in the vaccine acceptance by the vaccine type (figure 6) with a strong 'R' square value (R Squared = 0.974 (Adjusted R Squared = 0.973) (Figure 8 in the Appendix).

Table 2. Descriptive statistics of the percentage of vaccines administered

Product	Mean Statistic +/- (Std. Error of mean)	95% Confidence Interval
AstraZeneca	50.927 +/- 4.6258	41.419 - 60.436
Modena	50.822 +/- 5.0502	40.441 - 61.202
Pfizer/Biontech	86.285 +/- 2.1052	81.957 - 90.612
Average %	62.231 +/- 2.9438	

Figure 3. Descriptive statistics of the percentage of vaccines administered

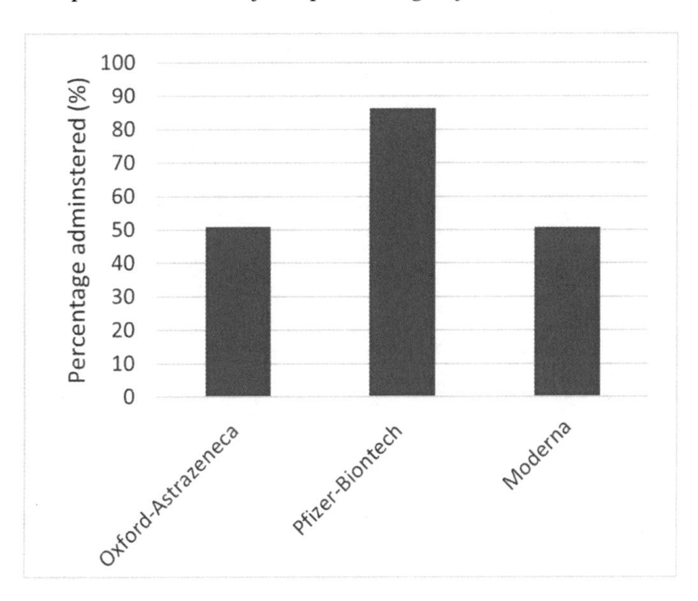

Table 3. ANOVA analysis compared to the vaccine doses received

		Sum of Squares	df	Mean Square	F	Sig.
Total dose administered	Between Groups	77145352756208.100	82	940796984831.806	20902.012	.000
	Within Groups	90019754.500	2	45009877.250		
	Total	77145442775962.600	84			
Vaccine Categories	Between Groups	149.294	82	1.821	.910	.662
	Within Groups	4.000	2	2.000		
	Total	153.294	84			

There exists a significant difference between the received and the administered vaccines by the member states. Compared to distributed doses, the administered doses were significantly lower than the control (p=0.00) at 95% CI table 3.

The stem plot shows the mean statistics and the deviations of the various vaccine platforms in the region. There exists great variation in the administered Modena and AstraZeneca vaccines in the region compared to that of the Pfizer-Biontech and the three other less distributed vaccines (Figure 4).

Figure 4. Stem plot

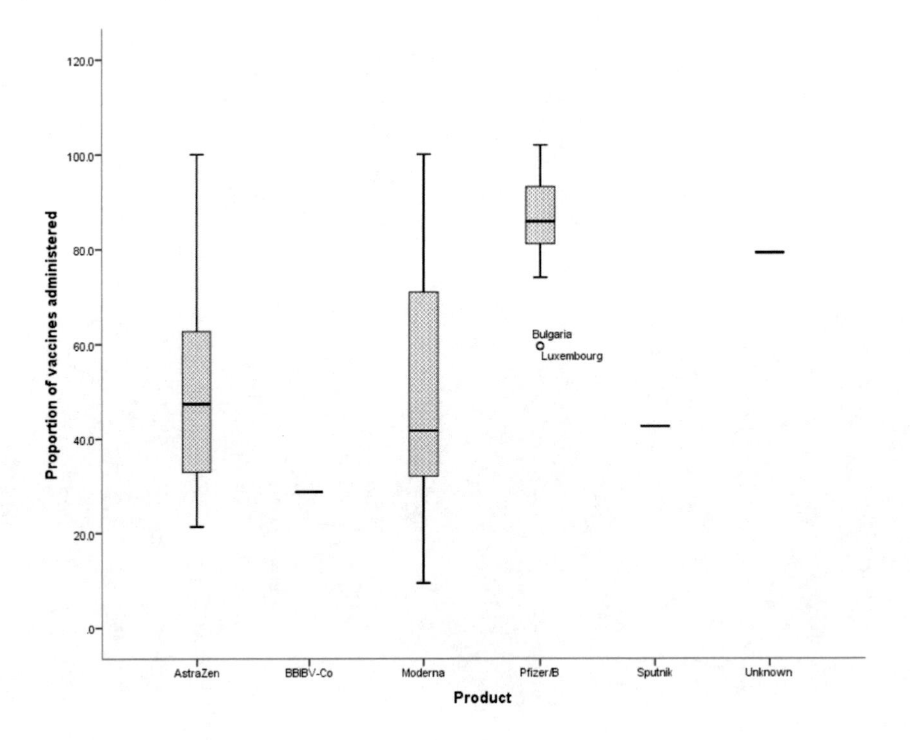

Over 1 million Pfizer vaccines have already been administered in the region while the acceptance of AstraZeneca, BBIBV-CorV vaccines administered compared to doses distributed are on the low side (Figure 5A; left). The second graph (Figure 5B; right). shows the marginal means of the administered vaccines from the univariate analysis of variances. The corrected model was statistically significant (p=0.00). The uncorrected model also showed statistically significant difference with p=0.034 with spearman's correlation analysis.

Figure 5. Administered vaccines

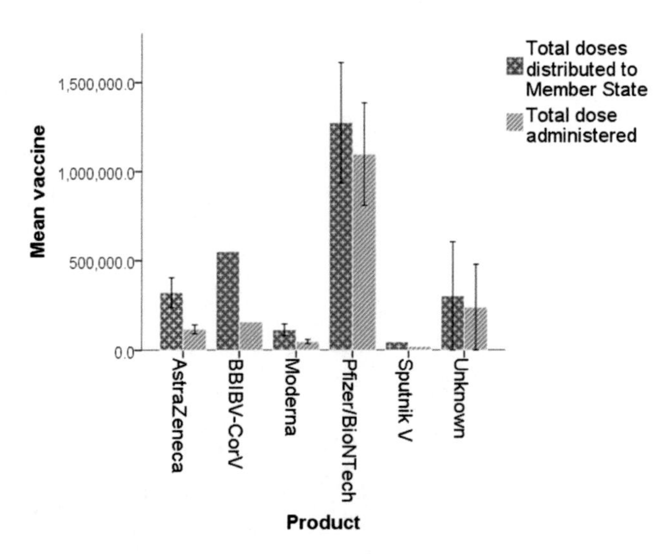

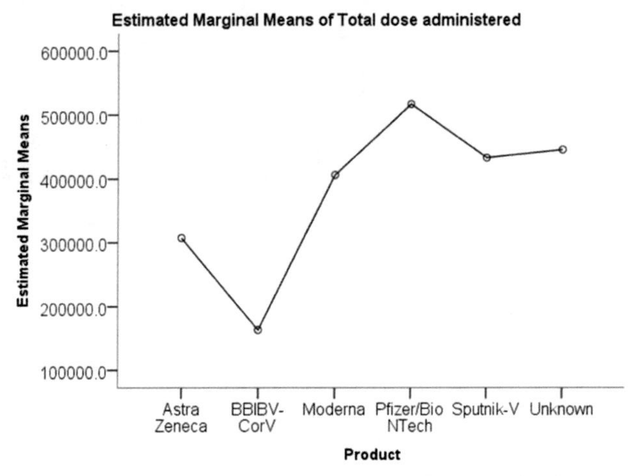

The acceptance of the COVID-19 vaccines are very high in countries like Denmark (100%) and Lithuania (100%) with 100 percent utilization of all the received vaccines. On the centrally, the administered rates are low in countries including Poland, France, Germany, Italy, and Spain. These four countries accounts for over 50% of the unused vaccines in the Eu member states (Figure 5). This findings confirms the previous report on COVID vaccine hesitancies(Boffey, 2021), (Lazarus et al., 2021a),(Etzioni-Friedman & Etzioni, 2020).

Figure 6. Country performance of the distributed and administered vaccines
Germany, France and Italy respectively received the highest number of vaccines as compared to the rest of the countries.

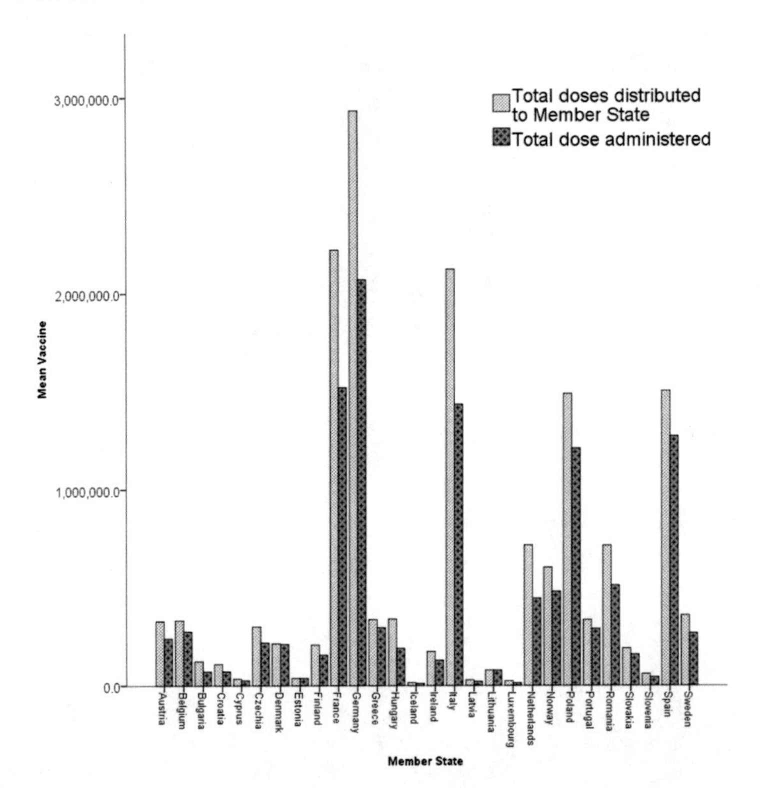

Figure 7. Automatic lineal model. Vaccine type significantly influenced on the administration of the vaccine in the study area
R Squared = .974 (Adjusted R Squared = .973).

Model Building Summary

Target: Total dose administered

	Step
	1
Information Criterion	3,515.307
Effect Product_transformed	✓

The model building method is Forward Stepwise using the Information Criterion.
A checkmark means the effect is in the model at this step.

DISCUSSION

The availability of safe and effective vaccine alone does not save lives; it is the inoculation plus other public health measures that do. Recent reports suggest the growing trend in vaccine preferential bias in parts of the world but not much in Europe. Defined by the WHO, 'Vaccination is a simple, safe, and effective way of protecting people against harmful diseases, before they come into contact with them''. (WHO, 2014). Vaccines use the body's natural immune system to build resistance to specific infections prior to contact to the pathogen. As important as vaccines are, it must be made clear that having safe and effective vaccines alone to not guarantee protection, it is the immunization plus other health measures that ensures protection. It is therefore important to attach a particular importance to factors that influences vaccine uptake. There has been numerous studies on vaccine hesitancy and acceptability in the past and factors such as trust of the vaccine's safety and efficacy are of particular importance (Lazarus et al., 2021a), and these factors are shared globally (Ehde et al., 2021, Gan et al., 2021). These previously identified factors need a more critical consideration by policy makers to promote vaccine uptake. It must be stated that since the vaccine trials were not initially planned head-to-head, a mere comparison of the clinical trials alone of the various vaccine platforms would be a great mistake. These trials were performed at different phases of the pandemic either before or during the confirmation of the variant strains such as the B.1.1.7 of the UK and South Africa, the B.1.351 of the Brazil, California which are more virulent than the formal (CDC, 2020). It is worth noting that all these vaccines are doing best what they ought to do; that is to be safe and to activate the immunes system to fight against diseases and death. People have experienced flu after receiving flu shots in the past, however the assurance after receiving flu vaccine is protection from serious flu during the flu season. Similarly, the current corona vaccines that are safe and nearly 100% assurance of protection from serious COVID-19 and or mortality from the disease should receive similar attention if the populace would like to return to the near normal in the shortest possible time.

Findings from the present study shows that the acceptance of the COVID-19 vaccine is generally lower than predicted in previous studies that investigated the wiliness of acceptance COD-19 vaccines if they are available. Average acceptance rate of 62.231% +/- 2.9438% was observed in the present study which is lower than reported previous studies. In a large global survey published in nature, 71.5% of participants (n=13,426) reported their wiliness to take a COVID-19 vaccine when available while 48.1% reported of taken it based on their employer's recommendation (Lazarus et al., 2021b). They however observed differences in acceptance rates ranged from almost 90% (in China) to less than 55% (in Russia). High acceptance rate of about 90% in the China and Indonesia has been reported in different than France, 78% (Dror et al., 2020)(Harapan et al., 2020) and other parts of the world (Lazarus et al., 2021b)(Harapan et al., 2020). In a multi-state European survey, acceptance rate of 73.9% (7664) has been reported with participants from Denmark, France, Germany, Italy, Portugal, the Netherlands, and the UK (Neumann-Böhme et al., 2020a). The observed lower acceptance rate of 62.231% +/- 2.9438% in the present study (Table 2, Figure 2) is lower compared to the reported wiliness rate (73.9%) to vaccinate with COVID-19 vaccines prior to the availability of the vaccines in the region.

High differences in the acceptance rate were also observed in the present study between the vaccine variants. Among the most popular vaccines in the region during the study, a high acceptance rate of 86.285 +/- 2.1052% was observed for Pfizer/Biontech vaccine while lower rates of 50.927 +/- 4.6258% for AstraZeneca vaccine and 50.822 +/- 5.0502% for Modena and less than 50% for BBIBV-CorV vaccine

(Table 2) were observed. It could be observed that Pfizer/Biontech vaccine received higher uptake than the pre general COVID-19 vaccination surveys in the region 77.3% (Neumann-Böhme et al., 2020a). However, the rates observed in the present study for both Modena and AstraZeneca is much lower (about 51%) compared to previous pre-vaccination surveys (Neumann-Böhme et al., 2020a, Freeman et al., 2020). Major factors such as misinterpretation and unfair-comparison of the clinical trials data of the present major vaccines in the region, conspiracy beliefs that foster mistrust, efficacy, and fear of both long- and short-term side effects could be responsible for the lower vaccine up-take observed in the present study. The biasness in the uptake observed in the present study between Pfizer/Biontech and the other vaccine groups could be hugely due to the differences in their phase's III safety and efficacy data. It must be noted that, both Modena and Pfizer/Biontech are RNA vaccines, but the uptake is higher for Pfizer/Biontech which recorded phase III trial efficacy of about 95% compared to 94% for Modena (Table 1). Again, Pfizer/Biontech also recorded a 100% in averting server COVID-19 in its 43,000 participants in the phase III trials.

Country comparison in the present study (Figure 5) shows lower utilization rates for countries like Poland, France, Germany, Italy, and Spain accounting for nearly 50% of all unused vaccines. Previously, lower rates of 53.7% for Italy (Vecchia et al., 2020), 58.9% for France (Lazarus et al., 2021b) and 68.4 for Germany have been reported which corresponds to the rates observed in the present study. It is worth noting that, the clinical trials of some COVID-19 vaccine candidates were put on partial hold due to the report of a serious adverse event (Mahase, 2020). While there are concerns of the lack of or insufficient publicity of trial data or extremely limited data of some candidates including the Russian Sputnik vaccine prior to general public use (Burki, 2020). Again, an area of consideration is the need to clear the misconception of the growing concern about future risk of worsening diseases' pathogenesis through antibody-dependent enhancement (ADE) after immunization which was observed in the SARS-COV 1 epidemic's vaccine candidates in *in vitro* studies (Yip et al., 2016, Yip et al., 2014). However, the risk of ADE is usually picked up during pre-clinical and large scale clinical trials phase observed as could be observed in HIV-1 vaccine candidate (Staprans et al., 1995), FIV vaccine candidates (Maj et al., 1992) and EIAV vaccine candidates (Raabe et al., 1999). It must be stated that, proper adjuvant selection may significantly influence the vaccine's associated ADE risks.

CONCLUSION

Vaccines train the immune system to create antibodies a particular disease. Though data on how long the obtained immunity from the various COVID-19 vaccine platforms will wan/persist are lacking, the available data indicate their ability to safely protect the population from serious COD-19 and mortality from the disease. Misinformation and misunderstanding of the incompatibility of the various phase III trials has led to rejection and low acceptance of certain COVID-19 vaccine platforms in the EU region. As a fact, vaccine hesitancy remains an insistent global threat. The present study observed negative preferential bias towards AstraZeneca and Modena vaccines (50% acceptance rate) compared to Pfizer vaccines (over 80% acceptance rate) in the EU region. The finding shows there exists a significant challenge in achieving the high vaccination coverage required to control the pandemic and return to near normal life. These call for structured health education in order to promote vaccine uptake and to promote effective control of the pandemic is urgent. These observations are of concern and needs much consideration since it slows down the control measures and the lingering of the pandemic. Such educations should put some level of emphasis on the safety, efficacy, sufficiency, and availability of Trials data and education on the ADE as reported in various viral vaccine trials.

AUTHOR STATEMENTS

The present study did not made use of any animal or human subjects in any phase of the study requiring ethical permission. However, permission for the use of the data from the European Center for Disease Control (ECDC) was granted based on the conditions of use (research and noncommercial purposes) by ECDC. No funding was received from any external sources, and it was privately funded by the researchers. The researchers have no competing interests in carrying out this present study.

REFERENCES

Sauramäki, J. M., Adusei-Mensah, F., Hakalehto, J., Armon, R., & Hakalehto, E. (2022). 7 Pandemic situation and safe transportation, storage, and distribution for food catering and deliveries. In E. Hakalehto (Ed.), Microbiology of Food Quality: Challenges in Food Production and Distribution During and After the Pandemics (pp. 149–172). De Gruyter. .

Adebamowo, C., Bah-Sow, O., & Binka, F. (2014). Randomised controlled trials for Ebola: Practical and ethical issues. *Lancet*, *384*(9952), 1423–1424.

Adusei-Mensah, F., Hakalehto, E., & Tikkanen-Kaukanen, C. (2021). Microbiological and Chemical Safety of African Herbal and Natural Products. In E. Hakalehto (ed.) Challenges in Food Production and Distribution During and After the Pandemic. Degruyter.

Adusei-Mensah, F., Kauhanen, J., & Tikkanen-Kaukanen, C. (2022). The Need for a Paradigm Shift in the Existing Strategies for Effective COVID-19 Control. *Online Journal of Contemporary Medicine*.

AstraZeneca. (2021). *A Phase III Randomized, Double-blind, Placebo-controlled Multicenter Study in Adults, to Determine the Safety, Efficacy, and Immunogenicity of AZD1222, a Non-replicating ChAdOx1 Vector Vaccine, for the Prevention of COVID-19 (Clinical Trial Registration No. NCT04516746)*. clinicaltrials.gov. https://clinicaltrials.gov/ct2/show/NCT04516746

Boffey, D. (2021, February 25). Revealed: Four in five Oxford Covid jabs delivered to EU not yet used. *The Guardian*. https://www.theguardian.com/world/2021/feb/25/acceptance-pro blem-as-most-oxford-covid-jabs-delivered-to-eu-not-yet-used

Burki, T. K. (2020). The Russian vaccine for COVID-19. *The Lancet. Respiratory Medicine*, *8*(11), e85–e86. doi:10.1016/S2213-2600(20)30402-1 PMID:32896274

CDC. (2020, February 11). COVID-19 and Your Health. Centers for Disease Control and Prevention. CDC. https://www.cdc.gov/coronavirus/2019-ncov/transmission/varia nt.html

CDC. (2022). History of Ebola Virus Disease (EVD) Outbreaks. CDC.

de Figueiredo, A., Simas, C., Karafillakis, E., Paterson, P., & Larson, H. J. (2020). Mapping global trends in vaccine confidence and investigating barriers to vaccine uptake: A large-scale retrospective temporal modelling study. *Lancet*, *396*(10255), 898–908. doi:10.1016/S0140-6736(20)31558-0 PMID:32919524

Dror, A. A., Eisenbach, N., Taiber, S., Morozov, N. G., Mizrachi, M., Zigron, A., Srouji, S., & Sela, E. (2020). Vaccine hesitancy: The next challenge in the fight against COVID-19. *European Journal of Epidemiology*, *35*(8), 775–779. doi:10.100710654-020-00671-y PMID:32785815

Ehde, D. M., Roberts, M. K., Herring, T. E., & Alschuler, K. N. (2021). Willingness to obtain COVID-19 vaccination in adults with multiple sclerosis in the United States. *Multiple Sclerosis and Related Disorders*, *49*, 102788. doi:10.1016/j.msard.2021.102788 PMID:33508570

Etzioni-Friedman, T., & Etzioni, A. (2020). Adherence to Immunization: Rebuttal of Vaccine Hesitancy. *Acta Haematologica, 1–5*. doi:10.1159/000511760 PMID:33202404

EUCDC. (2021). *COVID-19 Vaccine Tracker.* European Centre for Disease Prevention and Control. https://qap.ecdc.europa.eu/public/extensions/COVID-19/vaccin e-tracker.html#distribution-tab.

European Centre for Disease Prevention and Control (EUCDC). (2023). *Ebola outbreak in Uganda, as of 3 January 2023.* Europa.

Fauci, A. S. (2014). Ebola–underscoring the global disparities in health care resources. *The New England Journal of Medicine, 371*(12), 1084–1086. doi:10.1056/NEJMp1409494 PMID:25119491

Fink, S. (2015). Ebola spreads in sex prompt a CDC warning. *New York Times.*

Fisher-Hoch, S. P., Khan, J. A., Rehman, S., Mirza, S., Khurshid, M., & McCormick, J. B. (1995). Crimean Congo-haemorrhagic fever treated with oral ribavirin. *Lancet, 346*(8973), 472–474. doi:10.1016/S0140-6736(95)91323-8 PMID:7637481

Fowler, R., Fletcher, T., Fischer, W. II, Lamontagne, F., Jacob, S., Brett-Major, D., Lawler, J. V., Jacquerioz, F. A., Houlihan, C., O'Dempsey, T., Ferri, M., Adachi, T., Lamah, M.-C., Bah, E. I., Mayet, T., Schieffelin, J., McLellan, S. L., Senga, M., Kato, Y., & Bausch, D. (2014). Caring for critically Ill patients with Ebola virus disease. Perspectives from West Africa. *American Journal of Respiratory and Critical Care Medicine, 190*(7), 733–737. doi:10.1164/rccm.201408-1514CP PMID:25166884

Freeman, D., Loe, B. S., Chadwick, A., Vaccari, C., Waite, F., Rosebrock, L., Jenner, L., Petit, A., Lewandowsky, S., Vanderslott, S., Innocenti, S., Larkin, M., Giubilini, A., Yu, L.-M., McShane, H., Pollard, A. J., & Lambe, S. (2020). COVID-19 vaccine hesitancy in the UK: The Oxford coronavirus explanations, attitudes, and narratives survey (Oceans) II. *Psychological Medicine*, 1–15. doi:10.1017/S0033291720005188 PMID:33305716

Gan, L., Chen, Y., Hu, P., Wu, D., Zhu, Y., Tan, J., Li, Y., & Zhang, D. (2021). Willingness to Receive SARS-CoV-2 Vaccination and Associated Factors among Chinese Adults: A Cross Sectional Survey. *International Journal of Environmental Research and Public Health, 18*(4), 1993. doi:10.3390/ijerph18041993 PMID:33670821

Gerussi, V., Peghin, M., Palese, A., Bressan, V., Visintini, E., Bontempo, G., Graziano, E., De Martino, M., Isola, M., & Tascini, C. (2021). Vaccine Hesitancy among Italian Patients Recovered from COVID-19 Infection towards Influenza and Sars-Cov-2 Vaccination. *Vaccines*, *9*(2), 172. doi:10.3390/vaccines9020172 PMID:33670661

Harapan, H., Wagner, A. L., Yufika, A., Winardi, W., Anwar, S., Gan, A. K., Setiawan, A. M., Rajamoorthy, Y., Sofyan, H., & Mudatsir, M. (2020). Acceptance of a COVID-19 Vaccine in Southeast Asia: A Cross-Sectional Study in Indonesia. *Frontiers in Public Health*, *8*, 381. doi:10.3389/fpubh.2020.00381 PMID:32760691

Jenkins, R. A., Torugsa, K., & Markowitz, L. E. (2000). Willingness to participate in HIV-1 vaccine trials among young Thai men. *Sexually Transmitted Infections*, *76*(5), 386–392. doi:10.1136ti.76.5.386 PMID:11141858

Joffe, S. (2014). Evaluating novel therapies during the Ebola epidemic. *Journal of the American Medical Association*, *312*(13), 1299–1300. doi:10.1001/jama.2014.12867 PMID:25211645

Johnson, M. O. (2000). Personality correlates of HIV vaccine trial participation. *Personality and Individual Differences*, *29*(3), 459–467. doi:10.1016/S0191-8869(99)00206-8

Kim, J. H., Marks, F., & Clemens, J. D. (2021). Looking beyond COVID-19 vaccine phase 3 trials. *Nature Medicine*, *27*(2), 205–211. doi:10.103841591-021-01230-y PMID:33469205

Krosin, M. T., Klitzman, R., Levin, B., Cheng, J., & Ranney, M. L. (2006). Problems in comprehension of informed consent in rural and peri-urban Mali, West Africa. *Clinical Trials*, *3*(3), 306–313. doi:10.1191/1740774506cn150oa PMID:16895047

Lazarus, J. V., Ratzan, S. C., Palayew, A., Gostin, L. O., Larson, H. J., Rabin, K., Kimball, S., & El-Mohandes, A. (2021a). A global survey of potential acceptance of a COVID-19 vaccine. *Nature Medicine*, *27*(2), 225–228. doi:10.103841591-020-1124-9 PMID:33082575

Lazarus, J. V., Ratzan, S. C., Palayew, A., Gostin, L. O., Larson, H. J., Rabin, K., Kimball, S., & El-Mohandes, A. (2021b). A global survey of potential acceptance of a COVID-19 vaccine. *Nature Medicine*, *27*(2), 225–228. doi:10.103841591-020-1124-9 PMID:33082575

Mahase, E. (2020). Covid-19: Oxford researchers halt vaccine trial while adverse reaction is investigated. *BMJ (Clinical Research Ed.)*, *370*, m3525. doi:10.1136/bmj.m3525 PMID:32907856

Mj, H., R, O., G, R., Jc, N., & O, J. (1992). Enhancement after feline immunodeficiency virus vaccination. *Veterinary Immunology and Immunopathology*, *35*(1–2), 191–197. doi:10.1016/0165-2427(92)90131-9 PMID:1337397

Moderna. (2020). *Moderna Announces Primary Efficacy Analysis in Phase 3 COVE Study for Its COVID-19 Vaccine Candidate and Filing Today with U.S. FDA for Emergency Use Authorization.* Moderna, Inc. https://investors.modernatx.com/news-releases/news-release-details/moderna-announces-primary-efficacy-analysis-phase-3-cove-study/

Mupapa, K., Massamba, M., Kibadi, K., Kuvula, K., Bwaka, A., Kipasa, M., Colebunders, R., & Muyembe-Tamfum, J. J. (1999). Treatment of Ebola hemorrhagic fever with blood transfusions from convalescent patient. *The Journal of Infectious Diseases*, *179*(s1), S18–S23. doi:10.1086/514298 PMID:9988160

Neumann-Böhme, S., Varghese, N. E., Sabat, I., Barros, P. P., Brouwer, W., van Exel, J., Schreyögg, J., & Stargardt, T. (2020a). Once we have it, will we use it? A European survey on willingness to be vaccinated against COVID-19. *The European Journal of Health Economics*, *21*(7), 977–982. doi:10.100710198-020-01208-6 PMID:32591957

Neumann-Böhme, S., Varghese, N. E., Sabat, I., Barros, P. P., Brouwer, W., van Exel, J., Schreyögg, J., & Stargardt, T. (2020b). Once we have it, will we use it? A European survey on willingness to be vaccinated against COVID-19. *The European Journal of Health Economics: HEPAC: Health Economics in Prevention and Care*, *21*(7), 977–982. doi:10.100710198-020-01208-6 PMID:32591957

Paul, E., Steptoe, A., & Fancourt, D. (2021). Attitudes towards vaccines and intention to vaccinate against COVID-19: Implications for public health communications. *The Lancet Regional Health - Europe, 1*, 100012. doi:10.1016/j.lanepe.2020.100012

Pfizer Inc. (n.d.). *Pfizer and BioNTech Conclude Phase 3 Study of COVID-19 Vaccine Candidate, Meeting All Primary Efficacy Endpoints.* Pfizer. https://www.pfizer.com/news/press-release/press-release-detail/pfizer-and-biontech-conclude-phase-3-study-covid-19-vaccine

Qiu X, Wong G, Audet J, Bello A, Fernando L, et al. (2014). Reversion of advanced Ebola virus disease in nonhuman primates with ZMapp. *Nature 514*(7520):47–53.

Raabe, M. L., Issel, C. J., & Montelaro, R. C. (1999). In vitro antibody-dependent enhancement assays are insensitive indicators of in vivo vaccine enhancement of equine infectious anemia virus. *Virology*, *259*(2), 416–427. doi:10.1006/viro.1999.9772 PMID:10388665

Siettos, C., Anastassopoulou, C., Russo, L., Grigoras, C., & Mylonakis, E. (2015). Modeling the 2014 Ebola Virus Epidemic – Agent-Based Simulations, Temporal Analysis and Future Predictions for Liberia and Sierra Leone. *PLoS Currents*, *7*. doi:10.1371/currents.outbreaks.8d5984114855fc425e699e1a18cdc 6c9 PMID:26064785

Simon, A. E., Wu, A. W., Lavori, P. W., & Sugarman, J. (2007). Preventive misconception: Its nature, presence, and ethical implications of research. *American Journal of Preventive Medicine*, *32*(5), 370–374. doi:10.1016/j.amepre.2007.01.007 PMID:17478261

Staprans, S. I., Hamilton, B. L., Follansbee, S. E., Elbeik, T., Barbosa, P., Grant, R. M., & Feinberg, M. B. (1995). Activation of virus replication after vaccination of HIV-1-infected individuals. *The Journal of Experimental Medicine*, *182*(6), 1727–1737. doi:10.1084/jem.182.6.1727 PMID:7500017

The Moderna COVID-19 (mRNA-1273) vaccine: What you need to know. (n.d.). WHO. https://www.who.int/news-room/feature-stories/detail/the-moderna-covid-19-mrna-1273-vaccine-what-you-need-to-know

Vecchia, C. L., Negri, E., Alicandro, G., & Scarpino, V. (2020). Attitudes towards influenza vaccine and a potential COVID-19 vaccine in Italy and differences across occupational groups, September 2020. *Environmental Health*, *111*(6), 445–448. doi:10.23749/mdl.v111i6.10813 PMID:33311419

Voysey, M., Costa Clemens, S. A., Madhi, S. A., Weckx, L. Y., Folegatti, P. M., Aley, P. K., Angus, B., Baillie, V. L., Barnabas, S. L., Bhorat, Q. E., Bibi, S., Briner, C., Cicconi, P., Clutterbuck, E. A., Collins, A. M., Cutland, C. L., Darton, T. C., Dheda, K., & Dold, C. (2021).Single-dose administration and the influence of the timing of the booster dose on immunogenicity and efficacy of ChAdOx1 nCoV-19 (AZD1222) vaccine: A pooled analysis of four randomised trials. *Lancet*. doi:10.1016/S0140-6736(21)00432-3 PMID:33617777

WHO (2014). *Ground zero in Guinea: The Ebola outbreak smoulders - undetected - for more than 3 months. A retrospective on the first cases of the outbreak*. WHO.

WHO. (2021). *Coronavirus disease (COVID-19): Vaccines*. WHO. https://www.who.int/news-room/q-a-detail/coronavirus-disease-(covid-19)-vaccines

WHO. (n.d.). Vaccines and immunization: What is vaccination? Retrieved March 9, 2021, from https://www.who.int/news-room/q-a-detail/vaccines-and-immunization-what-is-vaccination

Yip, M. S., Leung, H. L., Li, P. H., Cheung, C. Y., Dutry, I., Li, D., Daëron, M., Bruzzone, R., Peiris, J. S., & Jaume, M. (2016). Antibody-dependent enhancement of SARS coronavirus infection and its role in the pathogenesis of SARS. *Hong Kong Medical Journal, Xianggang Yi Xue Za Zhi, 22*(3 Suppl 4), 25–31.

Yip, M. S., Leung, N. H. L., Cheung, C. Y., Li, P. H., Lee, H. H. Y., Daëron, M., Peiris, J. S. M., Bruzzone, R., & Jaume, M. (2014). Antibody-dependent infection of human macrophages by severe acute respiratory syndrome coronavirus. *Virology Journal, 11*(1), 82. doi:10.1186/1743-422X-11-82 PMID:24885320

APPENDIX

Table 4. ANOVA[a]

Model		Sum of Squares	df	Mean Square	F	Sig.
1	Regression	9.724	1	9.724	4.632	.034[b]
	Residual	184.731	88	2.099		
	Total	194.456	89			
a. Dependent Variable: Product						
b. Predictors: (Constant), Total dose administered						

Table 5. Univariate Analysis of variance table

Tests of Between-Subjects Effects					
Dependent Variable: Total dose administered					
Source	**Type III Sum of Squares**	**df**	**Mean Square**	**F**	**Sig.**
Corrected Model	75176379371710.270[a]	6	12529396561951.710	496.324	.000
Intercept	69379049655.741	1	69379049655.741	2.748	.101
TDosesReceived	56312128370120.984	1	56312128370120.984	2230.678	.000
Product	586230979722.406	5	117246195944.481	4.644	.001
Error	1969063404252.318	78	25244402618.619		
Total	91318156498552.000	85			
Corrected Total	77145442775962.580	84			
a. R Squared = .974 (Adjusted R Squared = .973)					

Figure 8. Univariate Analysis of variance table plot

Estimated Means

Target: Total doses distributed to Member State

Estimated means charts for the top ten significant effects (p<.05) are displayed.

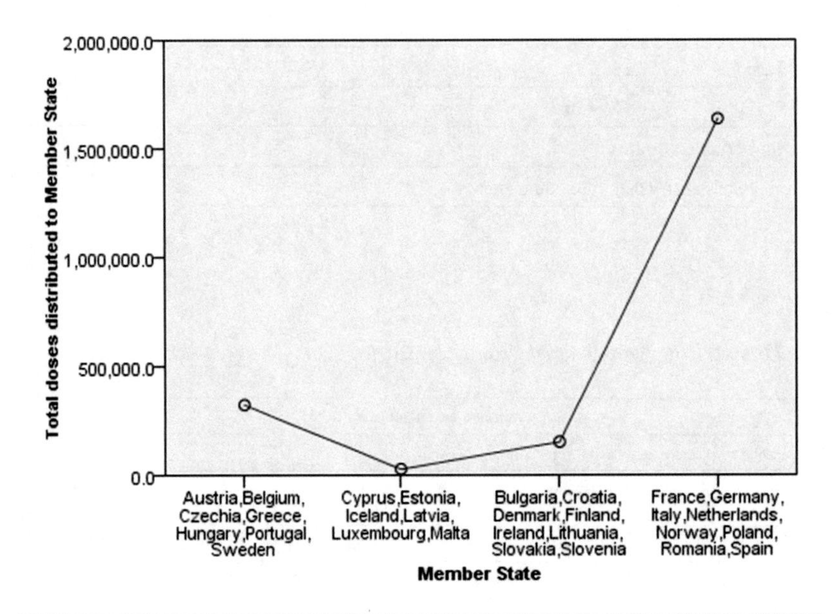

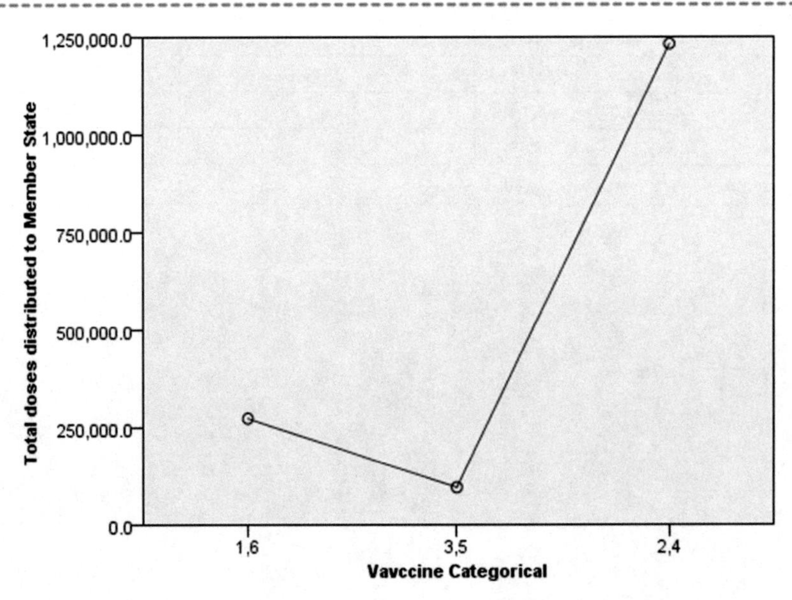

Chapter 13
An Enhanced Gabor Filter Based on Heat-Diffused Top Hat Transform for Retinal Blood Vessel Segmentation

Sonali Dash
https://orcid.org/0000-0002-6153-2655
Chandigarh University, India

Priyadarsan Parida
GIET University, India

Gupteswar Sahu
Raghu Engineering College, India

ABSTRACT

Precise retinal blood vessels segmentation is a vital assignment to diagnose many pathological ailments. Here, an efficient approach has been presented for the segmentation of retinal vessels that includes pre-processing, segmentation, and the post-processing stage. In the pre-processing stage, the retinal images are denoised and restored with the connected vessel lines by utilizing anisotropic diffusion filter. In the next step, retinal images are enhanced by using top hat transform. Further, Gabor filters of various orientations are applied on top hat transformed images to obtain different characteristics of the retinal images. Finally, hysteresis thresholding is applied for the segmentation. The accomplishment of the recommended methodology is inspected with other competitive combined methodologies based on median filter and Gabor filter using different performance indicators. The approach can be used effectively for diagnosis of different ocular disorders, like diabetic retinopathy and glaucoma, which can be followed by different surgical procedures for further treatment.

DOI: 10.4018/978-1-6684-6957-6.ch013

INTRODUCTION

In the healthcare industry, biomedical images are the primary data source and, simultaneously, utmost hard for analysis. Artificial Intelligence (AI) is a technique to automatically analyse and prevent the elevated risks of developing chronic conditions and help patients to avoid long-term health problems (Mohanty, Parida, & Patra, 2021, 2022; Parida, 2020; Rout & Parida, 2020; Rout, Parida, & Patnaik, 2021). As these automated structures become widespread in the healthcare industry, they may bring about progressive changes for radiologists, clinicians, ophthalmologists, and even patients using imaging technology to monitor the treatments. Thus, it is vital to develop an appropriate prediction model and link carefully for measurable events such as clinical parameters and patient outcomes to analyse the severity of the disease. This permits clinicians to obtain warnings about potential measures before they occur, making more choices about how to progress with a decision to prevent the disease's progression.

Since last many years, retinal images are widely utilized by ophthalmologists for the recognition and examination of various pathological states. Fundus photographs, similarly known as retinal photography are recorded accurately utilizing CCD (Charged Coupled Devices) cameras. These high precision cameras are capable of recording the inner surface of the eye at the micrometre level. The recorded image provides direct information regarding the presence of normal and abnormal features in the retina. The normal features comprise the fovea, optic disk, and vascular network. There exist various types of abnormal features like micro aneurysm, hard exudates, haemorrhage, and neovascularization that lead to diabetic retinopathy (DR). The manual approach of analysing and detecting of blood vessels is a very hard task as the blood vessels in the retinal images are complex and have low level contrast. In addition, each image does not display the sign of diabetic retinopathy. Henceforth, blood vessels information taken by measuring manually, for instance branching pattern, width, length, and tortuosity, turn out to be a time-consuming task. Consequently, it rises the time between diagnosis and treatment. This may affect the efficiency of the ophthalmologists. Thus, automatic approaches for the extraction and computation the vessels in retinal images are required for saving the task of the ophthalmologists and to support in describing the identified vessels and detecting the false positives.

There are various types of filters utilized in the literature for fundus image segmentation, among them Gabor filter, matched filter, homomorphic filter, bilateral filter, guided filter are often used. Later many extensions of these traditional filters are recommended by various authors and that proved to be performed better than the original filters. Few of the extended recommended techniques are discussed in the section literature survey.

This work suggests an efficient methodology for automatic detection and segmentation process of retinal blood vessel. Even though in literature various methods are proposed for segmentation of retinal blood vessel, still accurate blood vessel extraction is a challenging task owing to vessel width variation and low-quality retinal images. In this work, an unsupervised segmentation approach by jointly combining anisotropic diffusion filter, top hat filter and Gabor filter followed by hysteresis thresholding and morphological cleaning is recommended for retinal vessel extraction. The combinations that are used in this work are 1) Median filter and Gabor filter that is a conventional approach, 2) Anisotropic diffusion filter and Gabor filter is for comparison purpose 3) Anisotropic diffusion filter, Top hat filter and Gabor filter is the suggested approach.

The proposed approach may be summarized as per the following steps:

i. Initially, the fundus image is filtered with the usage of Anisotropic diffusion filter to reduce the noise components present in the image.
ii. The filtered image is further filtered using Top hat filter and Gabor filter for preserving the essential features.
iii. Further, Hystersis thresholding is applied to extract the vessels from the non-vessel regions.
iv. Finally, the Morphological cleaning operation is applied on the extracted vessel image to remove the unwanted regions.

The proposed approach may be used as an initial step for advanced diabetic retinopathy particularly for Vitrectomy. Similarly, after glaucoma diagnosis, some surgical procedures like Laser therapy, Filtering surgery, minimally invasive glaucoma surgery can be done for the treatment of the patients. Here, the diagnosis may be done via intelligent image analysis where a decision can be made for the particular surgical procedure.

Retinal imaging technology is rapidly advancing and can provide ever-increasing amounts of information about the structure, function and molecular composition of retinal tissue in humans in vivo. Most importantly, this information can be obtained rapidly, non-invasively and in many cases using Food and Drug Administration-approved devices that are commercially available. Technologies such as optical coherence tomography have dramatically changed our understanding of retinal disease and in many cases have significantly improved their clinical management. Since retina is an extension of the brain and shares a common embryological origin with central nervous system, there has also been intense interest in leveraging the expanding armamentarium of retinal imaging technology to understand, diagnose and monitor neurological diseases. This is particularly appealing because of the high spatial resolution, relatively low-cost and wide availability of retinal imaging modalities such as fundus photography or OCT compared to brain imaging modalities such as magnetic resonance imaging or positron emission tomography. Retinal imaging methodologies are extensively used to analyses several neurodegenerative diseases like sporadic late onset alzheimer's Disease, Parkinson's Disease and Huntington's Disease. Autosomal Dominant Alzheimer's Disease and cerebrovascular small disease, where the application of retinal imaging holds promise.

Apart from the above discussed diseases that can be identified from retinal imaging, the practice of diagnose of retinal imaging has changed more rapidly in the last several months than it has over few decades. This has been due to the coronavirus disease 2019 (COVID-19) pandemic. COVID-19 has grasped minimum of 124 countries and has developed as a worldwide health warning. The comprehension of the COVID virus, its epidemiology, transferral, and inferences for ophthalmology is continuously expanding. The objectives of this viewpoint are to address various important questions which are extremely crucial for ophthalmologists. We have considered one case study done by Wu et al. and discussed. They have studied case series of 38 patients with COVID-19 from a hospital in Hubai area and reported only 1 patient coming-out with conjunctivitis, but 31.6% of the cohort had indications of conjunctival hyperemia, chemosis, epiphora, or increased secretions during their illness. Ocular symptoms were more acute with serious pneumonia patients.

Based on the above discussion it has been revealed that the analysis of fundus images of COVID-19 affected patients and asymptomatic patients using machine learning has become a major challenge for the researchers than to study the other diseases. Retinal image assessment utilizing machine learning could have possible applications in the management of COVID-19.

This chapter is further lined up as follows. Section 2 demonstrates literature survey of few conventional approaches. In Section 3 suggested technique for image segmentation is described in detail. Section 4 presents the simulation results and discussions. Section 5 gives the conclusion.

LITERATURE REVIEW

Numerous works have been suggested for detection of ophthalmological disorders like diabetic retinopathy, hypertension, glaucoma, heart diseases of the 2D complex vessel network. A primary ophthalmological disease is diabetic retinopathy, which is caused by variations in blood vessels. These changes in blood vessels may cause blindness.

In recent years, several techniques have been recommended to extract retinal blood vessels. The retinal blood vessel segmentation approaches are commonly classified into two classes like supervised learning methods, and unsupervised learning methods. Chaudhuri et al. (Chaudhuri et al., 1989) suggested a new approach for retinal blood vessel segmentation using two-dimensional matched filter. Sofka et al. (Sofka and Stewart, 2006) introduced a multiscale matched filter for retinal vessel centre line extraction. Soares et al.(Soares et al., 2006) proposed a vessel segmentation technique by utilizing the Gabor filter and supervised classification. Rangayyan et al. (Rangayyan et al., 2007) have suggested a novel approach to detect the blood vessels in the retina utilizing Gabor filters. The same authors Rangayyan et al. (Rangayyan, 2008) have suggested a new method to detect the blood vessels in the retina by employing multiscale Gabor filters. Osareh et al. (Osareh and Shadgar, 2008) have recommended a new methodology of extracting retinal blood vessels utilizing Gabor filters and Support Vector Machines. Recently in 2018, Aslan et al. (Aslan, Ceylan and Durdu, 2018) have recommended segmentation of retinal blood vessel by utilizing extreme learning machines for Gabor filter. Farokhian et al. (Farokhian et al., 2017) have introduced a new approach to automatically select the parameters of Gabor filters through imperialism competitive algorithm for the segmentation of retinal vessel. Kharghanian et al. (Kharghanian and Ahmadyfard, 2012) have recommended a new method to extract features of the retinal blood vessel segmentation utilizing Gabor filter. Chaudhari et al. (Chaudhari, Rahulkar and Patil, 2014) have used wavelets of Gabor with linear mean squared error classifier for retinal blood vessel segmentation. In this proposed method a multiscale, multi-dimensional Gabor wavelet transform is used. This wavelet transform is utilizing supervised classification algorithm called linear square error. Minimum response is obtained at different scales. The vascular structure is determined by the vessel tracking method. Fraz et al. (Fraz et al., 2012) have suggested a supervised approach for blood vessel segmentation using gradient vector field, morphological transformation, line strength measures, and Gabor filter outputs.

The ridge-based vessel segmentation approach is recommended by Staal et al.(Staal et al., 2004), where vessel are assumed to be elongated structures and extracted images are used to be primitives to conduct line images. They have considered each part of the line element as local coordinates. Then, K-Nearest Neighbour classifier is used to choose the best element among the computed features at every pixel. Jiang et al. (Xiaoyi Jiang and Mojon, 2003) have suggested an adaptive local thresholding utilizing verification based multi threshold probing algorithm. This suggested method assumes a given binary image is formed from some threshold, so that any region of any binary image can be accepted as an object by classification procedure. The same operation is performed for different thresholds and at last results are combined to find the final segmentation (Xiaoyi Jiang and Mojon, 2003). Azzopardi et al. (Azzopardi et al., 2015) have proposed an innovative technique based on fusion of shifted filter responses [COSFIER] for the automatic segmentation. Strisciuglio et al. (Strisciuglio et al., 2015) have recommended a new approach for vessel detection, which is a delineation method based on BCOSFIRE and Generalized Matrix Learning Vector Quantization (GMLVQ). This technique is suggested mainly for detection of tiny vessels in fundus images on DRIVE and STARE database. Bao et al. (Bao et al., 2015) have proposed a segmentation technique for retinal images established on cake filter on STARE dataset. This cake filter is mainly used for directivity and orthogonality because retinal vessels spread in all directions, which requires a filter with more than one direction and orthogonality. Chaudhuri et al. (Chaudhuri et al., 1989) have recommended detecting the blood vessels in retinal images utilizing two-dimensional matched filters. To detect the vascular network from fundus images a fusion of morphological filters and cross curvature evaluation method is introduced by Zana et al. (Zana and Klein, 2001) and Kochner et al. (Kochner et al., 1998) have recommended a technique to detect retinal blood vessels which also includes edge detection based on steerable filters. Mendonca et al. (Mendonca and Campilho, 2006) have recommended a new technique based on directional filters and iterative region growing method. Tan et al. (Tan et al., 2016) have suggested a new method for blood vessel segmentation utilizing a centripetal parameterized Catmull-Rom spline. Al-Diri et al. (Al-Diri, Hunter and Steel, 2009) have recommended a new algorithm to segment and to measure retinal vessels based on growing a "Ribbon of Twins" active contour technique that utilizes two pairs of contours to capture all vessel edges by retaining width constancy. Martinez-Perez et al. (Martinez-Perez et al., 2007) have recommended an approach for automatically segmentation of blood vessels based on multiscale feature extraction. Retinal blood vessel is extracted and segmented utilizing homomorphic filters for normalising the illumination that is suggested by Dash et al. (Dash, Senapati, et al., 2021). The Coye filter is combined with discrete wavelet transform for improving the performance of vessel segmentation and which is recommended by Dash and Senapati (Dash and Senapati, 2020). The performance of the matched filter is improved by integrating with first order Gaussian derivative and particle swarm optimization and that is proposed by Subudhi et al. (Subudhi, Pattnaik and Sabut, 2016). Frangi-filter, matched filter and Gabor filter are jointly combined by Memari et al. for the noise reduction in the fundus images and to improve the performance measures (Memari et al., 2019). The mached filter is integrated with local features and extended to multiscale matched filter by Alsaeed et al. (AlSaeed, 2020). Optimal filter parameters for a Gaussian matched filter are selected by using particle swarm optimization and it is proposed by Sreejini and Govindan (Sreejini and Govindan, 2015). A thick and thin vessel of retinal blood vessels are detected by integrating curvelet transform and jerman filter and is recommended by Das et al. (Dash, Verma, et al., 2021). Matched filter is combined with guided filter for enhancing the fundus images. This method is suggested by Dash et al. (Dash et al., 2022). The original median filter is extended as an Improved Median Filter (IMF), Hybrid Median Filter (HMF), and Weighted

Median Filter (WMF) for vessel segmentation (Dash and Sahu, 2019; Parida, Dash and Bhoi, 2020). Bahadar Khan et al. (BahadarKhan, A Khaliq and Shahid, 2016) have suggested a new approach for retinal vessel segmentation by morphological hessian-based approach and denoising utilizing region-based otsu thresholding. Bahadar Khan et al. (Khan et al., 2019) have given a detailed review on retinal blood vessel extraction techniques and its challenges.

Coronavirus-2019 disease (COVID-19) has occurred very recently due to which many researches work related to this has not been suggested. Globally all the researchers are working on this disease. However, few researchers have reported that the retinal arteries and veins are dilated in COVID-19 patients with the veins significantly larger both in severe and non-severe cases. Few case studies associated to retinal images that are affected by COVID-19 patients are presented below.

Coronavirus disease-2019 (COVID-19) has been associated with affecting different parts of the body, and ophthalmological changes have been associated with ocular external diseases such as conjunctivitis (Wu et al., 2020), or retinal vasculature damage consequences such as cotton wool spots, which are the manifestation of disturbed axonal transport, and haemorrhages (Khan et al., 2019).

Caporossi et al. (Caporossi et al., 2021) have studied 28 eyes of 15 adults affected by ARDS COVID-19 (3 women and 12 men, aged 39-82 years), intubated in the intensive care unit (ICU) of Careggi Hospital, Florence, Italy. They have captured the retinal images using a fundus camera (Visuscout 100, Carl Zeiss Meditech AG, Germany). They have found that all the eyes are showing no vascular lesions at the macular area, but at the retinal mid-periphery, 4 patients have shown vascular lesions such as intraretinal microvascular abnormalities (IRMA), arterial saccular dilation, cotton wool spots at the vascular arcades and microhaemorrhages in more than one quadrant. Figures. 1 (a) to (d) are representing the defective retinal images captured by the authors (Marinho et al., 2020).

Figure 1. Retinal findings of four patients with COVID-19 ARDS intubated in an ICU. (a) two cotton wool spots at the inferior retinal arcade. (b) Red free imaging representing arteriolar saccular dilatation on an arteriovenous shunt area (IRMA). (c) Colour fundus picture representing a peripheral cockade haemorrhage related to an IRMA area and a microhaemorrhage. (d) Colour fundus picture representing a flame-shaped haemorrhage at the mid-periphery.

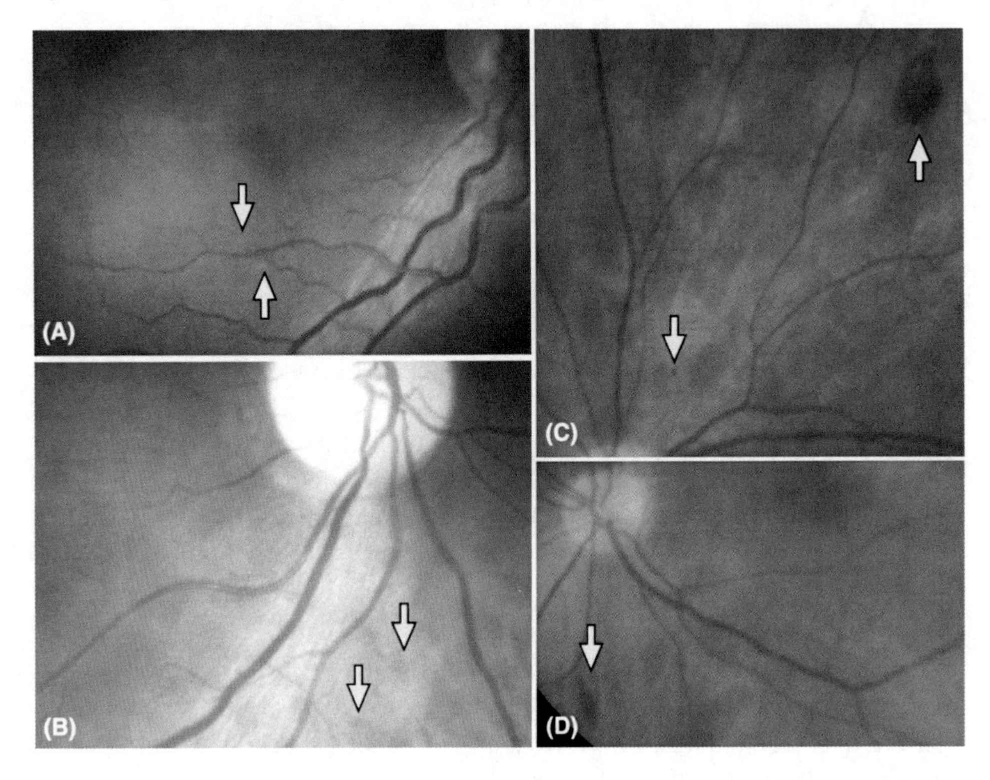

In another case study Invernizzia et al. (Invernizzi et al., 2020) have checked the retinal finding in terms of Mean arteries diameter (MAD) and Mean veins diameter (MVD) in COVID-19 patients and compared with unexposed subjects with multiple linear regression including age, sex, ethnicity, body mass index, smoking/alcohol consumption, hyperlipidaemia, hypertension, and diabetes.

They have considered 54 patients and 133 unexposed subjects for testing. Retinal findings in COVID-19 contained: haemorrhages (9.25%), cotton wools spots (7.4%), dilated veins (27.7%), tortuous vessels (12.9%). both MAD and MVD are higher in COVID patients compared to unexposed subjects (Rangayyan et al., 2007). In one more review report Bertoli et al. have mentioned that subtle retinal changes like hyperreflective lesions in the inner layers on optical coherence tomography (OCT), cotton-wool spots, and microhaemorrhages (Bertoli et al., 2020).

As the COVID-19 disease is very recent and the datasets of fundus images are still not available, consequently, till now there is no research have been recommended using machine learning techniques.

However, there is plenty of advanced machine learning techniques are suggested worldwide on the publicly available datasets. Numerous suggested techniques related to classification and segmentation of fundus images can be found on the recent review papers as cited (Bertoli et al., 2020; Invernizzi et al., 2020).

One project was going on at University of Lincoln and named as Retinal Vascular Modelling, Measurement and Diagnosis (REVAMMAD) project in which they have addressed the problem of diagnosing some of the most globally significant chronic medical conditions and vascular diseases including diabetes, hypertension, dementia and stroke, by focusing on the detailed analyses of changes caused to the blood vessels by utilising fundus images. The project was started in 01/04/2013 and ended in 31/03/2017 by prof. Andrew Hunter (Soomro et al., 2019). In another project researcher have developed a new retinal image and vasculature assessment software (RIVAS), a comprehensive software package designed for computerized analysis of retinal images utilizing machine learning methods for automatic analysis of the fundus images (Perona and Malik, 1990; Krissian et al., 2000; Gang, Chutatape and Krishnan, 2002; Heneghan et al., 2002; Kashani et al., 2021).

Since the retinal blood vessel has been acknowledged as an indispensable element in both ophthalmological and cardiovascular disease diagnosis, the accurate segmentation of the retinal vessel tree and classification of fundus imaging have become the prerequisite step for automated or computer aided diagnosis systems.

Blood vessel segmentation is a topic of high interest in medical image analysis since the analysis of vessels, detecting the cotton-wool spots, and micro haemorrhages are crucial for diagnosis, treatment planning and execution, and evaluation of clinical outcomes in different fields, including laryngology, neurosurgery and ophthalmology. Automatic or semi-automatic vessel segmentation and classification of fundus images and can support clinicians in performing tasks. Various medical imaging techniques are currently utilized in clinical practice and an appropriate selection of the segmentation and classification algorithm is mandatory to deal with the adopted imaging technique characteristics (e.g. resolution, noise and retinal image contrast).

Even though a lot of researches have been done and published on this area by many people, still the retinal findings of COVID-19 patients address several key questions that are particularly critical for ophthalmologists that are yet to be addressed. There are, however, several retinal findings of uncertain. While it is also clear that patients who are asymptomatic or pre-symptomatic patients have not been quantified. Intensive care unit patients, due to risk factors like invasive mechanical ventilation, prone position, and multi-resistant bacterial exposure, may develop ocular complications like ocular surface disorders, secondary infections, and less frequently acute ischemic optic neuropathy and intraocular pressure elevation. However, the risk of retinal toxicity with short-term high-dose use antimalarials is still unknown. Ocular side effects have also been reported with other investigational drugs like lopinavir-ritonavir, interferons, and interleukin-1. Several treatment strategies are recently under investigation for COVID-19, but none of them have been proved to be safe and effective till date.

Therefore, it is highly necessary for ophthalmologist to diagnose promptly. Retinal examination offers a unique opportunity to analyse vessels in vivo. Fundus examination is quick, not expensive and relatively non-invasive. If the fundus image data of COVID-19 patients are confirmed, retinal veins diameter could represent a useful parameter to monitor the inflammatory response and/or the endothelial damage in COVID-19.

Consequently, retinal changes should be further investigated in prospective studies to understand their possible applications in the diagnosis and management of COVID-19. The above study has motivated for fast and accurate diagnosis is possible through recommending new algorithms utilizing Machine Learning and Artificial Intelligence.

Analysis of blood vessel plays an important part in various clinical areas, like laryngology, oncology, ophthalmology, and neurosurgery, both for diagnosis, treatment planning and execution, and for the treatment outcome evaluation and follow up.

As the COVID-19 pandemic evolves and spreads worldwide, more information emerges how the virus affects the body. What was once a respiratory illness has now become a systemic infection, affecting multiple organs. Recently, a new study published in the journal Eclinical Medicine shows that the severe acute respiratory syndrome coronavirus 2 (SARS-CoV-2), the virus that causes the coronavirus disease (COVID-19), targets the retina.

A team of researchers at the Eye Clinic, Luigi Sacco Hospital, ASST Fatebenefratelli-Sacco, and the Department of Infectious Diseases in Italy aimed to determine if the COVID-a9 disease affects the retina since the disease has been linked to microvascular alterations. The researchers have analysed the retina of COVID-19 patients within 30 days from the start of the symptoms.

The team excluded patients admitted to the intensive care unit and those with retinal disorders, including diabetic retinopathy. Study participants completed questionnaires explaining their ocular symptoms. Overall, 54 patients and 133 unexposed participants were included in the study. The findings show that people with COVID-19 had retinal findings of haemorrhages, cotton wool spots, dilated veins, and tortuous vessels. Additionally, after the team measured the mean arteries diameter (MAD) and mean veins diameter (MVD) among the participants, they found that both MAD and MVD were higher in patients with COVID-19 than unexposed participants. Figure 2 shows the retinal findings in COVID-19 patients.

Figure 2. Retinal findings in patients with COVID-19 Results from the SERPICO-19 study.

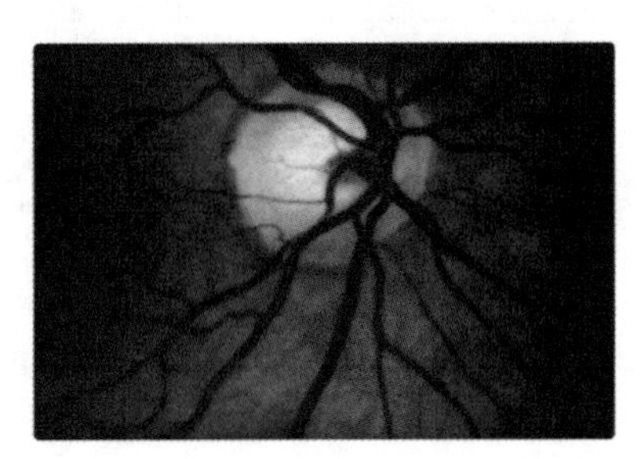

Therefore, it is concluded that COVID-19 can affect the retina. Retinal veins' diameter seems directly correlated with the disease severity.

This has motivated the researchers to suggest a novel methodology for analysing the fundus images with advanced image processing and artificial intelligence, computer vision-based techniques that can be extended for clinical practices for fast and precise identification of the diseases and also to monitor and control the COVID-19 patients.

Gabor filters are playing a fundamental role in understanding of retinal vessel segmentation. Gabor filter can further be considered and enhanced for achieving accurate extraction of retinal blood vessels. Consequently, Gabor filter is chosen for fundus image analysis by combining with anisotropic diffusion filter and top-hat filter.

PROPOSED METHOD

This work demonstrates an unsupervised approach to extract the retinal blood vessels based on hysteresis thresholding method. The recommended approach to extract the retinal blood vessels comprises of three steps described as follows:

Pre-Processing

As the retinal image suffers from non-uniform illumination and lower contrast, an effective pre-processing step is crucial before segmentation. In the pre-processing step the green channel of the RGB retinal image is used. The reason of selecting only the green channel is that it carries higher luminance than the red and blue channel.

Anisotropic Diffusion

Initially, anisotropic diffusion filter is applied on the green channel of the retinal image for denoising and to restore the connected vessel lines. In addition, it also removes noisy lines. The most principal aspect of retinal blood vessel segmentation is to retain and improve edges also local fine structures and simultaneously decrease the noise. To minimize the image noise, numerous methods have been suggested utilizing procedures for example linear and non-linear filtering. In linear spatial filtering, like Gaussian filtering, the constituents of a pixel are specified by the value of the weighted average of its close neighbors. This filtering helps in decreasing noise amplitude fluctuations and also reduces sharp particulars like lines or edges, and the resultant image look like a blurred image (Gang, Chutatape, & Krishnan, 2002). Nonlinear filters can be used to delete this unwanted effect. The frequent approach is median filtering. In this filtering the value the median of the neighbourhood pixels is calculated as output of the filter. This process preserves edges, however, the resolution is dropped by suppressing fine details (Krissian et al., 2000). To overcome this drawback of median filter, Perona and Malik (Perona and Malik, 1990) have established an anisotropic diffusion technique, a multiscale smoothing, and the edge finding method, that is a strong approach in image processing. The anisotropic diffusion is motivated from the heat diffusion equation by presenting a diffusion function that relies on the norm of the gradient of the image.

The basic anisotropic diffusion equation is given as:

$$I_t = div(c(x,y,t)\nabla I) = c(x,y,t)\Delta I = \nabla c.\nabla I \tag{1}$$

where div is the divergence operator, Ñ and Δ are the gradient and Laplacian operators correspondingly in regard to the space variables. The blurring takes place distinctly in every region with no interaction between regions. The region boundaries remain sharps.

Then for edge enhancement Perona and Malik have simplified the divergence operator expression as follows.

$$div\left(c(x,y,t)\nabla I = \frac{\partial}{\partial x}\left(c(x,y,t)I_x\right)\right) \tag{2}$$

Top Hat Transform

In digital image processing, top-hat transform is utilized to extract minute features and particulars from a specified image. There are two types of top-hat transforms exist such as white top-hat transform and black top-hat transform. The white top-hat transform is explained as the difference between the input image and its opening by some structuring element. Top-hat transforms are utilized for many image processing assignments like extraction of features, equalization of background, enhancing the image, and many more. In this work white top-hat transform is utilized for retinal blood vessel enhancement. The white top-hat transform yields an image, comprising those components of an input image that are lower than the structuring element, and are brighter than their surroundings. Top-hat transformed images comprise only non-negative values at all pixels. Let P is the grayscale image and s(x) be a grayscale structuring element then white Top-hat transformof P is defined as follow.

$$M(P)_{tophat} = P - (P \circ s) \tag{3}$$

Gabor Filter

As Gabor is the one that carries the property of directionality, thus, Gabor filters of various wavelengths and orientations are applied on the top hat-enhanced image to achieve different characteristics of images.

Gabor filter is a linear filter used for the detection of edge and is best appropriate for texture representation such as texture enhancement and feature extraction. The ability of Gabor filter is that it can differentiate oriented characteristics and fine tuning to accurate frequencies. The Gabor filter kernel is derived as

$$g(x,y) = \frac{1}{2\pi\sigma_x\sigma_y}\exp\left[-\frac{1}{2}\left(\frac{x^2}{\sigma_x^{\ 2}} + \frac{y^2}{\sigma_y^{\ 2}}\right)\right]\cos\left(2\pi f_0 x\right) \tag{4}$$

where σx and σy are the standard deviation values in the x *a*nd y *d*irections, and f0 is the frequency of the modulating sinusoid.

Gabor filters are seen as special kind of band pass filter which allows a specific band of frequencies to pass and blocks all other bans of frequencies. Gabor expansion is a time frequency analysis technique that combines both the time/space and frequency information. Gabor filter can be considered as orientation-based edge detectors. In the proposed method, the parameters that are selected for Gabor filter are σx=1.09, σy=1.09, and f0=2$_\pi$.

A Gabor filter bank with 8 different orientation ($0 \leq \theta \leq 180$) is generated. The retinal image is convolved with all 8 filters and the maximum response is recorded.

Segmentation Using Hysteresis Thresholding

In the next step, hysteresis thresholding is carried out for retinal vessel segmentation. Hysteresis thresholding approach as predicted by canny is utilized for segmentation (Heneghan et al., 2002). Thresholding is applied on Gabor filter responses $Iim_{f.}$ The special properties of the hysteresis thresholding are discussed below.

Two levels are utilized in hysteresis thresholding, lower and higher level. Pixel is set to one if the gray scale value above higher level, as with ordinary thresholding. Though, pixels that will have a gray scale exceeding lower level and are associated to pixels with gray scale values exceeding higher level are also set to 1. Isolated pixels above lower level are also set to 0. Hence, thin dark vessels exceeding the lower level that are associated to bright vessels exceeding higher level are comprised in the vasculature mask.

The final and last step is to yield binary output mask of the vasculature. To achieve this thresholding operation is performed on the images I_{imf}. In this method Hysteresis thresholding is applied because it exploits the connectedness appropriately which is highly required for the vasculature for its tree-like structure.

Particularly two levels, lower level T_l and higher-level T_h are used in the process of Hysteresis thresholding. Same as in ordinary thresholding here also the pixels with grayscale value higher than T_h are set to 1. On the other hand, pixels which are having grayscale value above T_l and are connected to pixels with grayscale values above T_h are similarly fixed to 1. Isolated pixels above T_l are set to 0 (as are all pixels below T_l). Therefore, thin dark vessels higher than T_l, which are linked to bright vessels greater than T_h, are incorporated in the vasculature mask. By utilizing morphological processing hysteresis, thresholding can easily be employed. Two binary images I_l and I_h are generated. I_l is generated by thresholding with T_l and I_h is generated by thresholding with T_h. Then I_h is reconstructed into I_l (I_h is the marker image and I_l the mask image). The equation for hysteresis thresholding is given as below.

$$H_{(T_l,T_h)(I_H)} = R_{[T_l,T_m](I_H)}\left[T_{(T_h,T_m)(I_H)}\right] \quad (5)$$

Global thresholding technique possess limited information about the neighborhood of the vessel; hence they can result in poor detection of thin vessels, small disconnected vessels and other distortions. To address these a local thresholding approach, which will take in to account the influence of neighboring vessel pixels can be implemented. Heneghan et al. in [46] have applied Hysteresis Thresholding to extract the vessels from the back ground. The Hysteresis thresholding segments the image using two threshold values T_{low} and T_{High}. Pixel values higher than T_{High}, are set to 1 and lower than T_{low} are set to '0', pixel value higher than T_{low}, and having at least one neighborhood pixel great than T_{High} is also set '1', other isolated pixels greater than T_{low} are set to '0'. Unlike mean C thresholding, Hysteresis thresholding takes into account the connected ness between neighboring pixels. Since the vessels are tree like structure the consideration of neighborhood relation improves segmentation result. Step for hysteresis thresholding are as follows:

(i) Two threshold values T_{low} and T_{High} are selected experimentally, with constrain $I_{min} < T_{low} < T_{High} < I_{max}$. Where I_{min} and I_{max} are minimum and maximum intensity value of the enhanced image.

(ii) Every pixel is compared with T_{low} and T_{High}

- If the pixel intensity > T_{High}, it is replaced by '1'
- Else If the pixel intensity < T_{low}, it is replaced by '0'
- Else If the pixel intensity > T_{low}, and has at least one pixel in its eight neighborhood > T_{High}, then also that pixel is set to '1'
- Else the pixel is replaced by '0'.

Post-Processing

In the final step, morphological cleaning operation is performed, as the images achieved from the segmentation method consists of some non-vessel that are eliminated using morphological cleaning operation. In this operation six neighbors comprising pixels are characterized as vessel. Figure 3 shows the block diagram of the suggested work. The input image is subjected to 3 different filtering operations (Anisotrpic Diffusion filter, Top-hat filter and Gabor filter) followed by Hysteris thresholding and morphological cleaning operation to extract the vessels from the input fundus image.

Figure 3. Block diagram of proposed approach.

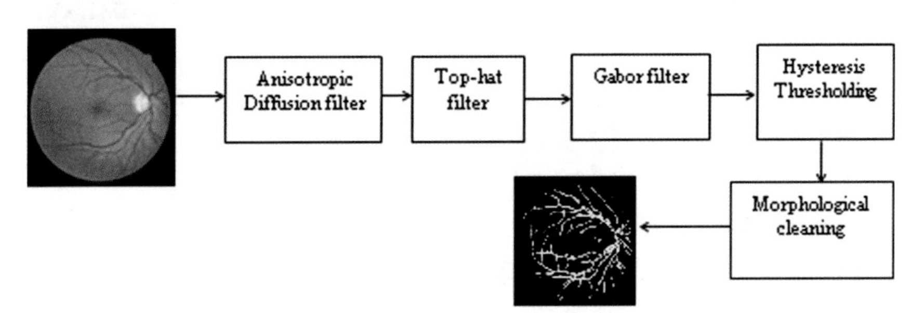

The various intermediate outputs of the proposed approach are demonstrated in Figure 4. In Figure 4, various images obtained from different filters such as image extracted from green channel, median filter, integrated model of Gabor and median filters, anisotropic diffusion filter, integrated model of Gabor and anisotropic diffusion filter, top hat transform, and integrated model of Gabor, anisotropic diffusion, and top hat filters are clearly represented. Figure. 4 (a) represents the original image, Figure. 4 (b) represents the image extracted from green channel, Figure. 4 (c) represents the output image of the median filter, Figure. 4 (d) shows the output image of the Gabor filter integrated with median filter, Figure. 4 (e) shows the output image of the anisotropic diffusion filter, Figure. 4 (f) shows the output image of the Gabor filter integrated with anisotropic diffusion filter, Figure. 4 (g) shows the output image of the Top hat filter, and Figure. 4 (h) shows the output image of the Gabor filter integrated with Top hat filter.

Figure 4. (a) Original retinal image, (b) Image extracted from green channel, (c) Median filter, (d) Gabor filter integrated with Median filter, (e) Anisotropic diffusion filter, (f) Gabor filter integrated with Anisotropic diffusion filter, (g) Top hat filter, (h) Gabor filter integrated with Anisotropic diffusion filter and top-hat filter.

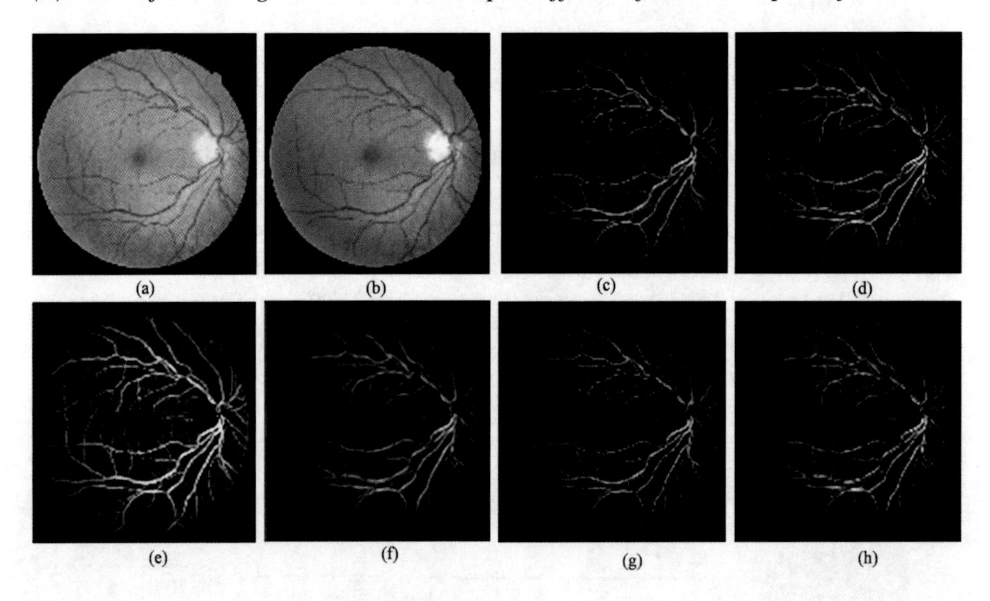

RESULTS AND DISCUSSIONS

The experimentation work is carried out in MATLAB 2017 environment using a PC with Core i3 processor and 8G RAM. As already described, the suggested method is an unsupervised segmentation method, and DRIVE database is utilized for the assessment of the suggested method. Further precisely, the DRIVE dataset consists of 40 retinal images, out of which for training 20 are used and for testing 20 images are used. A Canon CR5 3CCD camera is utilized for the capturing of the retinal images with a 458 field of view (FOV) and with colour channel 8 bits, and are of size 565×584 pixels. For each test and train set ground truth images are available that are hand-labelled by a human expert. The key aim of utilizing the DRIVE dataset is to carry the relative studies based on segmentation of the retinal blood vessels that will be relevant to the medical ground.

Four metrics are employed for comparing the performance of the recommended method with that of other retinal vessel segmentation approaches. Table 1 represents the details of true positive (TP), false positive (FP), true negative (TN), and false negative (FN) as calculated. For true count of pixels as vessel for segmented and ground truth images is identified as TP, and if the pixels are calculated as non-vessel, then identified as TN. Then again, FN is identified when the pixel is counted as non-vessel in segmented image and vessel in ground truth image, and the opposite count is known as FP.

Table 1. Contingency vessels classification.

	Vessel Present	**Vessel Absent**
Vessel Detected	True Positive (TP)	False Positive (FP)
Vessel Non-detected	False Negative (FN)	True Negative (TN)

From Table 1 the following performance measures are derived.

To analyses and quantify the method's efficiency the segmented result is compared with the ground truth and several performance measures like sensitivity (Sen), accuracy (Acc) and specificity (Spec) are calculated. The accuracy is defined as the ability of algorithm to differentiate the vessel and non-vessel pixels correctly. To estimate the accuracy, one has to calculate the proportion of true positive and true negative in all evaluated cases. Mathematically, it is defined as:

$$\text{Accuracy} = \frac{\text{TP} + \text{TN}}{\text{TP} + \text{FN} + \text{TN} + \text{FP}} \tag{6}$$

The sensitivity of a algorithm is its ability to find the non-vessel pixels cases correctly. Mathematically, it is stated as:

$$\text{Sensitivity} = \frac{\text{TP}}{\text{TP} + \text{FN}} \tag{7}$$

Specificity is the quantity of non-vessel pixels which are precisely marked as itself.

$$\text{Specificity} = \frac{\text{TN}}{\text{TN} + \text{FN}} \tag{8}$$

where TP, TN, FP and FN are defined as follows.

True positive (TP) = number of times pixel is correctly identified as a vessel.
False positive (FP) = number of times pixel is incorrectly identified as vessel.
True negative (TN) = number of times pixel is correctly identified as background.
False negative (FN) = number of times pixel is incorrectly identified as background.

The correct number of vessels classified to the complete number of vessel with reference to the ground truth is known as sensitivity. The complete non-vessels divided by total number of non-vessel in the ground truth image is known as specificity. The potentiality for estimation of the classification of the resultant images to the ground truth image is known as accuracy.

Table 2. Performance measures for the traditional Gabor with median filter.

Image	Sensitivity	Accuracy	Specificity
Retina1	0.620245	0.939863	0.959215
Retina2	0.605001	0.924955	0.961458
Retina3	0.621470	0.919604	0.951508
Retina4	0.588581	0.933074	0.975067
Retina5	0.600871	0.938731	0.963655
Retina6	0.601071	0.931009	0.955507
Retina7	0.599032	0.934594	0.957336
Retina8	0.615767	0.928375	0.966862
Retina9	0.640103	0.930930	0.975696
Retina10	0.606463	0.931461	0.962401
Retina11	0.590716	0.925236	0.941078
Retina12	0.647034	0.936905	0.962409
Retina13	0.605832	0.930354	0.960937
Retina14	0.681036	0.924303	0.975701
Retina15	0.638901	0.935926	0.958821
Retina16	0.604768	0.920766	0.956098
Retina17	0.598486	0.923808	0.954722
Retina18	0.605837	0.928448	0.965349
Retina19	0.612656	0.924100	0.962272
Retina20	0.639069	0.938367	0.961331
Average	**0.616147**	**0.9300405**	**0.9613712**

Initially, the experiment is carried out for the traditional median and Gabor filter. The performance measures obtained from the traditional approach from each retinal image are represented in Table 2. Afterwards the values of the performance measures are averaged to achieve a single performance measure. The traditional approach delivers average of sensitivity, accuracy, and specificity as 0.6161, 0.9300, and 0.9613 respectively.

Table 3. Performance measures for the traditional Gabor with Anisotropic filter.

Image	*Sensitivity*	*Accuracy*	*Specificity*
Retina1	0.640727	0.956993	0.964053
Retina2	0.642202	0.953585	0.965685
Retina3	0.655337	0.924438	0.963524
Retina4	0.607572	0.953556	0.978432
Retina5	0.612481	0.951113	0.974432
Retina6	0.648929	0.955521	0.965454
Retina7	0.631932	0.95757	0.962656
Retina8	0.642221	0.945943	0.966658
Retina9	0.66916	0.956027	0.977285
Retina10	0.620599	0.951546	0.969433
Retina11	0.628104	0.933133	0.956075
Retina12	0.683889	0.951603	0.964067
Retina13	0.619683	0.950969	0.967951
Retina14	0.716123	0.941687	0.979769
Retina15	0.655501	0.942246	0.963579
Retina16	0.622937	0.93276	0.95351
Retina17	0.613134	0.932363	0.950872
Retina18	0.637125	0.941048	0.96548
Retina19	0.661905	0.941618	0.96511
Retina20	0.665815	0.958543	0.969397
Average	**0.6437688**	**0.9466131**	**0.966171**

Secondly, to improve the performance of Gabor filter for extraction of the retinal images it is combined with anisotropic filter. The performance measures obtained from the suggested approach from each retinal image are represented in Table 3, which are averaged to get the single performance measure. The integrated anisotropic and Gabor filter approach delivers average of sensitivity, accuracy, and specificity as 0.6437, 0.9466, and 0.9661respectively.

From Table 4, it is observed that there is a good increment in the sensitivity. Further, there is a slight improvement in accuracy and specificity. Thus, to improve the performance measure further Gabor filter is integrated with top hat filter and anisotropic filter. The performance measures obtained from the suggested approach from each retinal image are represented in Table 4, which are averaged to get the single performance measure. The suggested Gabor filter integrated with anisotropic and top hat filter approach delivers average of sensitivity, accuracy, and specificity as 0.6645, 0.9503, and 0.9697 respectively. It demonstrates the proposed approach achieves a higher accuracy as compared to many state-of-art methods while retaining comparable sensitivity and specificity value.

Table 4. Performance measures for the traditional Gabor with Anisotropic and top hat filter.

Image	Sensitivity	Accuracy	Specificity
Retina1	0.651135	0.955575	0.96795
Retina2	0.663241	0.958358	0.967518
Retina3	0.668712	0.939557	0.96655
Retina4	0.62393	0.945271	0.979906
Retina5	0.63646	0.944259	0.977109
Retina6	0.659271	0.948194	0.96827
Retina7	0.649493	0.947404	0.968762
Retina8	0.653594	0.945704	0.968631
Retina9	0.67815	0.947162	0.978798
Retina10	0.657265	0.956131	0.971652
Retina11	0.64846	0.9523	0.959437
Retina12	0.708206	0.94651	0.968378
Retina13	0.638099	0.948588	0.968833
Retina14	0.732195	0.949758	0.978663
Retina15	0.6684	0.956353	0.968087
Retina16	0.658738	0.935694	0.977762
Retina17	0.647945	0.946709	0.958175
Retina18	0.66877	0.958306	0.966275
Retina19	0.689376	0.957291	0.964802
Retina20	0.689939	0.967498	0.968577
Average	**0.664569**	**0.950331**	**0.969707**

From the detail assessment of the results, it is noted that by applying the integrated model top hat filter with anisotropic filter then with Gabor filter the performance measures of the retinal images are increased remarkably than the traditional median filter and Gabor filter segmentation approach. Figure 5 shows the segmented images obtained from various approaches.

Figure 5. Segmentation images of different methods (a) Original image, (b) Ground truth image of the first observer, (c) Median filter with Gabor filter, (d) Anisotropic diffusion filter with Gabor filter, (e) proposed method based on top hat filter, Anisotropic diffusion filter, and Gabor filter.

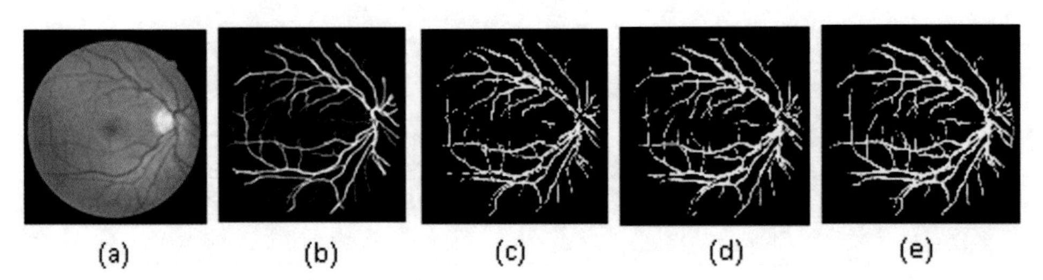

The performance of the proposed method on DRIVE dataset is compared with other approaches with reference to sensitivity, specificity and accuracy: Soares et al. (Soares et al., 2006), Rangayyan et al. (Rangayyan, 2008), Osareh et al. (Osareh and Shadgar, 2008), Aslan et al. (Aslan, Ceylan and Durdu, 2018), Farokhian et al. (Farokhian et al., 2017), Kharghanian et al. (Kharghanian and Ahmadyfard, 2012), Chaudhari et al. (Chaudhari, Rahulkar and Patil, 2014), Staal et al. (Staal et al., 2004), Jiang et al. (Xiaoyi Jiang and Mojon, 2003), Chaudhuri et al. (Chaudhuri et al., 1989), Tan et al. (Tan et al., 2016), Martinez-Perez et al. (Martinez-Perez et al., 2007), Dash et al. (Dash, Senapati, et al., 2021), Dash and Senapati (Dash and Senapati, 2020), Subudhi et al. (Subudhi, Pattnaik and Sabut, 2016), Memari et al. (Memari et al., 2019), AlSaeed et al. (AlSaeed, 2020), Sreejini and Govindan (Sreejini and Govindan, 2015), Dash et al. (Dash, Verma, et al., 2021), and Dash et al. (Dash et al., 2022). Table 5 illustrates the performance of our approach against the above approaches on DRIVE database.

In Table 5, results of both supervised and unsupervised techniqes for vessel segmentation are discussed. The hidden features of the retinal image are utilized in unsupervised method for segmentation. This method does not need any huge database for training. However, supervised approach uses prior information to decide a pixel as a vessel or not. Utilizer interaction is needed to determine the rule for each pixel to provide the training data for each pixel during classification. Based on the training data from various classes the classification is performed. It is shown in table 5 that sensitivity is varying from 0.3451 to 0.965 for both supervised and unsupervised methods. Mostly the aim of the authors are to improve the traiditional methods by enhancing the segmentation accuracy. In this work the aim is to improve the performance of the original Gabor filter and that is achieved. The proposed approach improves all the three performance matrices as compared to the original Gabor filter.

Table 5. The performance comparative analysis with different approaches for DRIVE dataset.

Methods Supervised/ unsupervised	Supervised/Unsupervised	Sensitivity	Accuracy	Specificity
(Soares et al., 2006)	Supervised	--	94.67	--
(Rangayyan, 2008)	Unsupervised	--	96.00	--
(Osareh and Shadgar, 2008)	Supervised	0.9650	96.75	97.10
(Aslan, Ceylan and Durdu, 2018)	Unsupervised	--	94.59	--
(Farokhian et al., 2017)	Unsupervised	0.6933	93.92	97.77
(Kharghanian and Ahmadyfard, 2012)	Unsupervised	--	94.69	--
(Chaudhari, Rahulkar and Patil, 2014)	Supervised	--	86.79	--
(Staal et al., 2004)	Supervised	--	93.44	--
(Xiaoyi Jiang and Mojon, 2003)	Unsupervised	0.6478	0.9222	0.9625
(Chaudhuri et al., 1989)	Supervised	0.6168	0.9284	0.9741
(Tan et al., 2016)	Unsupervised	--	0.93	--
(Martinez-Perez et al., 2007)	Supervised	--	0.96	--
(Dash, Senapati, et al., 2021)	Unsupervised	0.7203	0.9581	0.9871
(Subudhi, Pattnaik and Sabut, 2016)	Unsupervised	0.3451	0.911	0.9716
(Memari et al., 2019)	Unsupervised	0.761	0.961	0.981
(AlSaeed, 2020)	Unsupervised	0.6312	0.9353	0.9817
(Sreejini and Govindan, 2015)	Unsupervised	0.7132	0.9633	0.9866
(Dash, Verma, et al., 2021)	Unsupervised	0.7528	0.9600	0.9933
(Dash et al., 2022)	Unsupervised	0.7043	0.9613	0.9890
Gabor filter + Median filter		0.6161	0.9300	0.9613
Gabor filter + Anisotropic diffusion filter		0.6437	0.9466	0.9661
Proposed Method		0.6645	0.9503	0.9697

This work also presents a comparison of the quality of enhancement by comparing few parameters as discussed below.

After the image is enhanced, it is important to evaluate the quality of enhancement. The most accurate assessment is through the human observer, who makes use of the image. This type of evaluation is called as subjective evaluation. However, these are also several objective evaluation methods, which can assess the image quality that is close to subjective evaluation, without human intervention. Often the image enhancement process is application oriented. For fundus image the enhancement should result a clear distinction between the vessel and background. So here we have used Contrast Improvement Index (CII), Peak signal to noise ratio (PSNR), Entropy and AMBE parameters for quality assessment of enhanced image.

Contrast Improvement Index (CII)

CII is defined as the ratio of the contrast values for the retinal vessel in the enhanced image and the original image.

$$CII = \frac{C_{en}}{C_I} \tag{9}$$

C_{en} and C_I is the contrast of the vessels in the enhanced image and original image respectively.

$$\text{Here } C_I = \left|\frac{V - B}{V + B}\right| \tag{10}$$

V: average gray values of the retinal vessels
B: average gray values of non-vessel regions

It is obvious that a larger value of *CI* means a larger difference between the retinal vessel intensity and background intensity. Ce_n is also calculated similarly. It is to be noted that the manually segmented vessel image should be available. From the manual segmented image, the vessel point and background points are found, and the intensity of the corresponding points in the enhanced image gives the gray value of vessel and background respectively. The higher the value of CII, better is the contrast enhancement.

PSNR (Peak Signal to Noise Ratio)

PSNR formally defines the quality of the resultant image after the application of any enhancement technique on it. Higher the PSNR value, better is the quality of enhanced image.

So PSNR is defined as:

$$PSNR = 10log\frac{MAX^2}{MSE} \tag{11}$$

Here the maximum gray value is MAX=255.

$$Mean\ square\ error\left(MSE\right)=\frac{1}{R*W}\sum_{i=1}^{R}\sum_{j=1}^{W}\left(I_{en}-I\right)^{2} \tag{12}$$

R and W: size of image.

Entropy

Entropy measures the content or information of an image. Higher the entropy value indicated richness of the details in the image. The average information content or entropy of an image is defined as:

$$H\left(I\right)=-\sum_{i=0}^{255}p\left(i\right)*log\left(p\left(i\right)\right) \tag{13}$$

Here p(i) is the probability density function of ith intensity value in the image I.

Absolute Mean Brightness Error (AMBI)

It is an indicator of how much brightness is preserved in the enhanced image.

$$AMBI=\frac{\left|E\left[I\right]-E\left[I_{en}\right]\right|}{L} \tag{14}$$

Here E[.] denotes the expected mean. The factor L i.e. the maximum intensity value is divided to normalize AMBI value. Lower the AMBI value better is the brightness preservation.

The objective quantification of the proposed method also gives similar results. Table 6, shows the contrast improvement index for various methods. Though the Gabor transform integrated with median filter-based method achieves better contrast as compared to other, but it is clear from figure 4 that the visual quality of the image is very poor as compared to other methods. The proposed method shows a good contrast improvement index as well as the best visual quality. So the proposed method is the winner in improving the contrast, as compared to the other methods. This demonstrates that the integrated model anisotropic diffusion, top hat and Gabor achieve very good contrast between vessels and background as compared to state of art methods. Table 6 illustrates the contrast improvement index for various methods.

From the Table 6 it can be well remarked that the Top hat approach outperforms all other approach but when it is combined with Anisotropic and Gabor it provides a comparable result as compared to other state of art techniques.

Table 6. Comparison of Contrast Improvement Index of Different Methods.

	Gabor and Median	Anisotropic Diffusion	Anisotropic and Gabor	Top hat	Anisotropic, top hat and Gabor
Image 1	2.816508	1.769716	0.71645	5.771075	3.137294
Image 2	2.371785	1.564098	0.726119	2.664533	3.538993
Image 3	2.293146	1.98249	0.802377	3.039403	3.002407
Image 4	1.670603	1.402398	0.690015	2.088422	3.7925
Image 5	3.208751	2.216307	0.657827	2.891888	3.341351
Image 6	2.655487	1.687453	0.733893	3.618734	3.009283
Image 7	1.60204	1.352651	0.720493	2.573632	3.632808
Image 8	2.764224	1.804074	0.725592	4.391297	4.084498
Image 9	4.741458	2.239358	0.630652	7.151067	5.435817
Image 10	2.353884	1.928652	0.690052	4.838993	3.587289
Image 11	2.028152	1.531284	0.684226	1.471898	2.832782
Image 12	2.931691	1.872271	0.67166	4.337389	3.176618
Image 13	2.622124	1.638282	0.730538	4.271677	6.128602
Image 14	2.479149	1.705244	0.725662	4.338926	3.80998
Image 15	1.431292	1.42676	0.532411	3.425839	3.644832
Image 16	3.083265	1.744403	0.677422	4.769799	3.152806
Image 17	3.258999	1.578381	0.45408	6.079814	3.520846
Image 18	3.328666	1.783138	0.573741	8.280012	3.76193
Image 19	2.099217	1.809764	0.752015	4.723004	2.627991
Image 20	3.261365	2.097654	0.681825	5.553551	3.734276
Average	2.577636	1.749799	0.685813	**4.230255**	3.512051

Table 7 illustrates the PSNR of different methods. PSNR is the estimated the quality of the enhanced image. Table 8 represents the entropy of enhanced image and their average values. Table 9 shows the average AMBE for the above methods. The integrated model anisotropic diffusion, top hat and Gabor show the lowest value among all. Since the lower the value of AMBE better is the brightness preservation. Integrated model anisotropic diffusion, top hat and Gabor enhanced image is considered to be a better technique among others. Even if the suggested method achieves better contrast while preserving the entropy, PSNR and AMBE value, but the time complexity is slightly higher.

Table 7. Comparison of PSNR value of Different Methods.

	Gabor and Median	Anisotropic Diffusion	Anisotropic and Gabor	Top hat	Anisotropic, top hat and Gabor
Image 1	11.64291	12.55811	9.576256	9.989443	13.49976
Image 2	12.34934	13.00619	9.164862	9.374304	12.66361
Image 3	9.019908	10.47386	12.67109	13.34713	11.37046
Image 4	11.08668	13.44096	10.59476	10.60545	11.63302
Image 5	9.588658	11.96307	11.82083	12.39932	10.38246
Image 6	11.34437	13.05633	10.02865	10.16656	14.30018
Image 7	11.17682	12.64788	10.35956	10.62699	11.40098
Image 8	10.37926	13.44385	11.13836	11.13123	9.534694
Image 9	12.71206	13.40561	8.690564	8.714004	14.79073
Image 10	9.469495	11.88296	12.04587	12.66943	10.88268
Image 11	12.07029	13.26608	9.593853	9.683226	13.70093
Image 12	11.0411	12.47433	10.1105	10.43116	11.21468
Image 13	12.49582	12.62692	8.99675	9.197796	16.57871
Image 14	10.98499	12.5807	10.28681	10.63349	11.67705
Image 15	8.561828	13.09159	13.82905	14.47828	11.77129
Image 16	12.47853	12.78994	8.916566	9.165258	13.58101
Image 17	14.00183	14.28581	8.435038	7.922273	15.57972
Image 18	12.72831	13.20691	8.786217	8.926826	14.7356
Image 19	9.332722	11.68632	12.2402	12.78724	12.56854
Image 20	10.46882	12.08596	10.73276	11.12548	12.46526
Average	11.14669	12.69867	10.40093	10.66874	12.71657

Table 8. Comparison of Entropy value of Different Methods.

	Gabor and Median	Anisotropic Diffusion	Anisotropic and Gabor	Top hat	Anisotropic, top hat and Gabor
Image 1	5.147796	5.543701	6.308325	3.779316	5.794434
Image 2	5.290474	5.691748	6.304226	3.806602	6.049035
Image 3	4.925515	5.22671	6.120222	3.685869	6.047888
Image 4	5.298393	5.97066	6.583059	3.280693	6.049699
Image 5	4.876951	5.202708	6.01992	3.922785	5.961215
Image 6	5.025544	5.543245	6.154972	3.186389	6.101943
Image 7	5.351165	6.005704	6.679293	3.703481	6.090764
Image 8	4.966005	5.440574	6.15374	3.34877	5.985368
Image 9	4.986482	5.342488	5.844981	3.204723	6.013996
Image 10	5.087448	5.445798	6.280047	3.865955	5.933658
Image 11	5.340999	5.892036	6.454464	3.565355	6.007174
Image 12	5.052942	5.423303	6.20627	3.483694	6.959046
Image 13	5.202212	5.711092	6.30749	3.425247	6.1384
Image 14	5.167951	5.575126	6.352832	3.452052	6.093914
Image 15	5.159646	5.754148	6.522505	4.052482	6.070447
Image 16	5.13033	5.515375	6.151842	3.560366	6.991197
Image 17	5.174512	5.664943	5.032187	3.092285	6.07234
Image 18	5.166673	5.546539	5.981961	3.537049	6.996617
Image 19	5.094041	5.449256	6.281492	3.441043	6.081625
Image 20	4.928385	5.283714	6.111214	3.489557	6.998575
Average	5.118673	5.561443	6.192552	3.544186	6.221867

Table 9. AMBE Comparison of various methods.

	Gabor and Median	Anisotropic Diffusion	Anisotropic and Gabor	Top hat	Anisotropic, top hat and Gabor
Image 1	0.214732	0.190383	0.277041	0.259692	0.15133
Image 2	0.197477	0.180125	0.289517	0.277473	0.157139
Image 3	0.300383	0.238181	0.196811	0.177124	0.192026
Image 4	0.241574	0.16921	0.243328	0.240994	0.191688
Image 5	0.279453	0.202233	0.215385	0.192765	0.226881
Image 6	0.226699	0.179743	0.262671	0.256844	0.120039
Image 7	0.239084	0.185798	0.251477	0.238333	0.195819
Image 8	0.255526	0.171044	0.231372	0.226424	0.245285
Image 9	0.17953	0.174314	0.306341	0.303805	0.109411
Image 10	0.286934	0.201332	0.20936	0.188135	0.214454
Image 11	0.210935	0.173295	0.274401	0.268865	0.143511
Image 12	0.233232	0.192198	0.261229	0.24894	0.201653
Image 13	0.194646	0.188616	0.294891	0.286386	0.056559
Image 14	0.235497	0.189461	0.25601	0.243729	0.180874
Image 15	0.32556	0.171574	0.167548	0.146048	0.188952
Image 16	0.18989	0.186274	0.298815	0.28718	0.141476
Image 17	0.150522	0.158508	0.314639	0.333853	0.089135
Image 18	0.182193	0.177544	0.303072	0.294854	0.114597
Image 19	0.292803	0.206466	0.204163	0.190131	0.217827
Image 20	0.249492	0.200149	0.243189	0.229269	0.165785
Average	0.234308	0.186822	0.255063	0.244542	0.165222

CONCLUSION

Retinal blood vessels are extracted by suggesting an unsupervised approach through Gabor filter followed by two another filters. Hysteresis thresholding is used for the segmentation. One filter that is anisotropic filter is utilized for denoising of the retinal images and the top-hat transform is applied for the vessel enhancement. Thus, by utilizing both denoising and enhancement prior to Gabor delivers better results than the original median and Gabor filters. The vessels are extracted more precisely with sensitivity, accuracy, and specificity as 0.6645, 0.9503, and 0.9697 respectively, that is better than the original approach when compared. The suggested work is only focused to improve the performance of the original Gabor filter. The results demonstrate that the suggested approach delivers better performance metrices than the original Gabor filter in terms of sensitivity, accuracy, and specificity.

The proposed method produces impressive enhanced image and also preserves the fine vessel details. This approach seems to be promising in improving the contrast as well as retaining the brightness of fundus images. Yet, few of the thin extracted vessels are showing irregularity at the walls.

In future this approach can also be extended for enhancement of real time data base and the assessment parameters can be fine-tuned through suitable modification in the objective function. This can be modified in different direction for enhancement of noisy image and very low contrast image which will make the algorithm robust, stable and more efficient. Moreover, it will enable new practical applications, where analysis of low contrast images in real-time is required, e.g. robotic microsurgery of the eye.

ACKNOWLEDGMENT

This research received no specific grant from any funding agency in the public, commercial, or not-for-profit sectors.

REFERENCES

Al-Diri, B., Hunter, A., & Steel, D. (2009). An Active Contour Model for Segmenting and Measuring Retinal Vessels. *IEEE Transactions on Medical Imaging*, *28*(9), 1488–1497. doi:10.1109/TMI.2009.2017941 PMID:19336294

AlSaeed, D. (2020). A Novel Blood Vessel Extraction Using Multiscale Matched Filters with Local Features and Adaptive Thresholding. *Bioscience Biotechnology Research Communications*, *13*(3), 1104–1113. doi:10.21786/bbrc/13.3/18

Aslan, M. F., Ceylan, M., & Durdu, A. (2018) Segmentation of Retinal Blood Vessel Using Gabor Filter and Extreme Learning Machines. In *2018 International Conference on Artificial Intelligence and Data Processing (IDAP)*, (pp. 1–5). IEEE. 10.1109/IDAP.2018.8620890

Azzopardi, G., Strisciuglio, N., Vento, M., & Petkov, N. (2015). Trainable COSFIRE filters for vessel delineation with application to retinal images. *Medical Image Analysis*, *19*(1), 46–57. doi:10.1016/j.media.2014.08.002 PMID:25240643

Bahadar, K., Khaliq, A., & Shahid, M. (2016). A Morphological Hessian Based Approach for Retinal Blood Vessels Segmentation and Denoising Using Region Based Otsu Thresholding. PLOS ONE, 11(7), e0158996. doi:10.1371/journal.pone.0158996

Bao, X.-R., Ge, X., She, L.-H., & Zhang, S. (2015). Segmentation of Retinal Blood Vessels Based on Cake Filter. *BioMed Research International*, *2015*, 1–11. doi:10.1155/2015/137024 PMID:26636095

Bertoli, F., Veritti, D., Danese, C., Samassa, F., Sarao, V., Rassu, N., Gambato, T., & Lanzetta, P. (2020). Ocular Findings in COVID-19 Patients: A Review of Direct Manifestations and Indirect Effects on the Eye. *Journal of Ophthalmology*, *2020*, 1–9. doi:10.1155/2020/4827304 PMID:32963819

Caporossi, T., Bacherini, D., Tartaro, R., VIrgili, G., Peris, A., & Giansanti, F. (2021). Retinal findings in patients affected by COVID 19 intubated in an intensive care unit. *Acta Ophthalmologica*, *99*(7), e1244–e1245. doi:10.1111/aos.14734 PMID:33377599

Chaudhari, H. P., Rahulkar, A. D., & Patil, C. Y. (2014). Segmentation of Retinal Vessels by the Use of Gabor Wavelet and Linear Mean Squared Error Classifier. *International Journal of Emerging Engineering Research and Technology*, *2*(2), 119–125.

Chaudhuri, S., Chatterjee, S., Katz, N., Nelson, M., & Goldbaum, M. (1989). Detection of blood vessels in retinal images using two-dimensional matched filters. *IEEE Transactions on Medical Imaging*, *8*(3), 263–269. doi:10.1109/42.34715 PMID:18230524

Dash, S., & Sahu, G. (2019) Retinal blood vessel segmentation by employing various upgraded median filters. In *Proceedings - International Conference on Intelligent Systems and Green Technology, ICISGT 2019*, (pp. 35–39). IEEE. 10.1109/ICISGT44072.2019.00023

Dash, S., & Senapati, M. R. (2020). Enhancing detection of retinal blood vessels by combined approach of DWT, Tyler Coye and Gamma correction. *Biomedical Signal Processing and Control*, *57*, 101740. doi:10.1016/j.bspc.2019.101740

Dash, S., Senapati, M. R., Sahu, P. K., & Chowdary, P. S. R. (2021). Illumination normalized based technique for retinal blood vessel segmentation. *International Journal of Imaging Systems and Technology*, *31*(1), 351–363. doi:10.1002/ima.22461

Dash, S., Verma, S., Kavita, Bevinakoppa, S., Wozniak, M., Shafi, J., & Ijaz, M. F. (2022). Guidance Image-Based Enhanced Matched Filter with Modified Thresholding for Blood Vessel Extraction. *Symmetry, 14*(2), 194. doi:10.3390ym14020194

Dash, S., Verma, S., Kavita, Khan, M. S., Wozniak, M., Shafi, J., & Ijaz, M. F. (2021). A hybrid method to enhance thick and thin vessels for blood vessel segmentation. *Diagnostics (Basel), 11*(11), 2017. doi:10.3390/diagnostics11112017 PMID:34829365

Farokhian, F., Yang, C., Demirel, H., Wu, S., & Beheshti, I. (2017). Automatic parameters selection of Gabor filters with the imperialism competitive algorithm with application to retinal vessel segmentation. *Biocybernetics and Biomedical Engineering, 37*(1), 246–254. doi:10.1016/j.bbe.2016.12.007

Fraz, M. M., Remagnino, P., Hoppe, A., Uyyanonvara, B., Rudnicka, A. R., Owen, C. G., & Barman, S. A. (2012). An Ensemble Classification-Based Approach Applied to Retinal Blood Vessel Segmentation. *IEEE Transactions on Biomedical Engineering, 59*(9), 2538–2548. doi:10.1109/TBME.2012.2205687 PMID:22736688

Gang, L., Chutatape, O., & Krishnan, S. M. (2002). Detection and measurement of retinal vessels in fundus images using amplitude modified second-order Gaussian filter. *IEEE Transactions on Biomedical Engineering, 49*(2), 168–172. doi:10.1109/10.979356 PMID:12066884

Heneghan, C. (2002). Characterization of changes in blood vessel width and tortuosity in retinopathy of prematurity using image analysis. *Medical Image Analysis, 6*(4), 407–429. doi:10.1016/S1361-8415(02)00058-0 PMID:12426111

Invernizzi, A., Torre, A., Parrulli, S., Zicarelli, F., Schiuma, M., Colombo, V., Giacomelli, A., Cigada, M., Milazzo, L., Ridolfo, A., Faggion, I., Cordier, L., Oldani, M., Marini, S., Villa, P., Rizzardini, G., Galli, M., Antinori, S., Staurenghi, G., & Meroni, L. (2020). Retinal findings in patients with COVID-19: Results from the SERPICO-19 study. *EClinicalMedicine, 27*, 100550. doi:10.1016/j.eclinm.2020.100550 PMID:32984785

Jiang, X., & Mojon, D. (2003). Adaptive local thresholding by verification-based multithreshold probing with application to vessel detection in retinal images. *IEEE Transactions on Pattern Analysis and Machine Intelligence, 25*(1), 131–137. doi:10.1109/TPAMI.2003.1159954

Kashani, A. H., Asanad, S., Chan, J. W., Singer, M. B., Zhang, J., Sharifi, M., Khansari, M. M., Abdolahi, F., Shi, Y., Biffi, A., Chui, H., & Ringman, J. M. (2021). Past, present and future role of retinal imaging in neurodegenerative disease. *Progress in Retinal and Eye Research*, *83*, 100938. doi:10.1016/j.preteyeres.2020.100938 PMID:33460813

Khan, K. B., Khaliq, A. A., Jalil, A., Iftikhar, M. A., Ullah, N., Aziz, M. W., Ullah, K., & Shahid, M. (2019). A review of retinal blood vessels extraction techniques: Challenges, taxonomy, and future trends. *Pattern Analysis & Applications*, *22*(3), 767–802. doi:10.100710044-018-0754-8

Kharghanian, R., & Ahmadyfard, A. (2012). Retinal Blood Vessel Segmentation Using Gabor Wavelet and Line Operator. *International Journal of Machine Learning and Computing*, *2*(5), 593–597. doi:10.7763/IJMLC.2012.V2.196

Kochner, B. (1998). Course tracking and contour extraction of retinal vessels from color fundus photographs: most efficient use of steerable filters for model-based image analysis. In K. M. Hanson (Ed.), *Medical Imaging 1998: Image Processing* (pp. 755–761)., doi:10.1117/12.310955

Krissian, K., Malandain, G., Ayache, N., Vaillant, R., & Trousset, Y. (2000). Model-Based Detection of Tubular Structures in 3D Images. *Computer Vision and Image Understanding*, *80*(2), 130–171. doi:10.1006/cviu.2000.0866

Marinho, P. M., Marcos, A. A. A., Romano, A. C., Nascimento, H., & Belfort, R. Jr. (2020). Retinal findings in patients with COVID-19. *Lancet*, *395*(10237), 1610. doi:10.1016/S0140-6736(20)31014-X PMID:32405105

Martinez-Perez, M. E., Hughes, A. D., Thom, S. A., Bharath, A. A., & Parker, K. H. (2007). Segmentation of blood vessels from red-free and fluorescein retinal images. *Medical Image Analysis*, *11*(1), 47–61. doi:10.1016/j.media.2006.11.004 PMID:17204445

Memari, N., Ramli, A. R., Saripan, M. I. B., Mashohor, S., & Moghbel, M. (2019). Retinal Blood Vessel Segmentation by Using Matched Filtering and Fuzzy C-means Clustering with Integrated Level Set Method for Diabetic Retinopathy Assessment. *Journal of Medical and Biological Engineering*, *39*(5), 713–731. doi:10.100740846-018-0454-2

Mendonca, A. M., & Campilho, A. (2006). Segmentation of retinal blood vessels by combining the detection of centerlines and morphological reconstruction. *IEEE Transactions on Medical Imaging*, *25*(9), 1200–1213. doi:10.1109/TMI.2006.879955 PMID:16967805

Osareh, A., & Shadgar, B. (2008) Retinal Vessel Extraction Using Gabor Filters and Support Vector Machines. in Communications in Computer and Information Science, (pp. 356–363). Springer. doi:10.1007/978-3-540-89985-3_44

Parida, P., Dash, J., & Bhoi, N. (2020). Retinal Blood Vessel Extraction from Fundus Images Using Enhancement Filtering and Clustering. *ELCVIA. Electronic Letters on Computer Vision and Image Analysis*, *19*(1), 38. doi:10.5565/rev/elcvia.1239

Perona, P., & Malik, J. (1990). Scale-space and edge detection using anisotropic diffusion. *IEEE Transactions on Pattern Analysis and Machine Intelligence*, *12*(7), 629–639. doi:10.1109/34.56205

Rangayyan, R. M.. (2007) Detection of Blood Vessels in the Retina Using Gabor Filters. in *2007 Canadian Conference on Electrical and Computer Engineering*, (pp. 717–720). IEEE. 10.1109/CCECE.2007.184

Rangayyan, R. M. (2008). Detection of blood vessels in the retina with multiscale Gabor filters. *Journal of Electronic Imaging*, *17*(2), 023018. doi:10.1117/1.2907209

Soares, J. V. B., Leandro, J. J. G., Cesar, R. M., Jelinek, H. F., & Cree, M. J. (2006). Retinal vessel segmentation using the 2-D Gabor wavelet and supervised classification. *IEEE Transactions on Medical Imaging*, *25*(9), 1214–1222. doi:10.1109/TMI.2006.879967 PMID:16967806

Sofka, M., & Stewart, C. V. (2006). Retinal Vessel Centerline Extraction Using Multiscale Matched Filters, Confidence and Edge Measures. *IEEE Transactions on Medical Imaging*, *25*(12), 1531–1546. doi:10.1109/TMI.2006.884190 PMID:17167990

Soomro, T. A., Afifi, A. J., Zheng, L., Soomro, S., Gao, J., Hellwich, O., & Paul, M. (2019). Deep Learning Models for Retinal Blood Vessels Segmentation: A Review. *IEEE Access: Practical Innovations, Open Solutions*, *7*, 71696–71717. doi:10.1109/ACCESS.2019.2920616

Sreejini, K. S., & Govindan, V. K. (2015). Improved multiscale matched filter for retina vessel segmentation using PSO algorithm. *Egyptian Informatics Journal*, *16*(3), 253–260. doi:10.1016/j.eij.2015.06.004

Staal, J., Abramoff, M. D., Niemeijer, M., Viergever, M. A., & van Ginneken, B. (2004). Ridge-Based Vessel Segmentation in Color Images of the Retina. *IEEE Transactions on Medical Imaging*, *23*(4), 501–509. doi:10.1109/TMI.2004.825627 PMID:15084075

Strisciuglio, N. (2015) Multiscale blood vessel delineation using B-COSFIRE filters. In Lecture Notes in Computer Science (including subseries Lecture Notes in Artificial Intelligence and Lecture Notes in Bioinformatics), pp. 300–312. Springer. doi:10.1007/978-3-319-23117-4_26

Subudhi, A., Pattnaik, S., & Sabut, S. (2016). Blood vessel extraction of diabetic retinopathy using optimized enhanced images and matched filter. *Journal of Medical Imaging (Bellingham, Wash.)*, *3*(4), 044003. doi:10.1117/1.JMI.3.4.044003 PMID:27981066

Tan, J. H., Acharya, U. R., Chua, K. C., Cheng, C., & Laude, A. (2016). Automated extraction of retinal vasculature. *Medical Physics*, *43*(5), 2311–2322. doi:10.1118/1.4945413 PMID:27147343

Wu, P., Duan, F., Luo, C., Liu, Q., Qu, X., Liang, L., & Wu, K. (2020). Characteristics of Ocular Findings of Patients with Coronavirus Disease 2019 (COVID-19) in Hubei Province, China. *JAMA Ophthalmology*, *138*(5), 575–578. doi:10.1001/jamaophthalmol.2020.1291 PMID:32232433

Zana, F., & Klein, J.-C. (2001). Segmentation of vessel-like patterns using mathematical morphology and curvature evaluation. *IEEE Transactions on Image Processing*, *10*(7), 1010–1019. doi:10.1109/83.931095 PMID:18249674

Chapter 14
Arrhythmia Recognition and Classification Using Kernel ICA and Higher Order Spectra:
SVM Method of Detection and Classification of Arrhythmia

Raghu N.
https://orcid.org/0000-0002-2091-8922
Jain University (Deemed), India

Kiran B.
https://orcid.org/0000-0002-6640-6703
Jain University (Deemed), India

Manjunatha K. N.
Jain University (Deemed), India

ABSTRACT

The conventional methodologies of arrhythmia identification are based on morphological features or certain transformation technique. These conventional techniques are partially successful in arrhythmia identification, because it treats heart as a linear structure. In this chapter, ECG based arrhythmia identification is assessed by employing MIT-BIH arrhythmia dataset. The proposed approach contains two major steps: feature extraction and classification. Initially, a combination of non-linear and linear feature extraction is carried-out using Principal Component Analysis, Kernel Independent Component Analysis and Higher Order Spectrum for achieving optimal feature subsets. The linear experiments on ECG data achieves high performance in noise free data and the non-linear experiments distinguish the ECG data more effectively, extract hidden information and also helps to attain better performance under noisy conditions. After finding the feature information, a binary classifier Support Vector Machine is employed for classifying the normality and abnormality of arrhythmia.

DOI: 10.4018/978-1-6684-6957-6.ch014

INTRODUCTION

The summation of cramping potential of the heart and diagnosis of numerous cardiac abnormalities like Arrhythmia is signified using ECG (Jung et al., 2017). The second most common heart disease first being Coronary Artery disease and one of the most common cardiac disorder is Arrhythmia which significantly effects the world's population percentage (Haldar NAH et al., 2017). Arrhythmia is a disorder from which almost around 15% of the world population suffers from (Khalea AF et al., 2015). Most of the causes of Arrhythmia are associated to cardiovascular diseases (Wang JS et al., 2013). Some of the life-threatening medical emergencies which may lead to sudden death or cardiac arrest or even hemodynamic collapse are Flutter and Ventricular Fibrillation which are classified under Arrhythmia. Visual observations of ECG signals are presently used for the detection of Arrhythmia by physicians (Kutlu Y et al., 2015). Instead of using human visual observations an automatic Arrhythmia detector would have many more benefits like it helps faster detection of Arrhythmia from the records of ECG and handles large database easily (Asl BM et al., 2018).

In present days the computerised detection of Arrhythmia has become a challenge in the medical field (Osowski S et al., 2008). The detection of Arrhythmia is still not accurate even after carrying out various researches for the enhancement of the accuracy for the classification of ECG signals (Mishra AK et al., 2010) and hence this research is for improvising the classification accuracy of the signals by implementing an effective scheme for the analysis of ECG database (Linhares, R et al., 2016). The widely used methods for the extraction of the features from an ECG signals are, mean, covariance, correlation, entropy features and many such methods (Thomas M et al., 2015). The combination of the linier and non-linier scheme such as PCA, KICA and HOS are used to explain and differentiate the ECG database. SVM method of classification is used for the classification of the outcome after comparison with other methods like Neutral Network (NN) classifiers and SVM-Radial Basis Function. This classified outcome results shows that the proposed scheme is more effective in the detection and classification of Arrhythmia (Nanjundegowda et al., 2018).

This Chapter consists of the following content. The classification methodology i.e SVM method which includes effective linear and non-linear features in section II. Correlative analysis between the proposed and the pre-existing methodology is presented in Section III. The conclusion is presented in Section IV.

Effective linier and non-linear components are put into practice together with the binary classifier SVM to overcome the drawbacks and for the further enhancement of the detection and classification of Arrhythmia.

PROPOSED METHODOLOGY

Different methods like QRS detection and sub-division, extraction of feature and the suggested automatic recognition system, classifiers are utilized (N. et al., 2020). The system's overall diagram is constructed and showed the below figure 1 and working of each part is explained in details in the preceding content.

Figure 1. Block diagram typically used to represent the suggested methods.

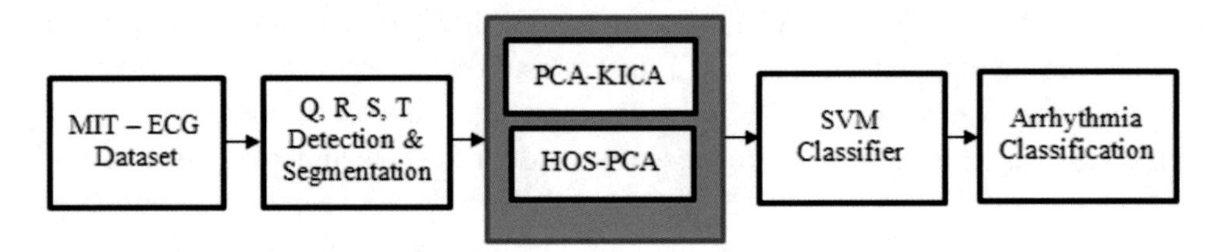

Materials and Procedures

The MIT BIH arrhythmia database was the source of the analysis employed in this article (Goldberger AL et al., 2006). The data has been collected at a frequency of 360 Hz. 10000 normal beats and 24989 abnormal beats were used in this study. The abnormal beats data were broken down into the following groups: 8069 Left Bundle Branch Blocks, 7126 Ventricular Premature Contractions, 2544 Atrial Premature Contractions, and 7250 Right Bundle Branch Blocks (VPC). Here is a brief explanation of several common ECG beats:

- Normal beat: P, QRS complex and T waves are present in the normal ECG signal. 120ms and 200ms is the interval range of the PR wave and for the normal heart it beats 60 to 100 times per minute.
- Right Bundle Branch Block (RBBB): The additional deflection in the QRS complex indicates a quick depolarization of the left ventricle followed by a later depolarization of the right ventricle.
- Left Bundle Branch Block (LBBB): The contraction of the left ventricle a little later than the right ventricle is resulted due to the delay in the activation of the left ventricle. The QRS complex overshoots a period of 120ms.
- Atrial Premature Contraction (APC): It is the heartbeat that beats too soon and comes from. The sinoatrial node controls the heart's beat during normal sinus rhythm; it is activated when the atria in another location depolarize before the sinoatrial node.

- Ventricular Premature Contraction (VPC): A problem will arise outside the sinoatrial node if the QRS complex widens and is not connected to the P wave that came before it or if the T wave is inverted.

The strategy used for classifying normal and abnormal types of heart beats that are automated is shown in the above figure that is figure 1. The functioning of each element the block is elaborated in the upcoming topics. De-ioninsing of wavelet using dB 6 wavelet is done to the ECG signals that have been collected from the MIT BIH Arrhythmia database (Raghu, N et al., 2020). Up to 6 levels of various sub bands are formed after the decomposition of the ECG. The frequency range of 0-2.8125 Hz is consisted in the 6th level approximation sub band. This band of frequency consists of baseline wander. And thus, the necessity of this sub band is unnecessary. The information in an ECG after 45hz is very less and insignificant. And hence the sub bands that store data are the detailed 3rd, 4th, and 5th levels. Hence the other sub bands other than these can be neglected. The denoised ECG can be obtained after the computation of the inverse-DWT. The denoised ECG is now exposed to QRS complex detection through the Pan Tompkins method.

The most vital peak physiologically is the QRS complex. An abridged d version of pan Thompkins algorithm helps in identifying the QRS complex (Zadeh AE et al., 2010). The determination of the QRS complex involves the moving of the average filtering, computation of derivatives, squaring and threshold operations (Elhaj FA et al., 2016). The information provided by the derivative operations are slope information, removal of the high frequency noise by the moving average operations, the enhancement of the high amplitude samples is done by squaring and the rectangular pulses which are responsible for the peaking of the R wave is provided by the threshold operations. After the R peak has been identified, the ECG is subdivided by obtaining 99 samples prior to the R peak and 100 samples following the R peak, both of which contain the R peak. Both the normal subdivisions of the ECG and the development of arrhythmia are aided by this.

Kernel Independent Component Analysis

In ICA, the hidden signals are recovered from a combination of observable signals; a mixture mechanism is not identified. Let's assume that in an ICA model, a vector from an unknown source S is not observed by itself but rather with a linear combination of numerous vectors, as stated by equation number. (1)

$$X(t) = AS(t) \tag{1}$$

Where, $X(t)$ is consists of observation matrices of m signal, $S(t)$ is signal source which is a separate component, while A is a mixed matrix of M and N. You can get S(t) from X for every time t and an unknown matrix A. (t). To estimate the model, a mixed matrix W solution is constructed. Equation represents the ICA solution of the mixed model using the observation signal X(t) following the W transform and the estimate value of the n source signal Y(t) (2).

$$Y(t) = WX(t) = WAX(t) \tag{2}$$

The characteristics that an ICA extracts are linear. Highly complicated nonlinear structures are not truly classified in an acceptable manner. As a result, we require a technique that offers a novel approach for the nonlinear analysis of ECG data, which can be accomplished via the Kernel method. A signal is mapped onto a high-dimensional space from a low-dimensional space, and the minimum value of the kernel contrast function is used to search in the dimensional space. This introduction of the kernel method in ICA is known as KICA, and it is primarily used for the Reconstruction within the Kernel Hilbert Space (RKHS), which is a nonlinear function in comparison. In the equation, the few different kernel function types are depicted (3), (4) and (5).

Linear Kernel: $K(x_i, x) = (x.x_i)$ (3)

Polynomial Kernel: $K(x_i, x) = ((x.x_i) + c)^d c \geq 0$ (4)

Radial basis function (RBF) Kernel: $K\left(x_i, x\right) = \exp\left(\dfrac{x_i - x^2}{2\sigma^2}\right) \sigma \geq 0;$ (5)

The RBF kernel was chosen as the kernel for this study. The following are the steps needed to perform the various ECG cycles via KCIA,

Step1: Decide how many sources there are by entering the data.
Step2: the separation matrix's initialization W
Step3: calculation of the source signals' estimated values, s i=Wx i, and their centred Gram matrices, K 1,.., K_m
Step4: determining the lowest eigen value $\lambda_F(K_1,\ldots,K_m)$ of the generalized characteristic vector equation $K\alpha=\lambda D\alpha$.
Step5: Use the equation to calculate the objective function *(6).*

$$C(w) = -\frac{1}{2} log_2 \lambda_F (K_1, \dots\dots\dots, K_m) \quad (6)$$

Step6: Reduce the goal function to a minimum and output *S*.

A set of assumed named set of signals which is independent is what composes any ECG cycle signal that is x_i. A set of signals which are not dependent on each other are obtained by the KICA decomposition of n cycles of the ECG single matrix $X = (X_1, X_2, \dots\dots, X_n)^T$. The extraction of the nonlinear featured vector, which is based on the collection of independent signal vectors employed in the creation of the feature subspace, provides the coefficient of each cycle of ECG signals projected in the direction of signal B. The equation (7) used for the identification of the projection coefficient vector uses the pseudo-inverse method.

$$A_i = x_i \times S^+ \quad (7)$$

S+ stands for the pseudo-inverse matrix of the independent component S, and A i for the feature vector of the recognised ECG single. The signal discrimination artefacts caused by muscle contraction, movement, and irregular breathing are reduced by KICA. The different artefacts are isolated using the blind source separation which decreases the influence of the artefacts on the classification.

High Order Spectrum

Higher Order Spectrum refers to the spectral representation of a signal's higher order moments (HOS). The third order statistics employed in this work is called bi-spectrum. The averaged by periodogram is used to calculate the bi spectrum B(f (1,) f 2) of a signal, which is the Fourier transform of the third order correlation. (8)

$$B(f_1,f_2) = E[X(f_1)X(f_2)X^*(f_1+f_2)] \quad (8)$$

Fourier transformation If the complex conjugation operator X(f)* is used to represent the signal x(nT), then E[.] is the average of all possible realisations of the random signal, commonly known as the expectation operator. Fast Fourier Transform (FFT) techniques are used to compute X(f), the discrete time Fourier transform, for deterministic sampled signals utilising discrete frequency samples. The range of the frequency f's normalised value is 0 to 1.

A complex valued function of two frequencies, the Bi spectrum produced by equation (8). Real signals have conjugate symmetric Fourier transforms. Asymmetry is seen in the bi spectrum as well. Assuming there is no bi spectral aliasing, the bi spectrum must be computed in its principal domains. The bi spectrum of a real valued signal is uniquely described by the triangle 0f $0 \leq f_2 \leq f_1 \leq f_1 + f_2 \leq 1$. This major domain, also known as the non-redundant region, is denoted by the symbol and is shown in figure. 2. The triangular section in figure contains the major domain, shown as. 2. In this literature, a variety of techniques using the HOS parameter, including cumulate and bi spectrum, are suggested.

Figure 2. Principal domain of bi-spectrum computation is shown inside the triangular.

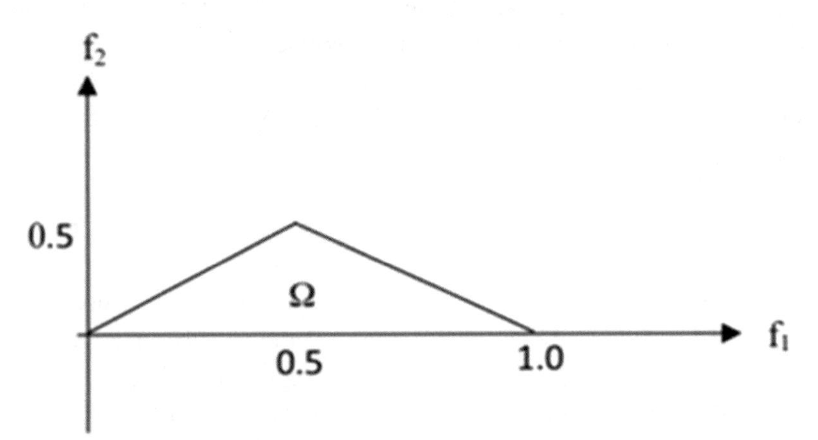

Principal Component Analysis

The dimensions of the data can be decreased and maximum utilization and extraction of the useful features of the ECG signals can be done by adoption the PCA which is a statistical methodology. The performance of PCA is the most effective when compared to the various techniques which are used for the detection and the classification of Arrhythmia, as the noises are spared effectively after factorizing the target signal. PCA also gives more prominence to the covariance and variance structure of the new variables $x_1, x_2, x_3, \ldots, x_p$. the magnitudes of these variables are higher compared to the other variables, as the new variables receive heavy weights.

By choosing variables on scales with wide ranges or using different measurement units, the can be avoided. Using n observations for each p-th main component of a random variable, let R be the sample correlation matrix. The pairings of R's Eigen-values and Eigen-vectors are provided as $(\varepsilon 1\, e1)$, $(\varepsilon 2, e2)$ $(\varepsilon 3, e_3)$, ……, $(\varepsilon p, ep)$. The ith sample principal component of a vector x= x1,x2 x3…,xp variable is given in the equation (9).

$$eiZ = ei1Z_1 + ei2Z_2 + \ldots eipZ_p,\ i = 1,2,3,\ldots,p \tag{9}$$

Where, $e_iZ = (e_{i1}, e_{i2}, e_{i3}, \ldots, e_{ip})$ represents i^{th} Eigen value and $Z = Z_1, Z_2, Z_3, \ldots, Z_p$ is the regular vector observation.

The sample covariance pairings are given as zero in main component, while n i represents the sample variance. Additionally, it is observed that the principal component's total sample variance is equal to the sum of sample variances for all standardised variables. The equation mathematically states the standardised vector observation (10).

$$Z_{k} = \frac{x_k - \overline{x}_k}{\sqrt{v_{kk}}}, k = 1, 2, 3, \ldots p \quad (10)$$

Where the sample variance of the variable x_k is represented by v_{kk} and the sample mean by x_k. Figure 3 compares the samples of various ECG signals.

Figure 3. Examples of various ECG signals.

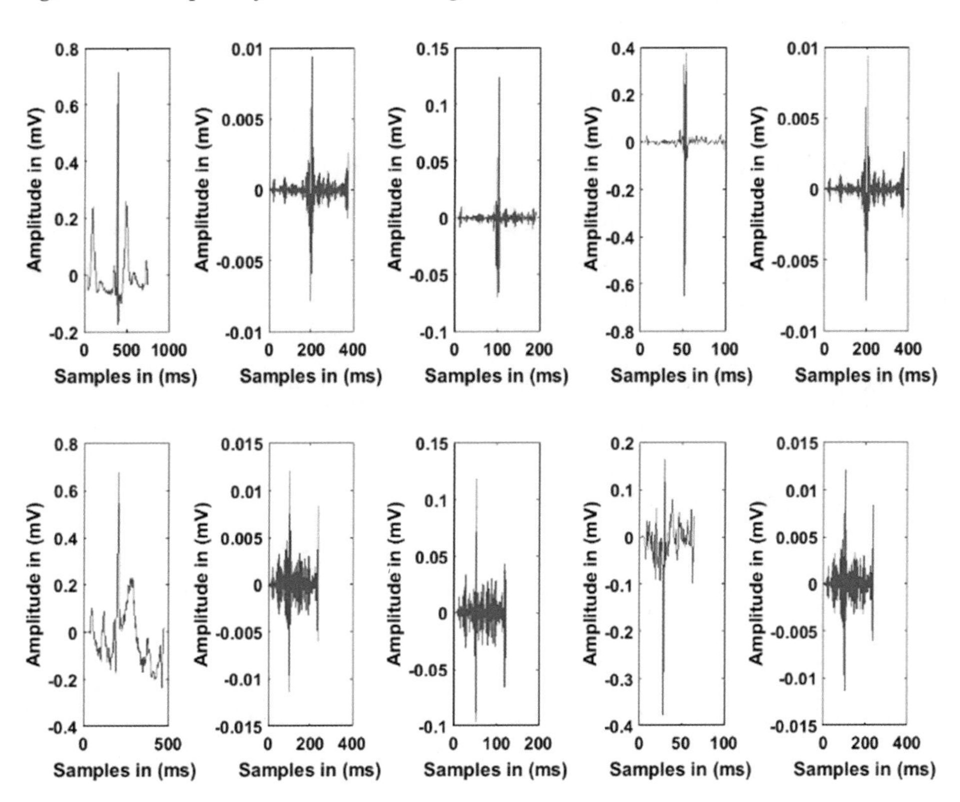

Support Vector Machine (SVM)

ECG is classified using SVM, which validates an effective mechanism to extract the parameters and the set of rules to carry out the classification. A separate hyperplane is used to represent SVM which is a discriminative classification approach. The main objective of SVM is to generate an optimum model after training the classifier using training data. Diverse applications such as, computer vision fields, bio-informatics and others use the SVM classifier as it is known for its high accuracy and the processing capacity for problems caused by high-dimensional data, like gene expressions.

SVM is the most effective classifier for two problems that relate to Vepnik-Chervonekis (VC) and structural principles. The model complexity is taken into account to determine notable generalisation ability. A linear discriminant function's general equation is w.x+b=0. to distinguish between noise-free samples and to capitalise on the distinction between two groups, an ideal hyperplane is needed. This is accomplished by Applying the equation satisfied (11),

$$pi[w.x+b] - 1 \geq 0,\ i=1,2,\ldots,N \tag{11}$$

The saddle point of a Lagrange function, used in the following equation with Lagrange multipliers and declining $\|\mathbf{w}\|^2$, is used to solve this optimization problem. The ideal discriminant function is mathematically described by equation (12),

$$f(x) = sgn\left\{\left(w^{*}x\right)+b^{*}\right\} = sgn\left\{\sum_{i=1}^{N}\alpha_i^{*}.pi\left(x_i^{*}.x\right)+b^{*}\right\}.......... \tag{12}$$

Then, substitute the interior product by a kernel function $k(x,x')$ in formula (13), to resolve the sizeable mathematical complexity moulded by the high parameters. In this way, the linear separate ability of the evaluated samples are improvised and the discriminant function can be re framed as,

$$f(x) = sgn\left\{\sum_{i=1}^{N}\alpha_i^{*}.pi.k\left(x_i^{*}.x\right)+b^{*}\right\}................ \tag{13}$$

Kernels can be classified into three different categories: linear, polynomial, and sigmoid kernels.

Experimental Outcome

For the experimental simulations required by this study to assess the performance effectiveness of the suggested algorithm, MATLAB (version 2017a) was used on a PC with a 3.2 GHz i5 processor. On the MIT-BIH Arrhythmia database, this proposed technique was compiled utilising NN and SVM-RBF classifiers. The comparative analyses were conducted with regard to the accuracy, sensitivity, and specificity.

Performance Evaluation

Appropriate achievement metrics like sensitivity and specificity are employed to understand the correlation between the input and output variables of the system. The following formulas, which are given in equation, provide sensitivity and specificity for classifying the normality and abnormality of arrhythmia illnesses (14) and (15).

$$Sensitivity = \frac{Number\ of\ TP}{Number\ of\ TP + Number\ of\ FN} \times 100 \ldots\ldots\ldots\ldots \quad (14)$$

$$Specificity = \frac{Number\ of\ TN}{Number\ of\ TN + Number\ of\ FP} \times 100 \ldots\ldots\ldots\ldots \quad (15)$$

In this case, TP stands for true positive, FP for false negative, TN for true negative, and FN for false negative.

The best assessment criterion for identifying the efficacy of the heart's normal and pathological actions is accuracy. The general equation for classification of normality and abnormalities of arrhythmia illnesses is shown in the equation (16).

$$Accuracy = \frac{TP + TN}{TP + TN + FP + FN} \times 100 \ldots\ldots\ldots\ldots\ldots\ldots\ldots\ldots\ldots \quad (16)$$

Experimental Results of MIT-BIH Arrhythmia Database

The MIT-BIH arrhythmia database was projected to be used for 80% of training and 20% of testing in this comparative analysis to compare the performance of the pre-existing system with that of the scheme proposed in this work. Table I demonstrates that the sensitivity of the suggested scheme is 99%, while the sensitivity of the existing techniques is 98.91% and 98.90%, respectively. In a similar vein, the proposed method's specificity is 99.08% while the previously used approaches only provide 97.85% and 98.90% specificity. The figure 4 provides a descriptive collation of the sensitivity and specificity in relation to the MIT-BIH arrhythmia database..

Table 1. Comparison of suggested and existing techniques' performance (sensitivity and specificity).

Classifiers	Features	Sensitivity (%)	Specificity (%)
SVM-RBF [16]	PCA-DWT + ICA-HOS	98.91%	97.85%
NN [16]	PCA-DWT + ICA-HOS	98.90%	98.90%
SVM [proposed]	**KICA-PCA PCA-HOS**	**99%**	**99.08%**

Figure 4. Comparing the sensitivity and specificity of new and existing techniques in a descriptive manner.

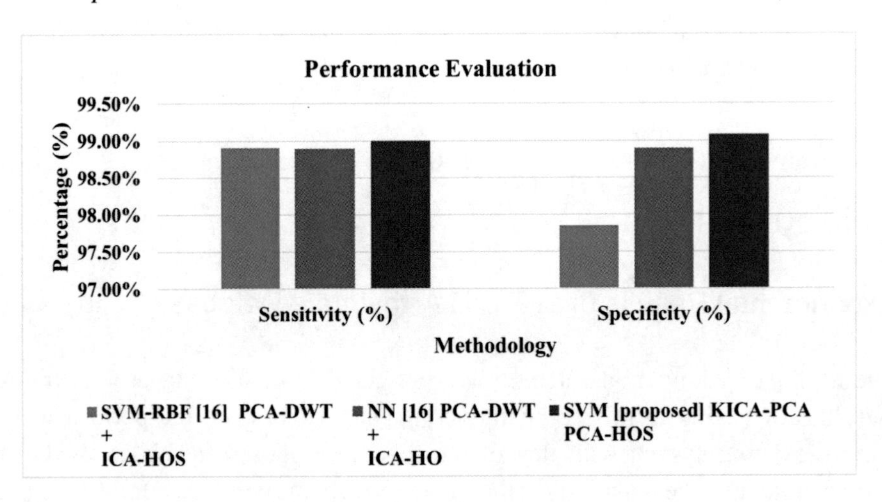

Table 2 compares the new approach's and the pre-existing approach's accuracy in classifying arrhythmias. Using the SVM-RBF and NN classification, the pre-existing systems PCA-DWT, ICA-HOS, PCA-DWT + ICA-HOS, and PCA-KICA demonstrate accuracy of 88.04%, 93.48%, 97.83%, 94.57%, 98.91%, 98.90%, 97.14%, and 98.5%. On the other hand, the suggested method, which employs KICA-PCA-PCA-HOS and SVM methodology, achieves a classification accuracy of 99.04%. The Tables I and II show how well the proposed method performed in comparison to the pre-existing ones on the MIT-BIH arrhythmia database. The figures 5 and 6 provide a descriptive comparison of the accuracy.

Table 2. Comparison of proposed and existing techniques' accuracy and performance.

Classifiers	Features	Classification accuracy
SVM-RBF [16]	PCA-DWT	88.04%
NN [16]		93.48%
SVM-RBF [16]	ICA-HOS	97.83%
NN [16]		94.57%
SVM-RBF [16]	PCA-DWT + ICA-HOS	98.91%
NN [16]		98.90%
SVM [17]	PCA-KICA	97.14%
NN		98.5%
NN	KICA-PCA PCA-HOS	99%
SVM [proposed]		**99.04%**

Figure 5. Comparison of suggested and existing methods' accuracy.

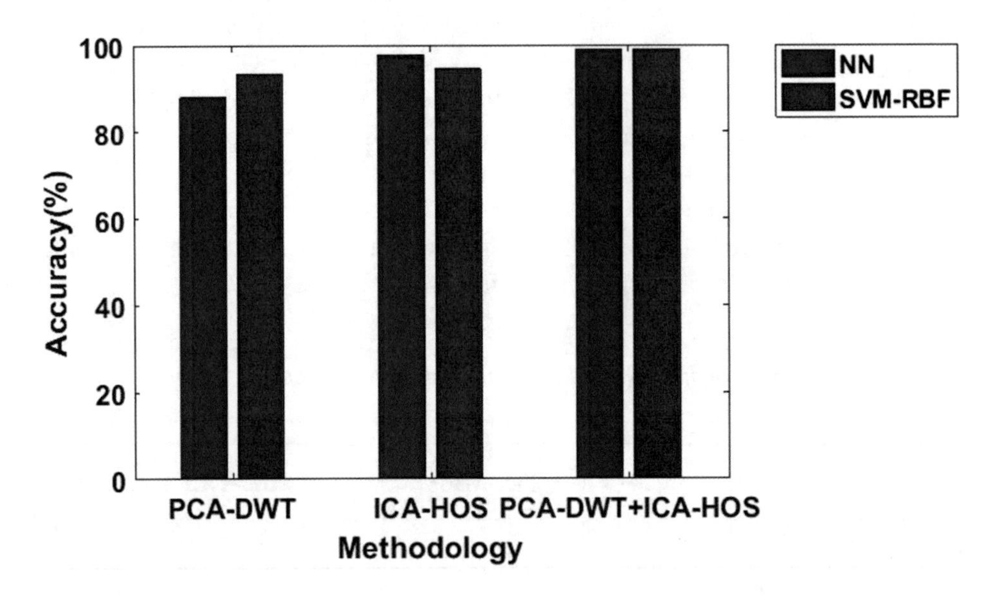

Figure 6. Comparison of the proposed and existing methodologies' accuracy.

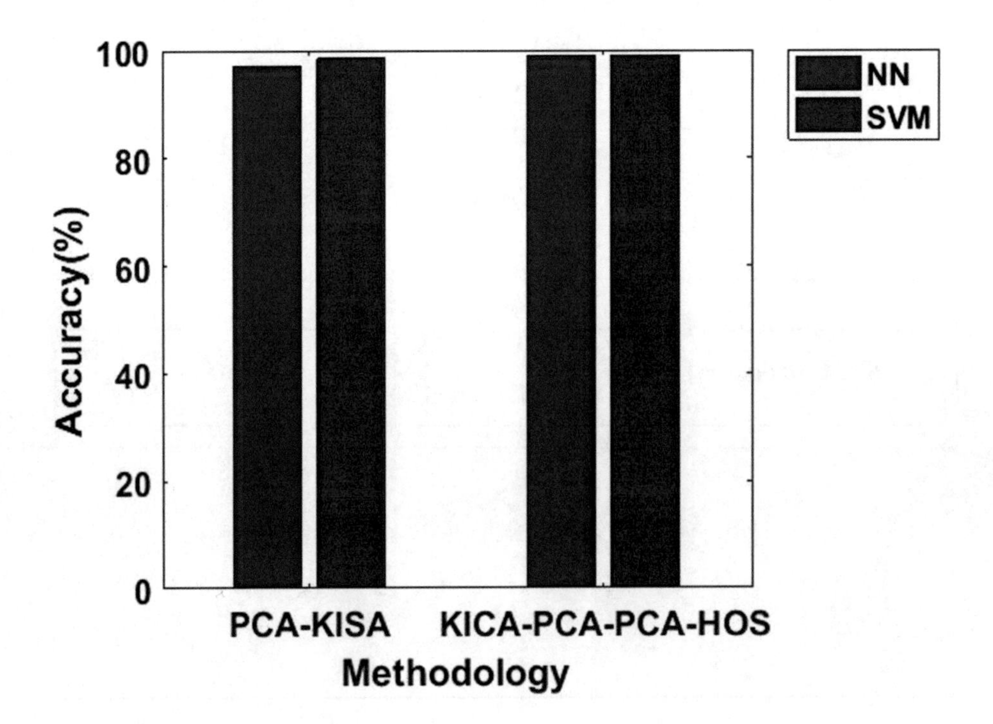

Comparative Evaluation

A comparison of the existing work and the proposed scheme is shown in Table III. A new arrhythmia detection technique that integrates the linear and non-linear features was proposed by Elhaj, et al. [16]. (PCA, DWT, ICA, HOS). After the characteristics were extracted, a binary classifier was used to categorise the ECG data. An open source database (the MIT-BIH arrhythmia database) was used to confirm the accuracy of the results, and it produced a 98.91% accuracy rate. An innovative technique that combines PCA-KICA (feature extraction) with SVM was released by A.E. Zadeh, et al. [17]. (classifier). The accuracy was 97.14% when compared to the baseline in this investigation, which used the MIT-BIH arrhythmia database.

Table 3. Analysis of proposed and existing work in comparison.

References	Database	Features considered	Classification method	Accuracy
F.A. Elhaj, *et al.* [16]	MIT-BIH arrhythmia database	PCA-DWT ICA-HOS	SVM-RBF	98.91%
A.E. Zadeh, *et al.* [17]	MIT-BIH arrhythmia database	PCA-KICA	SVM	97.14%
Proposed work	**MIT-BIH arrhythmia database**	**KICA-PCA PCA-HOS**	**SVM**	**99.04%**

CONCLUSION

The ECG signal-based arrhythmia disease prediction project is one of the most significant research initiatives in computer-aided health monitoring systems. The purpose of this study was to create a useful feature for classifying the normality and abnormality of arrhythmia disease using the MIT-BIH arrhythmia dataset. Non-linear and linear features (PCA, KICA, and HOS) are employed in this situation to provide the optimal feature subsets and to omit extraneous characteristics. The SVM classifier using this feature data is used to categorise the normality and abnormality of arrhythmia disease. In comparison to other available methods for arrhythmia identification, the proposed strategy provided effective performance with improvements in accuracy, sensitivity, and specificity of about 0.5–1% over the prior approaches. In the coming work, suitable feature extraction techniques will be integrated with binary learning classification methodologies to further improve the classification rate of arrhythmia illnesses.

REFERENCES

Asl, B. M., Setarehdan, S. K., & Mohebbi, M. (2008). Support vector machine-based arrhythmia classification using reduced features of heart rate variability signal. *Artificial Intelligence in Medicine*, *44*(1), 51–64. doi:10.1016/j.artmed.2008.04.007 PMID:18585905

Cherif, L. H., Debbal, S. M., & Bereksi-Reguig, F. (2010). Choice of the wavelet analyzing in the phonocardiogram signal analysis using the discrete and the packet wavelet transform. *Expert Systems with Applications*, *37*(2), 913–918. doi:10.1016/j.eswa.2009.09.036

Dash, S. K., & Rao, G. S. (2016, March). Robust multiclass ECG arrhythmia detection using balanced trained neural network. In *2016 International Conference on Electrical, Electronics, and Optimization Techniques (ICEEOT)* (pp. 186-191). IEEE. 10.1109/ICEEOT.2016.7754994

Elhaj, F. A., Salim, N., Harris, A. R., Swee, T. T., & Ahmed, T. (2016). Arrhythmia recognition and classification using combined linear and nonlinear features of ECG signals. Computer methods and programs in biomedicine, 127, 52-63. https://doi:10.1016/j.cmpb.2015.12.024

Gayathri, S., Suchetha, M., & Latha, V. (2012). ECG Arrhythmia Detection and Classification Using Relevance Vector Machine. *Procedia Engineering*, *38*, 1333–1339. doi:10.1016/j.proeng.2012.06.164

Goldberger, A. L. (2006). *Clinical Electrocardiography: A Simplified Approach* (7th ed.). Elsevier.

Haldar, N. A. H., Khan, F. A., Ali, A., & Abbas, H. (2017). Arrhythmia classification using Mahalan obis distance based improved Fuzzy C Means clustering for mobile health monitoring systems. *Neurocomputing*, *220*, 221–235. doi:10.1016/j.neucom.2016.08.042

Jung, W. H., & Lee, S. G. (2017). An arrhythmia classification method in utilizing the weighted KNN and the fitness rule. *IRBM*, *38*(3), 138–148. doi:10.1016/j.irbm.2017.04.002

Khalea, A. F., Owis, M. I., & Yassine, I. A. (2015). A novel technique for cardiac arrhythmia classification using spectral correlation and support vector machines. *Expert Systems with Applications*, *42*(21), 8361–8368. doi:10.1016/j.eswa.2015.06.046

Kutlu, Y., & Kuntalp, D. (2011). A multi-stage automatic arrhythmia recognition and classification system. *Computers in Biology and Medicine*, *41*(1), 37–45. doi:10.1016/j.compbiomed.2010.11.003 PMID:21183163

Linhares, R. R. (2016). Arrhythmia detection from heart rate variability by SDFA method. *International Journal of Cardiology*, *224*, 27–32. doi:10.1016/j.ijcard.2016.08.286 PMID:27611914

Luz, E. J. D. S., Nunes, T. M., De Albuquerque, V. H. C., Papa, J. P., & Menotti, D. (2013). ECG arrhythmia classification based on optimum-path forest. *Expert Systems with Applications*, *40*(9), 3561–3573. doi:10.1016/j.eswa.2012.12.063

Martis, R. J., Acharya, U. R., Prasad, H., Chua, C. K., Lim, C. M., & Suri, J. S. (2013). Application of higher order statistics for atrial arrhythmia classification. *Biomedical Signal Processing and Control*, *8*(6), 888–900. doi:10.1016/j.bspc.2013.08.008

Melin, P., Amezcua, J., Valdez, F., & Castillo, O. (2014). A new neural network model based on the LVQ algorithm for multi-class classification of arrhythmias. *Information Sciences*, *279*, 483–497. doi:10.1016/j.ins.2014.04.003

Mishra, A. K., & Raghav, S. (2010). Local fractal dimension based ECG arrhythmia classification. *Biomedical Signal Processing and Control*, *5*(2), 114–123. doi:10.1016/j.bspc.2010.01.002

N., R. (2020). Arrhythmia Detection Based on Hybrid Features of T-Wave in Electrocardiogram. In J. Thomas, P. Karagoz, B. Ahamed, & P. Vasant (Eds.), *Deep Learning Techniques and Optimization Strategies in Big Data Analytics* (pp. 1-20). IGI Global. . doi:10.4018/978-1-7998-1192-3.ch001

Nanjundegowda, R., & Meshram, V. (2018). Arrhythmia recognition and classification using kernel ICA and higher order spectra. *Int J Eng Technol*, *7*(2), 256–262. doi:10.14419/ijet.v7i2.9535

Osowski, S., Markiewicz, T., & Hoai, L. T. (2008). Recognition and classification system of arrhythmia using ensemble of neural networks. *Measurement*, *41*(6), 610–617. doi:10.1016/j.measurement.2007.07.006

Özbay, Y., & Tezel, G. (2010). A new method for classification of ECG arrhythmias using neural network with adaptive activation function. *Digital Signal Processing*, *20*(4), 1040–1049. doi:10.1016/j.dsp.2009.10.016

Raghu, N. (2020). Arrhythmia detection based on hybrid features of T-wave in electrocardiogram. In *Deep Learning Techniques and Optimization Strategies in Big Data Analytics* (pp. 1–20). IGI Global.

Thomas M, Das MK & Ari S (2015). Automatic ECG arrhythmia classification using dual tree complex wavelet based features. *262 International Journal of Engineering & Technology AEU-International Journal of Electronics and Communications, 69*) (4), 715-721. . doi:10.1016/j.aeue.2014.12.013

Wang, J. S., Chiang, W. C., Hsu, Y. L., & Yang, Y. T. C. (2013). ECG arrhythmia classification using a probabilistic neural network with a feature reduction method. *Neurocomputing*, *116*, 38–45. doi:10.1016/j.neucom.2011.10.045

Zadeh, A. E., Khazaee, A., & Ranaee, V. (2010). Classification of the electrocardiogram signals using supervised classifiers and efficient features. Computer methods and programs in biomedicine, 99(2), 179-194. doi:10.1016/j.cmpb.2010.04.013

Chapter 15
Prospective Health Impact Assessment on Nutritional mHealth Intervention on Maternal Mortality

Frank Adusei-Mensah
https://orcid.org/0000-0001-8237-5305
University of Eastern Finland, Finland

Kennedy J. Oduro
Cape Coast Teaching Hospital, Ghana

Dorcas Ofosu-Budu
University of Eastern Finland, Finland

ABSTRACT

The aim of the present case study is to assess prospectively the HIA of a proposed mobile health intervention to reduce MMR in 10-years. PHIA was carried out on a proposed mHealth intervention to MMR. In addition, an online feasibility pilot study was carried out involving 41 participants from September 1st, 2021, to January 2022. The intervention improved the well-being of pregnant women via education on good nutrition. It reduced MMR, travel costs, frequency of visits to healthcare centers, and increased equality in healthcare accessibility. Due to the reduced frequency of hospital visits, the risk of transportation and road accidents were noticed. About 88% of participants stated the intervention is feasible and worthwhile. While nearly 95% said they are eager and prepared to use the intervention when implemented. The intervention can improve the health of mothers, MMR, and reduce health inequality. Feasibility and willingness to use the new intervention were very high, hence the intervention should be tested on a larger population and in different geographical regions. .

DOI: 10.4018/978-1-6684-6957-6.ch015

INTRODUCTION

Health interventions are necessary to alleviate and improve the health of inhabitants in a community. Though there have been some improvements in healthcare services in Ghana, residents in rural communities are unable to experience the full benefits for diverse reasons. Consequently, they continue to face inadequate healthcare services, increasing health inequality among rural communities. All in all, women and children suffer more, and unacceptably, maternal and under-5 mortalities continue to be a public health concern globally. However, the rate is high in many middle-income and low-income countries (MLIC), especially in sub-Saharan Africa. So, there is an urgent need for a more easily accessible health intervention to reduce maternal mortality.

Maternal and under-5 mortality remains a great concern in many countries globally. However, over 86% of global maternal deaths occur in middle and low- and middle-income countries (LMIC) annually though they are mostly preventable (WHO, 2021b, WHO., 2014). In Colaci et al's study (2016), 99% of global maternal deaths occur in developing countries, usually in rural communities. About 50% of pregnant women in LMIC lack adequate care during child delivery resulting in high maternal mortality rates (MMR) (Moyer et al., 2013). For example, the prevalence of pregnancy-related hypertension is one of the leading causes of maternal mortality (Mudjari and Samsu, 2015). Nonetheless, most pregnant women in developing countries are oblivious to this knowledge and, hence, they are unable to detect it early or to seek medical attention during pregnancy. Although most organizations are determined to reduce the occurrence of maternal and under 5 mortalities, it continues to persist. This is unsurprising because, the top-three preventable factors that adversely affect most maternal mortality (MM) have been identified; inadequate antenatal care delivery, lack of maternal health awareness, and tribal belief systems (Colaci, et al., 2016). In 2015, WHO launched a strategy to end preventable maternal mortality (EPMM). The aim and target of the program were to reduce the global MMR to less than 70 per 100 000 live births by 2030 (SDGs 3.1) (WHO., 2014). Even though the prevalence has reduced, a lot needs to be done to further reduce the occurrence to its barest minimum. As the saying goes "knowledge is power", it has become prudent that pregnant women are educated and encouraged to attend antenatal services. They should also be informed about immunization against tetanus, iron and folate supplementation, voluntary counseling, testing for HIV, the importance of good nutrition, and resting. Due to the challenges in accessing healthcare, especially, in rural areas, the health education is partly hampered.

There is a need to devise other ways of monitoring, disseminating information and communicating with the women concerning their health and well-being. This has become necessary and imperative because it has been established that poor access to quality healthcare is a strong contributor to high maternal and under-5 mortality rates in developing countries especially sub-Saharan Africa (Adam et al., 2021). Furthermore, due to the shortage of doctors and other health professionals, interventions that will serve and monitor the health of many pregnant women but are not resource intensive are highly recommended. This will help healthcare professionals easily detect and identify women who are at risk and need urgent healthcare. Following the advancement of technology globally, there is a need to explore ways of communicating with others with ease. Generally, perinatal periods can be very demanding for mothers, especially new mothers. The period comes with emotional, physical, financial, and social adjustments to the new norms and expectations (Dol et al., 2020). Due to the overwhelming nature of pregnancy, it is imperative that pregnant women are monitored and provided with the needed information to ease their stress.

Considering the common use of mobile phones, they can be used as a tool for health professionals to communicate and monitor the health and well-being of their patients. Mobile phones use has been exploited in health interventions in some contexts but not much has been done for MMR control in Ghana. For instance, in an intervention, mHealth was observed to improve maternal health (Colaci et al., 2016;). There are however challenges to overcome in a mobile health intervention, eg high illiteracy rate in some rural areas of developing countries. However, despite the low literacy rate, mobile health applications still have the potential to improve maternal health. Hence, the objective of the current case project is to propose an mHealth intervention to reduce maternal mortality from the current 360/ 100,000 live births to 70 deaths per 100,000 live births in 10 years. A yearly target of reduction is 3%. Secondary to carry out pHIA on the proposed intervention.

Population health is determined by factors mostly outside the healthcare system (WHO, 2006). Health impact assessment (HIA) champions in identifying these factors in policies/ projects for better health for all by minimizing the negative impact. HIA uses "a combination of procedures; prospective, concurrent and or retrospective approaches to judge policy (Lock, 2000). Based on its global acceptability and credibility, prospective HIA was chosen for the present MMR intervention (Rogerson et al., 2020).

mHealth

The era of technological advancement has brought some vibes to different fields and industries. The wide and easy accessibility and simplicity of mobile phones make them a favourable gadget for delivering health-related interventions (Colaci et al., 2016). The use of mobile and wearable health information and sensing technologies (mHealth) has the potential to reduce the cost of health care and improve well-being in numerous ways (Kumar et al., 2013). It is essential for conditions whose mortality rates are high, especially in areas where health services are not easily accessible. Mobile health (mHealth), an aspect of electronic health (e-health) has been used in many countries for various health interventions. For example, mobile phone interventions have been used in areas like family planning, malaria, tuberculosis, maternal and public health, and human immunodeficiency virus (HIV) (Colaci et al., 2016). M-health including video conferencing, audio calls, and text messaging have been used in most developed countries like Finland in meeting health goals. Additionally, m-health has been used in diabetes, asthma, obesity, smoking cessation, and depression management (Kumar et al., 2013). In Finland, patient-doctor or patient-nurse audio/ video calls are used for some health issues without hospital visits increasing services equity (Pohjois-Suomen sosiaalialan osaamiskeskus, 2018).

Developing countries including Ghana have great opportunities for mHealth technologies due to the rising usage of mobile phones in the region in the last decade. Looking at the disparities in healthcare services among rural and urban residents in Ghana, it is important that m-health interventions are explored. According to Sey in 2011, in Ghana, people value their phones and consider them as an integral part of their lives because it serves multiple functions. For example, people transact financial businesses using their mobile phones, stay in touch with family and friends and use them for social media and other purposes. Therefore, it is commonplace to see people with mobile phones. Within a decade, the African population's phone usage had grown from 10% to 60% (1999 to 2008) and currently between 75% - 90% of the adult population (Aker & Mbiti, 2010, Amoakoh-Coleman et al., 2016). Accordingly, the power, availability, and usage of mobile phones in the region can be harnessed to improve health and reduce MMR. A similar intervention has been used in Rwanda on MMR with impressive outcome (Musabyimana et al., 2018). Furthermore, in some studies in Kenya, Madagascar, Rwanda and Nepal, mobile phones have proven to be efficient in reporting precise and complete data on the status of pregnant women thereby increasing follow-ups. Also, it has helped in the uptake of prenatal care and facility-based delivery rates (Karageorgos et al., 2018).

MATERIALS AND METHODS

The study made use of an elaborate outline of the pHIA methodology. Cross-sectional interviews (N=41) were collected to support the theory for the present intervention. To assess the potential benefits and negative health impacts of the planned intervention, we followed the guidelines for a rapid pHIA. A typical HIA has five steps including: screening, scoping, appraisal, reporting, evaluation and monitoring (Figure 1).

Research Design (HIA)

The present study made use of a mixed-method approach.

Figure 1. Flowchart of the HIA process

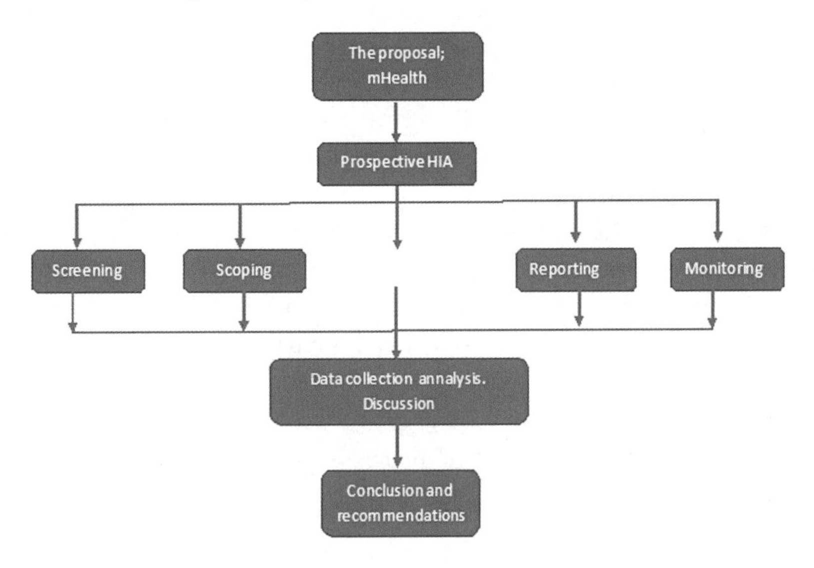

The Proposed Intervention

Ghana has high MMR of over 300/ 100,000 live births which is above WHO's recommended average of 70/ 100,000 live births (Ghana Health Service, 2016). Close to 1.47% women faces lifetime risk of maternal complications or at worst cases death due to preventable causes (Moyer et al., 2013, WHO et al., 2014). In a study to explore the predictors of maternal mortality in Ghana, evidence from the 2017 GMHS verbal autopsy data, they observed that bleeding during pregnancy, excessive bleeding during childbirth, and releasing a pregnant woman from the hospital ill and the use of traditional or herbal medicines for the illnesses contributed to the loss of life (Sumankuuro et al., 2020). For improved pregnancy outcome, it is beneficial for the pregnant woman to be in an adequate nutritional state. According to Wu and colleagues in 2012, poor nutrition during pregnancy has dire consequences on their health. It has been associated with anaemia, maternal haemorrhage, insulin resistance, and hypertensive disorders. As a result, nutritional education should be provided for pregnant women and mothers through different models, policies and programs in meeting the set MMR goals. The project hopes to achieve the set goals by an annual reduction of MMR by 3% for the next 10 years. We propose a mobile nutritional guide through a freely available app resource for nurses and nutritionists to guide pregnant women. Further, psychological counseling is needed to improve the well-being of these women due to the extra stress and burden that pregnancy poses. A holistic approach should therefore be considered as part of the intervention. The intervention involves the provision of 3 Nokia-7 phones to each of the 5 health centers and one Nokia-7 phone to each community center (125 community centers). Pregnant women who do not have personal phones can participate in the intervention via community center-based phones. A resource person from a mobile health solution app (GRAVID) will give technical training to the healthcare professionals/ dieticians, pregnant women and community heads during the early phase of the intervention (Akinseinde et al., 2016).

GRAVID is an Android open-source application tool for cost-effective development and widespread community coverage. GRAVID provides a monitoring tool for caregivers to track the progress of gravid women and children. Regular nutritional updates will be provided by health professionals (nutritionists, midwives) to enhance prenatal and postnatal periods of mothers and under-5-year children. GRAVID can be used by community health workers to collect field-based health data, send alerts and reminders, facilitate health education sessions, and conduct person-to-person communication (Akinseinde et al., 2016).

The Prospective HIA on the mHealth Intervention

Screening

The screening step served as a checklist for assessing the health impact on the target population and whether it should undergo HIA (WHO, 2021a) (**Figure** 1). The project aims to reduce MMR to 70 deaths per 100,000 live births per year in 10 years with an annual reduction of 3%. HIA could be applied to this intervention. MHealth interventions on hypertension (Wu et al., 2019), and RapidSMS messaging intervention in Rwanda with substantial health impact on mothers and children (Musabyimana et al., 2018). In addition, there are also endpoints in measuring the progress and the success of the present intervention. Annual surveys, evaluating MMR, and average birthweights of children before/after the intervention are critical endpoints in measuring the progress and to evaluate the success of the intervention. The intervention could be terminated at the end of the third year if no reduction in the MMR is observed.

Scoping

The scope of the assessment was established based on the aims and budget of the present intervention and a desktop literature review of similar interventions. Poor nutrition and eating habits have been identified as one of the contributing factors to MMR. The target group of this HIA is pregnant women during the antenatal, and post-natal periods and reside in Adansi North District of Ghana. These women have less access to health services and health information and relatively use fewer health services than men (Buor, 2004).

Appraisal

We performed a baseline assessment of the food production, nutritional state and assessment of health resources available to the local population. We evaluated the possible negative and positive health impacts of the target populations. The health outcomes and factors affecting the implementation of the intervention are presented (table 1). Efficient HIA depends on the availability of robust evidence of health impacts to predict the impact on the health of the affected population (Petticrew et al., 2004).

Reporting

The results of the pHIA are presented in the current paper (table 2). The HIA evaluated the impacts of the intervention on health and other parameters (alternative 1) compared with without the intervention (alternative 0), (table 2).

Monitoring

In monitoring the progress of the intervention, the use of health outcomes such as assessment of low birth weight, MMR, stillbirths, iron and folic acid consumption, and preterm birth assessment before and after the intervention are essential (figure1, table 1) (Patel et al., 2019).

HIA FINDINGS

Adansi North District is a district within the Ashanti Region of Ghana with 125 communities, a surface area of 1140 km^2 and 122,350 inhabitants as of 2015 (Ghana Health Service, 2016). The communities are mostly rural, and they are mostly into agricultural business (77%) (Adansi North District assembly, 2013). With enough food produced in the district, the women have the resources to eat healthily if they receive the right guidance from a health practitioner or dietician. However, the district is highly under-resourced with clinics/hospitals and healthcare providers (Ghana Health Service, 2016). Due to the limited care providers, the large surface area, and over 120 communities, it will be difficult to provide effective physical nutritional assistance to pregnant and postnatal women in targeting MMR.

Table 1. Potential positive and negative impacts of the intervention

Stakeholder	Positive impacts	Negative impacts
Individual	• Better nutrition, increased wellbeing of pregnant women and mothers • Savings on travel time and cost to health care centers • Equality in healthcare accessibility • Less hustle and reduced risk to road accidents • Better nutrition and reduced MMR • Better health condition for the newborn	• Additional cost for women in acquiring personal phones. • Reduced experience of face-to-face reception • Mental stress to learn and use the mobile app.
Family	• Less hustle and reduced risk to road accidents • Better nutrition and increased wellbeing of family members • Time savings and quality time together with family.	• Additional cost for women in acquiring own cell phones.
Health professionals and health care system	• Receive on-the-job training for new task • Lessen time cost to monitor clients • Less pregnancy complications due to poor nutrition • Reduced delivery complications • Less complications and savings on health resources	• More time for training • Additional financial resources to operate the service • Concerns on client's privacy issues
Community	• Reduce health inequality • Enhances equal access to healthcare • Good health and wellbeing of the residents	• Time cost on community heads for arranging and using the 'community phones'.
Society and state	• Long-term cost savings • Reduced pregnancy complications • Reduced delivery complications due to poor nutrition • Savings on health budget due to lessing of complications	• Financial cost • Addition resources for workers training, monitoring and maintaining the intervention

Key Health Issues

MMR is high in Ghana and above the global average (Der et al., 2013). Poor nutrition and inequalities in access to quality health services affect MMR (Houweling et al.,

2007). Diet during pregnancy affects the growth and development of the foetus and mother (US Institute of Medicine, Committee on Quality of Health Care in America, 2000). The intervention will offer nutritional guidance to pregnant women during antenatal and post-natal periods, and it is aimed at improving the health of the pregnant woman by increasing health service usage via mHealth platform.

Women's Views on mHealth Services (from Literature)

Pregnant women and women in the postnatal period are eager for mHealth interventions. Women believe mobile phone communication with health workers would be much easier and faster. They opined, mhealth would be pivotal for future antenatal care (Feroz et al., 2017).

Health Care Workers' Views on mHealth Services

Community health workers regard video content and teaching tools as an acceptable and feasible means to provide health promotion and education to their clients (Coetzee et al., 2018). M-health interventions have been used to track pregnant women to improve antenatal and delivery care, as well as facilitate referrals (Amoakoh-Coleman et al., 2016). However, some health professionals have misgivings about privacy and trustworthiness; they believe in mHealth services there is a shift of patient data from trusted to untrusted sources.

mHealth Interventions' Outcomes (From Literature)

M-Health-SMS-messaging interventions have been associated with increased utilization of health care in improving maternal and neonatal outcomes (Lee et al., 2016, Sondaal et al., 2016). In nutritional guidance, mHealth interventions can be used to improve adherence to taking micronutrient supplements in pregnancy. There has been a positive correlation between mhealth and women's antenatal visits, diet counselling, iron supplement and vitamin intake (Fedha, 2014).

Planning and Using mHealth Interventions

Technological, financial, illiteracy and low accessibility to mobile phones amongst rural women are potential threats to the intervention (Amoakoh-Coleman et al., 2016). Integrating into health care, using existing guidelines and stakeholder collaborations has been shown to increase acceptance of mHealth interventions (Sondaal et al., 2016). The contextual adaptability of the current intervention is the strength of the present intervention.

Table 2. Impact with and without the intervention.

Focus	Current policy continues (alternative 0)	mHealth is provided (alternative 1)
Mothers	• Maternal death continues	• Maternal death decreases • Mothers get healthier • Nutrition improves • No need to travel long distances for healthcare
Children	• Children under 5 years death continues • Motherless children increase	• Children under 5 years death decreases • Motherless children decrease • Children get healthier • Nutrition improves
Health care system	• Unequal health care services • Lack of resources in facilities • Long waiting times in health care facilities • More complications	• Personalized services • Equality in health care services • Timesaving
Society	• Low antenatal coverage • Logistics and poor road network • Costs will stay or increase	• Costs decrease

CONTROLLING MECHANISMS

To ensure that mechanisms are aligned and monitored, checks on weekly contact between the health practitioner the pregnant women, MMR before, during and after the intervention, supplement intake before, during and after the intervention are checkpoints for evaluating the success of the intervention. It is possible to see the impacts of the intervention in 2-3 years' time, hence if no progress in MMR is seen in the first 3 years after implementation, the intervention could be aborted.

The Feasibility Study

We present the findings of the feasibility study on the above-described intervention on 41 participants from the target population. The online feasibility pilot study was conducted from September 1st, 2021, to January 31st, 2022, via google forms. Participants were invited by email and mobile messaging. An electronic form via google documents was sent to the participants via email and or a link to the form via WhatsApp message and Facebook. Also, an open Facebook link was shared by the PI to recruit participants. The form included a section on consent to participate and a brief description of the study and its aim. It is therefore assumed that any participant who filled in the survey form consented to participate in the study. Only 41 participants completed the form and were included in the analysis. The return rate is difficult to estimate due to the open invitation on Facebook without precise knowledge of the total number of those who might have received the form but did not return it (the denominator).

Ethical Consideration

This pilot study was an online feasibility study carried electrically to ascertain the applicability of the intervention. At this stage, participants' consent was sort from all the participants prior to participate in the study. The background and the objective to the study was provided to participants for informed decision. Participants also had the voluntarily right to exit from the study at any given time without any current or future implications to them. Should a field study become possible, ethical clearance will be sort from the district and other authorizing bodies.

Empirical Results of the Feasibility Study

We present the results of the feasibility study on 41 participating pregnant and or nursing mothers from the target population.

Table 3. Results from the pilot study

THEME	SURVEY QUESTION	RESPONSE (%, N)
Prevalence of MR among participants	Do you know of/ heard of a woman who has lost her life through maternal mortality in Adansi north district of Ghana or in your local community?	Yes (51.20%, N=41)
		No (49.8%, N=41)
		Maybe (0%, N=41)
Applicability of mHealth intervention	Do you think video and audio calls by nurses to pregnant women and lactating mothers can improve adherence to taking essential micronutrient supplements in pregnancy?	Yes (80%, N=41)
		No (20%, N=41)
		Maybe (0%, N=41)
Health impact of the intervention	Do you think video and audio calls by nurses to pregnant women and lactating mothers can improve women's antenatal visits, diet counselling, in pregnancy and lactation state to enhance safe birth?	Yes (83%, N=41)
		No (0%, N=41)
		Maybe (17%, N=41)
Assessing the need for the intervention.	Do you hope for an intervention to reduce the maternal mortality situation in Ghana?	Yes (98%, N=41)
		No (0%, N=41)
		Maybe (2%, N=41)
Assessing the impact of diet on MMR.	Do you think poor nutritional status of the pregnant woman can negatively influence maternal mortality?	Yes (98%, N=41)
		No (0%, N=41)
		Maybe (2%, N=41)
Evaluating the overall impact of the intervention.	Do you think nutritional guidance from nurses through video and audio phone calls can help improve the nutritional status of pregnant women in rural areas to help reduce maternal and neonatal mortality?	Yes (76%, N=41)
		No (7%, N=41)
		Maybe (17%, N=41)
Applicability score	On a scale of 1 to 5, rate how you see mobile intervention as a potential in reducing maternal mortality in Ghana during and after the COVID-19 pandemic. 1 = low and 5=high.	3 = 21.6%, (N=41) 4 = 45.9%, (N=41) 5 = 24.3%, (N=41)
Feasibility assessment	On a scale of 1 to 5, how would you rate the feasibility of nutritional guidance from nurses via video and audio phone calls to help improve the nutritional status of pregnant women in rural areas to help reduce neonatal and maternal mortality in Ghana. 1 = low and 5=high.	3 = 29.3%, (N=41)
		4 = 34.1%, (N=41)
		5 = 24.4%, (N=41)
E-health: Usability of the intervention	Do you wish to receive reminders on nutritional supplementation, appointments related to nutrition, childcare and danger signs in pregnancy?	Yes (95%, N=41)
		No (0%, N=41)
		Maybe (5%, N=41)

DISCUSSION

Most MMR occur in rural areas with limited resources and high inequality of health utilization and healthcare resources (WHO & World Bank, 2014, Apanga & Awoonor-Williams, 2018). Low skilled birth attendance rate, socio-cultural factors, low antenatal coverage, logistics and poor road network have been linked to high MMR in rural areas of Ghana (Apanga & Awoonor-Williams, 2018, Kn et al., 2015,Witter & Adjei, 2007). In developing countries like Ghana with health infrastructural constraints, low doctor: patient and nurse: patient ratios, long waiting times in healthcare facilities, using remote intervention is an important choice to consider in reducing MMR in the country. Over half (51%) of the participants believed maternal mortality was common and high which findings confirms the report by Ghana health service in 2016 (Ghana Health Service, 2016). It also shows that it has been a more persistent problem in the region.

SDG 3 aims to achieve a global MMR of 70/100,000 live birth by 2030, requiring close to a 7.4% annual reduction in Ghana's MMR (WHO, 2021b, Gurusamy & Janagaraj, 2018). Poor nutrition, inequalities in access to quality health services and poverty negatively influence MMR. Foetal growth restriction and its associated increased risk of MMR and stillbirths have been associated with maternal malnutrition (Nnam, 2015). Undernutrition, foetal growth restrictions, wasting, and deficiencies of vitamin-A and zinc cause about 3,1 million child deaths annually (Black et al., 2013). Iron and calcium deficiencies contribute substantially to maternal deaths, preterm birth, and increased infant mortality (Black et al., 2013).

Mhealth has the power to reduce the number of healthcare visits, provide personalized service, and on-demand interventions. The health impacts of development projects in rural areas are significantly larger than in developed countries (Utzinger, 2004). The intervention will help in reducing health inequalities in the district, over 91.9% believe it has a high impact (N=41) (Table 3). This finding supports the previous reports (Utzinger, 2004). The unequal distribution of healthcare resources in the rural areas of Ghana is serving as a hindrance to healthcare for mothers in the remote parts of the country. Using mobile technology to reach mothers in these areas will reduce the MMR problem in the district (Table 1). In the present study, 88% believe it is feasible (N=41) and that m-health holds great potential in averting maternal mortality in low-income countries (Table 3). According to a study by Ryu, (2012), the removal of potential barriers holds great success for an m-health intervention (Table 3). The finding also supports the reports of previous surveys. Willcox et al reported that pregnant women prefer to receive and listen to audio messages (Willcox et al., 2015). Most of them wish to receive reminders on medication, appointments, and health education messages related to nutrition, childcare, and danger signs in pregnancy Feroz et al., 2017). They opined that these reminders would help them self-track their progress, danger signs, and positive health behaviors (Feroz et al., 2017). In the present study, over 80% believe the current intervention is feasible, will feel comfortable using it and it has a great health impact (Table 3). The current intervention promises a lot of positive returns to all stakeholders in reducing health inequality among women and children (Tables 1 & 3) with great potential to improve the existing service delivery structure in the target area. The project promises a great and sustainable way of controlling MMR in the target population. It will in addition serve as an easy and affordable means of controlling the health inequality problems in the marginalized community.

Major barriers worth considering are the need to increase the number of health care workers leading to an increase in the health care budget of the community. Despite the potential barriers to consider, close to 90% in the present study (moderately feasible=29.3%, feasible=34.1% and highly feasible =24.4%; totaling 88%) believe the proposed intervention is highly feasible (Table 3). Similar m-health intervention 'MyDayPlan'' was readily acceptable and deemed feasible by participants in previous studies (Degroote et al., 2020). A similar intervention targeting HIV in South Africa was considered feasible for the setting (Nachega et al., 2016). The intervention will come with training, technical and implementation costs. Also, the acquisition costs of the phones, application updates and language translation into the local language are worth considering. However, the individual benefit outweighs the cost of the intervention. A total of 91.9% of participants believe the present intervention can reduce MMR in the country. The applicability and acceptability rate observed for the present m-health intervention correlates well with previous studies in sub-Saharan region. Lee and colleagues (S. Lee et al., 2017) reported that a total of over 480 mHealth programs were implemented in sub-Saharan Africa in one decade between 2006 and 2016. Again, in that same study, they reported that the western regional countries with 16 countries accounted for more than one-fourth of 145 and 487 mHealth programs (S. Lee et al., 2017). Regarding the target group, possible barriers could be the attitudes toward mhealth service, and the desire to face-to-face service. Attitude, cost-effectiveness, priority issues, technological knowledge, data handling, and sustainability have been previously identified as barriers to mhealth intervention (Ryu, 2012). Lack of resources and the need for additional training on how to implement the mHealth intervention could be an additional barrier on the side of healthcare professionals.

Using a mobile app to provide remote guidance services to pregnant women will enormously impact in reducing the health inequality and MMR in the district. The proposed intervention has the potential to be implemented in any resource-limited communities globally in tackling one of the Cardinal Health issues facing women and children. M-health services for antenatal care would enhance information dissemination, service delivery, client contact and service uptake, and medical education in pregnancy (Fedha, 2014)(McNabb et al., 2015). In the present study, participants believed m-health is feasible in the local rural communities (95.5%, N=41), and 91.9% believe the present intervention would have a high impact (N=41) in averting or reducing maternal mortality in the community.

CONCLUSION AND RECOMMENDATIONS

The current intervention seeks to use a mobile app with text messaging, video conferencing and charting capabilities to tackle an important health problem in a rural community. The pHIA on the intervention can be applied in similar contexts or other health challenges globally. It has the potential to reduce death rates and improve the quality of life. About 90 of the participants believed the intervention was feasible and has a high potential to reduce maternal mortality. Furthermore, others stated it was handy and economically sustainable. Again, the current intervention has huge potential in reaching a wide population with over 97% of the participants endorsing the intervention as a potential to control maternal mortality. It is highly recommended that pregnant women attend antennal care where healthcare is easily accessible together with the m-health intervention. Barriers and opportunities to the intervention were raised and finally, the health impact was assessed. Based on the HIA and the empirical data, it is evident that the intervention has the potential to positively impact SDG 3 and improve health. Some of the barriers reported were fear of technology failure, difficulty in understanding and using the apps, lack of adequate information and misunderstanding. The intervention is recommended for further consideration and implementation. More so, people should be educated on how to use the apps. Health practitioners should be mindful of their medical vocabulary to avoid miscommunication and misunderstanding. Finally, and most importantly people should be encouraged to visit the hospitals and not over rely on the mHealth interventions alone.

Limitations

The current intervention could be replicated globally by overcoming the below limitations. The limited number of participants in the current study (41) is a limiting factor to consider when trying to directly implement the proposed intervention. We, therefore, recommend further studies in larger populations prior to implementation. Again, possible recruitment bias could have been introduced in the current study; most participants recruited were via direct messaging and potential participants without prior contact with the PI either by mobile or Facebook were less likely to be recruited. This could be avoided in future studies with enough funds by employing face-to-face interviews with randomization.

AUTHOR STATEMENTS

No funding was received for the paper. The authors have no conflicting interest in carrying out this research. Ethical clearance was not needed in carrying out this work and no human nor animal subjects were involved in the study.

ACKNOWLEDGMENT

The author would like to acknowledge the enormous support of Marika Kemppainen, Saija Koskiniemi and Karikumpu all at the School of Nursing, the University of Eastern Finland, Kuopio, Finland for their enormous support.

REFERENCES

Adam, A., Fusheini, A., & Kipo-Sunyehzi, D. D. (2021). A Collaborative Health Promotion Approach to Improve Rural Health Delivery and Health Outcomes in Ghana: A Case Example of a Community-Based Health Planning and Services (CHPS) Strategy. In Rural Health. IntechOpen.

Adansi North District assembly. (2013). *Adansi North District Medium Term Development Plan (2014 – 2017)*. ANDA.

Aker, J. C., & Mbiti, I. M. (2010). Mobile Phones and Economic Development in Africa. *The Journal of Economic Perspectives*, *24*(3), 207–232. doi:10.1257/jep.24.3.207

Akinseinde, A. S., Badejo, J. A., & Malgwi, R. L. (2016). GRAVID: An indigenous m-health tool for smart and connected communities. *2016 Future Technologies Conference (FTC)*, (pp. 1331–1334). 10.1109/FTC.2016.7821776

Amoakoh-Coleman, M., Borgstein, A. B.-J., Sondaal, S. F., Grobbee, D. E., Miltenburg, A. S., Verwijs, M., Ansah, E. K., Browne, J. L., & Klipstein-Grobusch, K. (2016). Effectiveness of mHealth Interventions Targeting Health Care Workers to Improve Pregnancy Outcomes in Low- and Middle-Income Countries: A Systematic Review. *Journal of Medical Internet Research*, *18*(8), e226. doi:10.2196/jmir.5533 PMID:27543152

Apanga, P. A., & Awoonor-Williams, J. K. (2018). Maternal Death in Rural Ghana: A Case Study in the Upper East Region of Ghana. *Frontiers in Public Health*, *6*, 101. doi:10.3389/fpubh.2018.00101 PMID:29686982

Black, R. E., Victora, C. G., Walker, S. P., Bhutta, Z. A., Christian, P., de Onis, M., Ezzati, M., Grantham-McGregor, S., Katz, J., Martorell, R., & Uauy, R.Maternal and Child Nutrition Study Group. (2013). Maternal and child undernutrition and overweight in low-income and middle-income countries. *Lancet*, *382*(9890), 427–451. doi:10.1016/S0140-6736(13)60937-X PMID:23746772

Buor, D. (2004). Gender and the utilisation of health services in the Ashanti Region, Ghana. *Health Policy (Amsterdam, Netherlands)*, *69*(3), 375–388. doi:10.1016/j.healthpol.2004.01.004 PMID:15276316

Coetzee, B., Kohrman, H., Tomlinson, M., Mbewu, N., Roux, I. L., & Adam, M. (2018). Community health workers' experiences of using video teaching tools during home visits—A pilot study. *Health & Social Care in the Community*, *26*(2), 167–175. doi:10.1111/hsc.12488 PMID:28872210

Colaci, D., Chaudhri, S., & Vasan, A. (2016). mHealth interventions in low-income countries to address maternal health: A systematic review. *Annals of Global Health*, *82*(5), 922–935. doi:10.1016/j.aogh.2016.09.001 PMID:28283147

Degroote, L., Van Dyck, D., De Bourdeaudhuij, I., De Paepe, A., & Crombez, G. (2020). Acceptability and feasibility of the mHealth intervention 'MyDayPlan' to increase physical activity in a general adult population. *BMC Public Health*, *20*(1), 1032. doi:10.118612889-020-09148-9 PMID:32600352

Der, E. M., Moyer, C., Gyasi, R. K., Akosa, A. B., Tettey, Y., Akakpo, P. K., Blankson, A., & Anim, J. T. (2013). Pregnancy Related Causes of Deaths in Ghana: A 5-Year Retrospective Study. *Ghana Medical Journal*, *47*(4), 158–163. PMID:24669020

Dol, J., Richardson, B., Murphy, G. T., Aston, M., McMillan, D., & Campbell-Yeo, M. (2020). Impact of mobile health interventions during the perinatal period on maternal psychosocial outcomes: A systematic review. *JBI Evidence Synthesis*, *18*(1), 30–55. doi:10.11124/JBISRIR-D-19-00191 PMID:31972680

Fedha, T. (2014). Impact of Mobile Telephone on Maternal Health Service Care: A Case of Njoro Division. *Open Journal of Preventive Medicine*, *4*(5), 365–376. doi:10.4236/ojpm.2014.45044

Feroz, A., Rizvi, N., Sayani, S., & Saleem, S. (2017). Feasibility of mHealth intervention to improve uptake of antenatal and postnatal care services in peri-urban areas of Karachi: A qualitative exploratory study. *Journal of Hospital Management and Health Policy*, *1*(4), 4. https://jhmhp.amegroups.com/article/view/3945. doi:10.21037/jhmhp.2017.10.02

Ghana Health Service. (2016). *The health sector in Ghana facts and figures 2015*. Ghana Health Service. https://www.ghanahealthservice.org/ghs-item-details.php?cid=5&scid=55&iid=134

Gurusamy, P. S. R., & Janagaraj, P. D. (2018). A Success Story: The Burden of Maternal, Neonatal and Childhood Mortality in Rwanda - Critical Appraisal of Interventions and Recommendations for the Future. *African Journal of Reproductive Health*, *22*(2), 9–16. doi:10.29063/ajrh2018/v22i2.1 PMID:30052329

Houweling, T. A. J., Ronsmans, C., Campbell, O. M. R., & Kunst, A. E. (2007). Huge poor-rich inequalities in maternity care: An international comparative study of maternity and child care in developing countries. *Bulletin of the World Health Organization*, *85*(10), 745–754. doi:10.2471/BLT.06.038588 PMID:18038055

Institute of Medicine (US) Committee on Quality of Health Care in America. (2000). *To Err is Human: Building a Safer Health System* (L. T. Kohn, J. M. Corrigan, & M. S. Donaldson, Eds.). National Academies Press. https://www.ncbi.nlm.nih.gov/books/NBK225182/

Karageorgos, G., Andreadis, I., Psychas, K., Mourkousis, G., Kiourti, A., Lazzi, G., & Nikita, K. S. (2018). The promise of mobile technologies for the health care system in the developing world: A systematic review. *IEEE Reviews in Biomedical Engineering*, *12*, 100–122. doi:10.1109/RBME.2018.2868896 PMID:30188840

Kn, A. (2015). Can she make it? Transportation barriers to accessing maternal and child health care services in rural Ghana. *BMC Health Services Research*, *15*(1), 333–333. doi:10.118612913-015-1005-y PMID:26290436

Kumar, S., Nilsen, W. J., Abernethy, A., Atienza, A., Patrick, K., Pavel, M., Riley, W. T., Shar, A., Spring, B., Spruijt-Metz, D., Hedeker, D., Honavar, V., Kravitz, R., Lefebvre, R. C., Mohr, D. C., Murphy, S. A., Quinn, C., Shusterman, V., & Swendeman, D. (2013). Mobile health technology evaluation: The mHealth evidence workshop. *American Journal of Preventive Medicine*, *45*(2), 228–236. doi:10.1016/j.amepre.2013.03.017 PMID:23867031

Lee, S., Cho, Y., & Kim, S.-Y. (2017). Mapping mHealth (mobile health) and mobile penetrations in sub-Saharan Africa for strategic regional collaboration in mHealth scale-up: An application of exploratory spatial data analysis. *Globalization and Health*, *13*(1), 63. doi:10.118612992-017-0286-9 PMID:28830540

Lee, S. H., Nurmatov, U. B., Nwaru, B. I., Mukherjee, M., Grant, L., & Pagliari, C. (2016). Effectiveness of mHealth interventions for maternal, newborn and child health in low- and middle-income countries: Systematic review and meta-analysis. *Journal of Global Health*, *6*(1), 010401. doi:10.7189/jogh.06.010401 PMID:26649177

Lock, K. (2000). Health impact assessment. *BMJ (Clinical Research Ed.)*, *320*(7246), 1395–1398. doi:10.1136/bmj.320.7246.1395 PMID:10818037

McNabb, M., Chukwu, E., Ojo, O., Shekhar, N., Gill, C. J., Salami, H., & Jega, F. (2015). Assessment of the Quality of Antenatal Care Services Provided by Health Workers Using a Mobile Phone Decision Support Application in Northern Nigeria: A Pre/Post-Intervention Study. *PLoS One*, *10*(5), e0123940. doi:10.1371/journal.pone.0123940 PMID:25942018

Moyer, C. A., Dako-Gyeke, P., & Adanu, R. A. (2013). Facility-based delivery and maternal and early neonatal mortality in sub-Saharan Africa: A regional review of the literature. *African Journal of Reproductive Health*, *17*, 30–43. PMID:24069765

Musabyimana, A., Ruton, H., Gaju, E., Berhe, A., Grépin, K. A., Ngenzi, J., Nzabonimana, E., Hategeka, C., & Law, M. R. (2018). Assessing the perspectives of users and beneficiaries of a community health worker mHealth tracking system for mothers and children in Rwanda. *PLoS One*, *13*(6), e0198725. doi:10.1371/journal.pone.0198725 PMID:29879186

Nachega, J. B., Skinner, D., Jennings, L., Magidson, J. F., Altice, F. L., Burke, J. G., Lester, R. T., Uthman, O. A., Knowlton, A. R., Cotton, M. F., Anderson, J. R., & Theron, G. B. (2016). Acceptability and feasibility of mHealth and community-based directly observed antiretroviral therapy to prevent mother-to-child HIV transmission in South African pregnant women under Option B+: An exploratory study. *Patient Preference and Adherence*, *10*, 683–690. doi:10.2147/PPA.S100002 PMID:27175068

Nnam, N. M. (2015). Improving maternal nutrition for better pregnancy outcomes. *The Proceedings of the Nutrition Society*, *74*(4), 454–459. doi:10.1017/S0029665115002396 PMID:26264457

Parry, J., & Stevens, A. (2001). Prospective health impact assessment: Pitfalls, problems, and possible ways forward. *BMJ (Clinical Research Ed.)*, *323*(7322), 1177–1182. doi:10.1136/bmj.323.7322.1177 PMID:11711414

Patel, A. B., Kuhite, P. N., Alam, A., Pusdekar, Y., Puranik, A., Khan, S. S., Kelly, P., Muthayya, S., Laba, T.-L., Almeida, M. D., & Dibley, M. J. (2019). M-SAKHI-Mobile health solutions to help community providers promote maternal and infant nutrition and health using a community-based cluster randomized controlled trial in rural India: A study protocol. *Maternal and Child Nutrition*, *15*(4), e12850. doi:10.1111/mcn.12850 PMID:31177631

Petticrew, M., Whitehead, M., Macintyre, S. J., Graham, H., & Egan, M. (2004). Evidence for public health policy on inequalities: 1: the reality according to policymakers. *Journal of Epidemiology and Community Health, 58*(10), 811–816. doi:10.1136/jech.2003.015289 PMID:15365104

Pohjois-Suomen sosiaalialan osaamiskeskus [Northern Finland's Center of Expertise in the Social Sector]. (2018). *Monipuoliset tuen muodot kotona asumiseen Lapissa – Toimivan kotihoidon käsikirja. Toimiva kotihoito Lappiin – Monipuoliset tuen muodot kotona asumiseen -hanke [Versatile forms of support for living at home in Lapland- Manual for functional home care. Functional home care in Lapland- Multifaceted forms of support for living at home project]*. Grano Oy, Helsinki.

Rogerson, B., Lindberg, R., Baum, F., Dora, C., Haigh, F., Simoncelli, A. M., Parry Williams, L., Peralta, G., Pollack Porter, K. M., & Solar, O. (2020). Recent Advances in Health Impact Assessment and Health in All Policies Implementation: Lessons from an International Convening in Barcelona. *International Journal of Environmental Research and Public Health, 17*(21), 7714. doi:10.3390/ijerph17217714 PMID:33105669

Ryu, S. (2012). Book Review: MHealth: New Horizons for Health through Mobile Technologies: Based on the Findings of the Second Global Survey on eHealth (Global Observatory for eHealth Series, Volume 3). *Healthcare Informatics Research, 18*(3), 231–233. doi:10.4258/hir.2012.18.3.231

Sey, A. (2011). 'We use it different, different': Making sense of trends in mobile phone use in Ghana. *New Media & Society, 13*(3), 375–390. doi:10.1177/1461444810393907

Sondaal, S. F. V., Browne, J. L., Amoakoh-Coleman, M., Borgstein, A., Miltenburg, A. S., Verwijs, M., & Klipstein-Grobusch, K. (2016). Assessing the Effect of mHealth Interventions in Improving Maternal and Neonatal Care in Low- and Middle-Income Countries: A Systematic Review. *PLoS One, 11*(5), e0154664. doi:10.1371/journal.pone.0154664 PMID:27144393

Sumankuuro, J., Wulifan, J. K., Angko, W., Crockett, J., Derbile, E. K., & Ganle, J. K. (2020). Predictors of maternal mortality in Ghana: Evidence from the 2017 GMHS Verbal Autopsy data. *The International Journal of Health Planning and Management, 35*(6), 1512–1531. doi:10.1002/hpm.3054 PMID:32901986

Utzinger, J. (2004). Health impact assessment: Concepts, theory, techniques, and applications. *Bulletin of the World Health Organization, 82*(12), 954–954.

WHO. UNICEF, UNFPA, The World Bank, & United Nations Population Division. (2014). Trends in maternal mortality: 1990 to 2013: Estimates by WHO, UNICEF, UNFPA, The World Bank and the United Nations Population Division. WHO.

WHO. (2021a). *Health impact assessment*. WHO. https://www.who.int/westernpacific/health-topics/health-impact-assessment

WHO. (2021b). *Maternal and reproductive health*. WHO. https://www.who.int/data/maternal-newborn-child-adolescent-ageing/advisory-groups/gama/activities-of-gama

WHO & World Bank. (2014). *Trends in Maternal Mortality: 1990 to 2013*. World Health Organization. http://VH7QX3XE2P.search.serialssolutions.com/?V=1.0&L=VH7QX3XE2P&S=AC_T_B&C=Trends%20in%20Maternal%20Mortality%20:%201990%20to%202013&T=marc&tab=BOOKS

WHO. (2006). *WHO Constitution, Basic Documents, Forty-fifth edition, Supplement, October 2006*. WHO. https://www.who.int/about/who-we-are/constitution

Willcox, J. C., van der Pligt, P., Ball, K., Wilkinson, S. A., Lappas, M., McCarthy, E. A., & Campbell, K. J. (2015). Views of Women and Health Professionals on mHealth Lifestyle Interventions in Pregnancy: A Qualitative Investigation. *JMIR mHealth and uHealth*, *3*(4). https://doi.org/10.2196/mhealth.4869

Witter, S., & Adjei, S. (2007). Start-stop funding, its causes and consequences: A case study of the delivery exemptions policy in Ghana. *The International Journal of Health Planning and Management*, *22*(2), 133–143. https://doi.org/10.1002/hpm.867

Wu, G., Imhoff-Kunsch, B., & Girard, A. W. (2012). Biological mechanisms for nutritional regulation of maternal health and fetal development. *Paediatric and Perinatal Epidemiology*, *26*, 4–26.

Wu, Y., Zhao, P., Li, W., Cao, M.-Q., Du, L., & Chen, J.-C. (2019). The effect of remote health intervention based on internet or mobile communication network on hypertension patients: Protocol for a systematic review and meta-analysis of randomized controlled trials. *Medicine*, *98*(9), e14707. https://doi.org/10.1097/MD.0000000000014707

APPENDIX

Table 4. The proposed budget for implementation (December 2022).

Code	Description	Quantity	Provider/ supplier	Duration/ Frequency	Estimated unit cost	Estimated cost
1	10 Nokia 2.3 phones for 5 health centers	10	Power, Finland	1 st month of the intervention	120 €	1200 €
2	125 Nokia 2.3 phones for 125 community centers	125	Power, Finland	1 st month of the intervention	120 €	15000 €
3	Training of health nurses and dieticians	1	Local GRAVID agents	4 hours	200 €	200 €
4	Community training for community heads and pregnant women, 3 communities per day	42	Nurses and local GRAVID agents	3 hours	200 €	8400 €
5	Mobile app	1	GRAVID	1 st month of the intervention	Open app	0.00 €
6	Miscellaneous	1	District authority	During the intervention	10%	2480 €
7	Total cost for the intervention					27280 €

Compilation of References

Aamir, K. M., Sarfraz, L., Ramzan, M., Bilal, M., Shafi, J., & Attique, M. (2021). A Fuzzy Rule-Based System for Classification of Diabetes. *Sensors (Basel)*, *21*(23), 8095. https://doi.org/10.3390/s21238095

Abbad Ur Rehman, H. L., Lin, C.-Y., Mushtaq, Z., & Su, S.-F. (2021). Performance analysis of machine learning algorithms for thyroid disease. *Arabian Journal for Science and Engineering*, *46*(10), 9437–9449. doi:10.100713369-020-05206-x

Abbas, Z., Rehman, M. U., Najam, S., & Rizvi, S. D. (2019, February). An efficient gray-level co-occurrence matrix (GLCM) based approach towards classification of skin lesion. In *2019 amity international conference on artificial intelligence (AICAI)* (pp. 317-320). IEEE.

Abbas, H. T., Alic, L., Erraguntla, M., Ji, J. X., Abdul-Ghani, M., Abbasi, Q. H., & Qaraqe, M. K. (2019). Predicting long-term type 2 diabetes with support vector machine using oral glucose tolerance test. *PLoS One*, *14*(12), e0219636. https://doi.org/10.1371/journal.pone.0219636

Abd-Eldayem, M. M. (2013). A proposed security technique based on watermarking and encryption for digital imaging and communications in medicine. *Egyptian Informatics Journal*, *14*(1), 1–13. doi:10.1016/j.eij.2012.11.002

Abedi, M., Marateb, H. R., Mohebian, M. R., Aghaee-Bakhtiari, S. H., Nassiri, S. M., & Gheisari, Y. (2021). Systems biology and machine learning approaches identify drug targets in diabetic nephropathy. *Scientific Reports*, *11*(1). https://doi.org/10.1038/s41598-021-02282-3

Adam, A., Fusheini, A., & Kipo-Sunyehzi, D. D. (2021). A Collaborative Health Promotion Approach to Improve Rural Health Delivery and Health Outcomes in Ghana: A Case Example of a Community-Based Health Planning and Services (CHPS) Strategy. In Rural Health. IntechOpen.

Adansi North District assembly. (2013). *Adansi North District Medium Term Development Plan (2014 – 2017)*. ANDA.

Adebamowo, C., Bah-Sow, O., & Binka, F. (2014). Randomised controlled trials for Ebola: Practical and ethical issues. *Lancet*, *384*(9952), 1423–1424.

Adusei-Mensah, F., Hakalehto, E., & Tikkanen-Kaukanen, C. (2021). Microbiological and Chemical Safety of African Herbal and Natural Products. In E. Hakalehto (ed.) Challenges in Food Production and Distribution During and After the Pandemic. Degruyter.

Adusei-Mensah, F., Kauhanen, J., & Tikkanen-Kaukanen, C. (2022). The Need for a Paradigm Shift in the Existing Strategies for Effective COVID-19 Control. *Online Journal of Contemporary Medicine.*

Agarwal, P., & Mehta, S. (2014). Nature-Inspired Algorithms: State-of-Art, Problems and Prospects. *International Journal of Computers and Applications*, *100*(14), 14–21. doi:10.5120/17593-8331

Aherrahrou, N., & Tairi, H. (2015). PDE based scheme for multi-modal medical image watermarking. *Biomedical Engineering Online*, *14*(1), 1–19. doi:10.118612938-015-0101-x PMID:26608730

Ahmed, R., Riaz, M. M., & Ghafoor, A. (2018). Attack resistant watermarking technique based on fast curvelet transform and Robust Principal Component Analysis. *Multimedia Tools and Applications*, *77*(8), 9443–9453. doi:10.100711042-017-5128-5

Ahsan, M., Luna, S. A. & Siddique, Z. (2022). *Machine-Learning-Based Disease Diagnosis: A Comprehensive Review.* MDPI: . doi:10.3390/healthcare10030541

Aker, J. C., & Mbiti, I. M. (2010). Mobile Phones and Economic Development in Africa. *The Journal of Economic Perspectives*, *24*(3), 207–232. doi:10.1257/jep.24.3.207

Akhtar, T. G., Gilani, S. O., Mushtaq, Z., Arif, S., Jamil, M., Ayaz, Y., Butt, S. I., & Waris, A. (2021). Effective Voting Ensemble of Homogenous Ensembling with Multiple Attribute-Selection Approaches for Improved Identification of Thyroid Disorder. *Electronics (Basel)*, *10*(23), 10. doi:10.3390/electronics10233026

Akinseinde, A. S., Badejo, J. A., & Malgwi, R. L. (2016). GRAVID: An indigenous m-health tool for smart and connected communities. *2016 Future Technologies Conference (FTC)*, (pp. 1331–1334). 10.1109/FTC.2016.7821776

Al Mamlook, R. E., Chen, S., & Bzizi, H. F. (2020, July). Investigation of the performance of machine learning classifiers for pneumonia detection in chest x-ray images. In *2020 IEEE International Conference on Electro Information Technology (EIT)* (pp. 098-104). IEEE. 10.1109/EIT48999.2020.9208232

Alan, A. I. (2021). Conversational Voice AI Platform. Alan. https://Alan.app/

Al-Diri, B., Hunter, A., & Steel, D. (2009). An Active Contour Model for Segmenting and Measuring Retinal Vessels. *IEEE Transactions on Medical Imaging*, *28*(9), 1488–1497. doi:10.1109/TMI.2009.2017941 PMID:19336294

Alharbi, A. H., & Hosni Mahmoud, H. A. (2022, May). Pneumonia transfer learning deep learning model from segmented X-rays. [). MDPI.]. *Health Care*, *10*(6), 987. PMID:35742039

Ali, A., Alrubei, M. A. T., Hassan, L. F. M., Al-Ja'afari, M. A. M., & Abdulwahed, S. H. (2020). Diabetes diagnosis based on KNN. *IIUM Engineering Journal, 21*(1), 175–181. doi:10.31436/iiumej.v21i1.1206

Ali, S., Jha, D., Ghatwary, N., Realdon, S., Cannizzaro, R., Salem, O. E., Lamarque, D., Daul, C., Riegler, M. A., Anonsen, K. V., Petlund, A., Halvorsen, P., Rittscher, J., de Lange, T., & East, J. E. (2021). PolypGen: A multi-center polyp detection and segmentation dataset for generalisability assessment. *ArXiv:2106.04463* https://arxiv.org/abs/2106.04463

Ali, M., Ahn, C. W., & Pant, M. (2016). Intelligent Watermarking Scheme Employing the Concepts of Block Based Singular Value Decomposition and Firefly Algorithm. *GCSR, 5*, 37–57.

Alizadehsani, R., Khosravi, A., Roshanzamir, M., Abdar, M., Sarrafzadegan, N., Shafie, D., Khozeimeh, F., Shoeibi, A., Nahavandi, S., Panahiazar, M., Bishara, A., Beygui, R. E., Puri, R., Kapadia, S., Tan, R.-S., & Acharya, U. R. (2021). Coronary artery disease detection using artificial intelligence techniques: A survey of trends, geographical differences and diagnostic features 1991–2020. *Computers in Biology and Medicine, 128*, 104095. doi:10.1016/j.compbiomed.2020.104095 PMID:33217660

Aljamaan, I., & Al-Naib, I. (2021). Prediction of Blood Glucose Level Using Nonlinear System Identification Approach. *IEEE Access: Practical Innovations, Open Solutions, 10*, 1936–1945. doi:10.1109/ACCESS.2021.3139578

Aljurayfani, M., Alghernas, S., & Shargabi, A. (2019). Medical Self-Diagnostic System Using Artificial Neural Networks. *International Conference on Computer and Information Sciences (ICCIS)*. IEEE. doi:10.1109/ICCISci.2019.8716386

Al-Naqeeb, A. B., & Nordin, M. J. (2017). Robustness Watermarking Authentication Using Hybridisation DWT-DCTand DWT-SVD. *Pertanika Science & Technology, 25*(0128-7680*)*, 73-86.

Alquran, H., Qasmieh, I. A., Alqudah, A. M., Alhammouri, S., Alawneh, E., Abughazaleh, A., & Hasayen, F. (2017, October). The melanoma skin cancer detection and classification using support vector machine. In *2017 IEEE Jordan Conference on Applied Electrical Engineering and Computing Technologies (AEECT)* (pp. 1-5). IEEE. 10.1109/AEECT.2017.8257738

AlSaeed, D. (2020). A Novel Blood Vessel Extraction Using Multiscale Matched Filters with Local Features and Adaptive Thresholding. *Bioscience Biotechnology Research Communications, 13*(3), 1104–1113. doi:10.21786/bbrc/13.3/18

Amato, F., López, A., Peña-Méndez, E. Vaňhara, P., Hampl, A., & Havel, J. (2013), Artificial neural networks in medical diagnosis. *Journal of Applied Biomedicine*. doi:10.2478/v10136-012-0031-x

Amirjahan, M., & Sujatha, D. N. (2016). *Comparative analysis of various classification algorithms for skin Cancer detection. PG & Research Department of Computer Science, Raja Doraisingam Govt*. Art College.

Amoakoh-Coleman, M., Borgstein, A. B.-J., Sondaal, S. F., Grobbee, D. E., Miltenburg, A. S., Verwijs, M., Ansah, E. K., Browne, J. L., & Klipstein-Grobusch, K. (2016). Effectiveness of mHealth Interventions Targeting Health Care Workers to Improve Pregnancy Outcomes in Low- and Middle-Income Countries: A Systematic Review. *Journal of Medical Internet Research*, *18*(8), e226. doi:10.2196/jmir.5533 PMID:27543152

Ani, R., Maria, E., Joyce, J. J., Sakkaravarthy, V., & Raja, M. A. (2017, March). Smart Specs: Voice assisted text reading system for visually impaired persons using TTS method. In *2017 International Conference on Innovations in Green Energy and Healthcare Technologies (IGEHT)* (pp. 1-6). IEEE., 10.1109/IGEHT.2017.8094103

Anyanwu, G. O., Nwakanma, C. I., Lee, J.-M., & Kim, D.-S. (2022). Optimization of RBF-SVM Kernel using Grid Search Algorithm for DDoS Attack Detection in SDN-based VANET. *IEEE Internet of Things Journal*, 1–1. doi:10.1109/JIOT.2022.3199712

Apanga, P. A., & Awoonor-Williams, J. K. (2018). Maternal Death in Rural Ghana: A Case Study in the Upper East Region of Ghana. *Frontiers in Public Health*, *6*, 101. doi:10.3389/fpubh.2018.00101 PMID:29686982

Ashisha, G. R., George, S. T., Mary, X. A., Sagayam, K. M., & Pramanik, S. (2022). Analysis of Diabetes disease using Machine Learning Techniques: A Review. *Research Square*. https://doi.org/10.21203/rs.3.rs-1572946/v1

Asif, M. A. (2020). Computer aided diagnosis of thyroid disease using machine learning algorithms. *In 2020 11th International Conference on Electrical and Computer Engineering* (pp. 222-225). IEEE.

Aslan, M. F., Ceylan, M., & Durdu, A. (2018) Segmentation of Retinal Blood Vessel Using Gabor Filter and Extreme Learning Machines. In *2018 International Conference on Artificial Intelligence and Data Processing (IDAP)*, (pp. 1–5). IEEE. 10.1109/IDAP.2018.8620890

Asl, B. M., Setarehdan, S. K., & Mohebbi, M. (2008). Support vector machine-based arrhythmia classification using reduced features of heart rate variability signal. *Artificial Intelligence in Medicine*, *44*(1), 51–64. doi:10.1016/j.artmed.2008.04.007 PMID:18585905

AstraZeneca. (2021). *A Phase III Randomized, Double-blind, Placebo-controlled Multicenter Study in Adults, to Determine the Safety, Efficacy, and Immunogenicity of AZD1222, a Non-replicating ChAdOx1 Vector Vaccine, for the Prevention of COVID-19 (Clinical Trial Registration No. NCT04516746)*. clinicaltrials.gov. https://clinicaltrials.gov/ct2/show/NCT04516746

Aversano, L. B., Bernardi, M. L., Cimitile, M., Iammarino, M., Macchia, P. E., Nettore, I. C., & Verdone, C. (2021). Thyroid disease treatment prediction with machine learning approaches. *Procedia Computer Science*, *192*, 1031–1040. doi:10.1016/j.procs.2021.08.106

Awotunde, J. B., Matiluko, O. E., & Fatai, O. W. (2014). Medical Diagnosis System Using Fuzzy Logic. *African Journal of Computing and ICT*, *7*(2), 99–106.

Ayan, E., & Ünver, H. M. (2019, April). Diagnosis of pneumonia from chest X-ray images using deep learning. In 2019 Scientific Meeting on Electrical-Electronics & Biomedical Engineering and Computer Science (EBBT) (pp. 1-5). IEEE. doi:10.1109/EBBT.2019.8741582

Ayan, E., Karabulut, B., & Ünver, H. M. (2022). Diagnosis of pediatric pneumonia with ensemble of deep convolutional neural networks in chest x-ray images. *Arabian Journal for Science and Engineering*, *47*(2), 2123–2139. doi:10.100713369-021-06127-z PMID:34540526

Azad, C., Bhushan, B., Sharma, R., Shankar, A., Singh, K. K., & Khamparia, A. (2021). Prediction model using SMOTE, genetic algorithm and decision tree (PMSGD) for classification of diabetes mellitus. *Multimedia Systems*. doi:10.1007/s00530-021-00817-2

Azzopardi, G., Strisciuglio, N., Vento, M., & Petkov, N. (2015). Trainable COSFIRE filters for vessel delineation with application to retinal images. *Medical Image Analysis*, *19*(1), 46–57. doi:10.1016/j.media.2014.08.002 PMID:25240643

Bahadar, K., Khaliq, A., & Shahid, M. (2016). A Morphological Hessian Based Approach for Retinal Blood Vessels Segmentation and Denoising Using Region Based Otsu Thresholding. PLOS ONE, 11(7), e0158996. doi:10.1371/journal.pone.0158996

Bakator, M., & Radosav, D. (2018). *Deep Learning and Medical Diagnosis: A Review of Literature.* MDPI. https://dx.doi.org/10.3390/mti2030047

Baliyan, M. (2020, July 1). *Self Organising Maps - Kohonen Maps.* GeeksforGeeks. https://www.geeksforgeeks.org/self-organising-maps-kohonen-maps/

Banu, G. R. (2016). A Role of decision Tree classification data Mining Technique in Diagnosing Thyroid disease. *International Journal on Computer Science and Engineering*, 64–70.

Bao, X.-R., Ge, X., She, L.-H., & Zhang, S. (2015). Segmentation of Retinal Blood Vessels Based on Cake Filter. *BioMed Research International*, *2015*, 1–11. doi:10.1155/2015/137024 PMID:26636095

Barone de Medeiros, I., Machado, M., José Damasceno, J., Machado Caldeira, A., dos Santos, R., & da Silva Filho, J. (2017) A Fuzzy Inference System to Support Medical Diagnosis in Real Time. *Science Direct.* doi:10.1016/j.procs.2017.11.356

Batista, E. D. (2021), Building Voice-First Flutter apps. [Video] Flutter Europe, Youtube. https://www.youtube.com/watch?v=L-c-ZyX-KtY

Begum, M., & Uddin, M. S. (2020). Digital image watermarking techniques: A review. *Information (Basel)*, *11*(2), 110. doi:10.3390/info11020110

Bellemo, V., Lim, G., Rim, T. H., Tan, G. S., Cheung, C. Y., Sadda, S., He, M., Tufail, A., Lee, M. L., Hsu, W., & Ting, D. S. W. (2019). Artificial intelligence screening for diabetic retinopathy: The real-world emerging application. *Current Diabetes Reports*, *19*(9), 1–12. doi:10.100711892-019-1189-3 PMID:31367962

Beniwal, S., Saini, U., Garg, P., & Joon, R. K. (2021). Improving performance during camera surveillance by integration of edge detection in IoT system. [IJEHMC]. *International Journal of E-Health and Medical Communications*, *12*(5), 84–96.

Bernal, J. J., Histace, A., Masana, M., Angermann, Q., Sánchez-Montes, C., Rodriguez, C., Hammami, M., Garcia-Rodriguez, A., Córdova, H., Romain, O., Fernández-Esparrach, G., Dray, X., & Sanchez, J. (2018, June 20). *Polyp Detection Benchmark in Colonoscopy Videos using GTCreator: A Novel Fully Configurable Tool for Easy and Fast Annotation of Image Databases*. Hal.science. https://hal.science/hal-01846141/

Bernal, J., Fernández, G., García-Rodríguez, A., & Sánchez, F. J. (2021). Polyp Segmentation in Colonoscopy Images. *Computer-Aided Analysis of Gastrointestinal Videos*, *151–154*, 151–154. Advance online publication. doi:10.1007/978-3-030-64340-9_19

Bernal, J., Sánchez, F. J., Fernández-Esparrach, G., Gil, D., Rodríguez, C., & Vilariño, F. (2015). WM-DOVA maps for accurate polyp highlighting in colonoscopy: Validation vs. saliency maps from physicians. *Computerized Medical Imaging and Graphics*, *43*, 99–111. doi:10.1016/j.compmedimag.2015.02.007 PMID:25863519

Bernal, J., Tajkbaksh, N., Sanchez, F. J., Matuszewski, B. J., Chen, H., Yu, L., Angermann, Q., Romain, O., Rustad, B., Balasingham, I., Pogorelov, K., Choi, S., Debard, Q., Maier-Hein, L., Speidel, S., Stoyanov, D., Brandao, P., Cordova, H., Sanchez-Montes, C, & Histace, A. (2017). Comparative Validation of Polyp Detection Methods in Video Colonoscopy: Results From the MICCAI 2015 Endoscopic Vision Challenge. *IEEE Transactions on Medical Imaging*, *36*(6), 1231–1249. doi:10.1109/TMI.2017.2664042 PMID:28182555

Bertoli, F., Veritti, D., Danese, C., Samassa, F., Sarao, V., Rassu, N., Gambato, T., & Lanzetta, P. (2020). Ocular Findings in COVID-19 Patients: A Review of Direct Manifestations and Indirect Effects on the Eye. *Journal of Ophthalmology*, *2020*, 1–9. doi:10.1155/2020/4827304 PMID:32963819

Bhattacharya, S. (2014). *Watermarking Digital Images Using Fuzzy Matrix Rules and Neighborhood Set. International Journal of Advanced Computing, Recent Science Publications*. ISSN.

Bhavsar, K. A., Abugabah, A., Singla, J., AlZubi, A., Bashir, A., & Nikita (2021). A Comprehensive Review on Medical Diagnosis Using Machine Learning. *CMC, 67*(2).

Bigdeli, A., Maghsoudi, A., & Ghezelbash, R. (2022). Application of self-organizing map (SOM) and K-means clustering algorithms for portraying geochemical anomaly patterns in Moalleman district, NE Iran. *Journal of Geochemical Exploration*, *233*, 106923. doi:10.1016/j.gexplo.2021.106923

Black, R. E., Victora, C. G., Walker, S. P., Bhutta, Z. A., Christian, P., de Onis, M., Ezzati, M., Grantham-McGregor, S., Katz, J., Martorell, R., & Uauy, R.Maternal and Child Nutrition Study Group. (2013). Maternal and child undernutrition and overweight in low-income and middle-income countries. *Lancet*, *382*(9890), 427–451. doi:10.1016/S0140-6736(13)60937-X PMID:23746772

Boffey, D. (2021, February 25). Revealed: Four in five Oxford Covid jabs delivered to EU not yet used. *The Guardian.* https://www.theguardian.com/world/2021/feb/25/acceptance-problem-as-most-oxford-covid-jabs-delivered-to-eu-not-yet-used

Britanak, V., & Rao, K. R. (2001). An efficient implementation of the forward and inverse MDCT in MPEG audio coding. *IEEE Signal Processing Letters*, *8*(2), 48–51. doi:10.1109/97.895372

Brown, C. A., Charles, P. D., Johnsen, W. A., & Chesters, S. (1993). Fractal analysis of topographic data by the patchwork method. *Wear*, *161*(1-2), 61–67. doi:10.1016/0043-1648(93)90453-S

Bukhari, M. M., Alkhamees, B. F., Hussain, S., Gumaei, A., Assiri, A., & Ullah, S. S. (2021). An Improved Artificial Neural Network Model for Effective Diabetes Prediction. *Complexity*, *2021*, 1–10. doi:10.1155/2021/5525271

Buor, D. (2004). Gender and the utilisation of health services in the Ashanti Region, Ghana. *Health Policy (Amsterdam, Netherlands)*, *69*(3), 375–388. doi:10.1016/j.healthpol.2004.01.004 PMID:15276316

Burki, T. K. (2020). The Russian vaccine for COVID-19. *The Lancet. Respiratory Medicine*, *8*(11), e85–e86. doi:10.1016/S2213-2600(20)30402-1 PMID:32896274

Caporossi, T., Bacherini, D., Tartaro, R., VIrgili, G., Peris, A., & Giansanti, F. (2021). Retinal findings in patients affected by COVID 19 intubated in an intensive care unit. *Acta Ophthalmologica*, *99*(7), e1244–e1245. doi:10.1111/aos.14734 PMID:33377599

Castiglioni, I., Rundo, L., Codari, M., Di Leo, G., Salvatore, C., Interlenghi, M., Gallivanone, F., Cozzi, A., D'Amico, N. C., & Sardanelli, F. (2021). AI applications to medical images: From machine learning to deep learning. *Physica Medica*, *83*, 9–24. https://doi.org/10.1016/j.ejmp.2021.02.006

CDC. (2020, February 11). COVID-19 and Your Health. Centers for Disease Control and Prevention. CDC. https://www.cdc.gov/coronavirus/2019-ncov/transmission/variant.html

CDC. (2022). History of Ebola Virus Disease (EVD) Outbreaks. CDC.

Chaitanya, K., Reddy, S., & Rao, G. (2014). Digital Color Image Watermarking In RGB Planes Using DWT-DCT-SVD Coefficients. *International Journal of Computer Science and Information Technologies*, *5*(2), 2413–2417.

Chaki, J., Thillai Ganesh, S., Cidham, S. K., & Ananda Theertan, S. (2020). Machine learning and artificial intelligence based Diabetes Mellitus detection and self-management: A systematic review. *Journal of King Saud University - Computer and Information Sciences.* doi:10.1016/j.jksuci.2020.06.013

Chakravorty, R., Liang, S., Abedini, M., & Garnavi, R. (2016, August). Dermatologist-like feature extraction from skin lesion for improved asymmetry classification in PH 2 database. In *2016 38th Annual International Conference of the IEEE Engineering in Medicine and Biology Society (EMBC)* (pp. 3855-3858). IEEE.

Chang, W. J., Chen, L. B., Hsu, C. H., Chen, J. H., Yang, T. C., & Lin, C. P. (2020). MedGlasses: A wearable smart-glasses-based drug pill recognition system using deep learning for visually impaired chronic patients. *IEEE Access: Practical Innovations, Open Solutions*, *8*, 17013–17024. doi:10.1109/ACCESS.2020.2967400

Chaubey, G. B., Bisen, D., Arjaria, S., & Yadav, V. (2021). Thyroid disease prediction using machine learning approaches. *National Academy Science Letters*, *44*(3), 233–238. doi:10.100740009-020-00979-z

Chaudhari, H. P., Rahulkar, A. D., & Patil, C. Y. (2014). Segmentation of Retinal Vessels by the Use of Gabor Wavelet and Linear Mean Squared Error Classifier. *International Journal of Emerging Engineering Research and Technology*, *2*(2), 119–125.

Chaudhary, A., & Garg, P. (2014). Detecting and diagnosing a disease by patient monitoring system. *International Journal of Mechanical Engineering And Information Technology*, *2*(6), 493–499.

Chaudhuri, S., Chatterjee, S., Katz, N., Nelson, M., & Goldbaum, M. (1989). Detection of blood vessels in retinal images using two-dimensional matched filters. *IEEE Transactions on Medical Imaging*, *8*(3), 263–269. doi:10.1109/42.34715 PMID:18230524

Chen, L.-C., Papandreou, G., Kokkinos, I., Murphy, K., & Yuille, A. L. (2018). DeepLab: Semantic Image Segmentation with Deep Convolutional Nets, Atrous Convolution, and Fully Connected CRFs. *IEEE Transactions on Pattern Analysis and Machine Intelligence*, *40*(4), 834–848. doi:10.1109/TPAMI.2017.2699184 PMID:28463186

Cherif, L. H., Debbal, S. M., & Bereksi-Reguig, F. (2010). Choice of the wavelet analyzing in the phonocardiogram signal analysis using the discrete and the packet wavelet transform. *Expert Systems with Applications*, *37*(2), 913–918. doi:10.1016/j.eswa.2009.09.036

Cho, J. W., Chung, H. Y., & Jung, H. Y. (2006, September). A robust blind audio watermarking using distribution of sub-band signals. In *International Workshop on Multimedia Content Representation, Classification and Security* (pp. 106-113). Springer. 10.1007/11848035_16

Chollet, F. (2017). Xception: Deep learning with depthwise separable convolutions. In *Proceedings of the IEEE conference on computer vision and pattern recognition* (pp. 1251-1258). 10.1109/CVPR.2017.195

Choubey, D. K., Paul, S., & Dhandhania, V. K. (2018). GA_NN: An Intelligent Classification System for Diabetes. *Advances in Intelligent Systems and Computing*, 11–23. doi:10.1007/978-981-13-1595-4_2

Choubey, D. K., Kumar, P., Tripathi, S., & Kumar, S. (2019). Performance evaluation of classification methods with PCA and PSO for diabetes. *Network Modeling and Analysis in Health Informatics and Bioinformatics*, *9*(1). https://doi.org/10.1007/s13721-019-0210-8

Chouhan, V., Singh, S. K., Khamparia, A., Gupta, D., Tiwari, P., Moreira, C., Damaševičius, R., & De Albuquerque, V. H. C. (2020). A novel transfer learning based approach for pneumonia detection in chest X-ray images. *Applied Sciences (Basel, Switzerland), 10*(2), 559. doi:10.3390/app10020559

Chouhan, V., Singh, S. K., Khamparia, A., Gupta, D., Tiwari, P., Moreira, C., & De Albuquerque, V. H. C. (2020). A novel transfer learning based approach for pneumonia detection in chest X-ray images. *Applied Sciences, 10*(2), 559.

Chow, S. (2009, November 5). *Pneumonia Classification.* News-Medical.net. https://www.news-medical.net/health/Pneumonia-Classification.aspx

Chowdary, G. J. (2021). Impact of machine learning models in pneumonia diagnosis with features extracted from chest x-rays using VGG16. [TURCOMAT]. *Turkish Journal of Computer and Mathematics Education, 12*(5), 1521–1530.

Chuang, H.-Y., Hofree, M., & Ideker, T. (2010). A Decade of Systems Biology. *Annual Review of Cell and Developmental Biology, 26*, 721–744. https://doi.org/10.1146/annurev-cellbio-100109-104122

Chu, D. K., Pan, Y., Cheng, S. M., Hui, K. P., Krishnan, P., Liu, Y., Ng, D. Y. M., Wan, C. K. C., Yang, P., Wang, Q., Peiris, M., & Poon, L. L. (2020). Molecular diagnosis of a novel coronavirus (2019-nCoV) causing an outbreak of pneumonia. *Clinical Chemistry, 66*(4), 549–555. doi:10.1093/clinchem/hvaa029 PMID:32031583

Cleaveland Clinic. (n.d.). *Aspiration Pneumonia: What It Is, Causes, Diagnosis, Treatment.* Cleveland Clinic. https://my.clevelandclinic.org/health/diseases/21954-aspiration-pneumonia

Coetzee, B., Kohrman, H., Tomlinson, M., Mbewu, N., Roux, I. L., & Adam, M. (2018). Community health workers' experiences of using video teaching tools during home visits—A pilot study. *Health & Social Care in the Community, 26*(2), 167–175. doi:10.1111/hsc.12488 PMID:28872210

Colaci, D., Chaudhri, S., & Vasan, A. (2016). mHealth interventions in low-income countries to address maternal health: A systematic review. *Annals of Global Health, 82*(5), 922–935. doi:10.1016/j.aogh.2016.09.001 PMID:28283147

Cruz, A. F. D., Norena, N., Kaushik, A., & Bhansali, S. (2014). A low-cost miniaturized potentiostat for point-of-care diagnosis. *Biosensors & Bioelectronics, 62*, 249–254. doi:10.1016/j.bios.2014.06.053 PMID:25016332

Cui, C., Cui, Y., Fu, Y., Ma, S., & Zhang, S. (2017). Microarray analysis reveals gene and microRNA signatures in diabetic kidney disease. *Molecular Medicine Reports.* doi:10.3892/mmr.2017.8177 PMID:29207157

Das, H., Naik, B., & Behera, H. S. (2018). Classification of Diabetes Mellitus Disease (DMD): *Progress in Computing, Analytics and Networking.* Springer Singapore.

Dash, S., & Sahu, G. (2019) Retinal blood vessel segmentation by employing various upgraded median filters. In *Proceedings - International Conference on Intelligent Systems and Green Technology, ICISGT 2019*, (pp. 35–39). IEEE. 10.1109/ICISGT44072.2019.00023

Dash, S. K., & Rao, G. S. (2016, March). Robust multiclass ECG arrhythmia detection using balanced trained neural network. In *2016 International Conference on Electrical, Electronics, and Optimization Techniques (ICEEOT)* (pp. 186-191). IEEE. 10.1109/ICEEOT.2016.7754994

Dash, S., & Senapati, M. R. (2020). Enhancing detection of retinal blood vessels by combined approach of DWT, Tyler Coye and Gamma correction. *Biomedical Signal Processing and Control*, *57*, 101740. doi:10.1016/j.bspc.2019.101740

Dash, S., Senapati, M. R., Sahu, P. K., & Chowdary, P. S. R. (2021). Illumination normalized based technique for retinal blood vessel segmentation. *International Journal of Imaging Systems and Technology*, *31*(1), 351–363. doi:10.1002/ima.22461

Dash, S., Verma, S., Kavita, Bevinakoppa, S., Wozniak, M., Shafi, J., & Ijaz, M. F. (2022). Guidance Image-Based Enhanced Matched Filter with Modified Thresholding for Blood Vessel Extraction. *Symmetry*, *14*(2), 194. doi:10.3390ym14020194

Dash, S., Verma, S., Kavita, Khan, M. S., Wozniak, M., Shafi, J., & Ijaz, M. F. (2021). A hybrid method to enhance thick and thin vessels for blood vessel segmentation. *Diagnostics (Basel)*, *11*(11), 2017. doi:10.3390/diagnostics11112017 PMID:34829365

de Figueiredo, A., Simas, C., Karafillakis, E., Paterson, P., & Larson, H. J. (2020). Mapping global trends in vaccine confidence and investigating barriers to vaccine uptake: A large-scale retrospective temporal modelling study. *Lancet*, *396*(10255), 898–908. doi:10.1016/S0140-6736(20)31558-0 PMID:32919524

De Oliveira Nogueira, T., Palacio, G. B. A., Braga, F. D., Maia, P. P. N., de Moura, E. P., de Andrade, C. F., & Rocha, P. A. C. (2022). Imbalance classification in a scaled-down wind turbine using radial basis function kernel and support vector machines. *Energy*, *238*, 122064. doi:10.1016/j.energy.2021.122064

Degroote, L., Van Dyck, D., De Bourdeaudhuij, I., De Paepe, A., & Crombez, G. (2020). Acceptability and feasibility of the mHealth intervention 'MyDayPlan' to increase physical activity in a general adult population. *BMC Public Health*, *20*(1), 1032. doi:10.118612889-020-09148-9 PMID:32600352

Der, E. M., Moyer, C., Gyasi, R. K., Akosa, A. B., Tettey, Y., Akakpo, P. K., Blankson, A., & Anim, J. T. (2013). Pregnancy Related Causes of Deaths in Ghana: A 5-Year Retrospective Study. *Ghana Medical Journal*, *47*(4), 158–163. PMID:24669020

Derevitskii, I. V., & Kovalchuk, S. V. (2020). Machine Learning-Based Predictive Modeling of Complications of Chronic Diabetes. *Procedia Computer Science*, *178*, 274–283. doi:10.1016/j.procs.2020.11.029

Deshmukh, T., & Fadewar, H. S. (2018). Fuzzy Deep Learning for Diabetes Detection. *Advances in Intelligent Systems and Computing*, 875–882. doi:10.1007/978-981-13-1513-8_89

Deshpande, S., & Shriram, R. (2016, September). Real time text detection and recognition on hand held objects to assist blind people. In *2016 International Conference on Automatic Control and Dynamic Optimization Techniques (ICACDOT)* (pp. 1020-1024). IEEE. 10.1109/ICACDOT.2016.7877741

Dewangan, A. kumar, & Agrawal, P. (2015). Classification of Diabetes Mellitus Using Machine Learning Techniques. *International Journal of Engineering and Applied Sciences, 2*(5), 257905. https://www.neliti.com/publications/257905/classification-of-diabetes-mellitus-using-machine-learning-techniques

Dey, N., Zhang, Y. D., Rajinikanth, V., Pugalenthi, R., & Raja, N. S. M. (2021). Customized VGG19 architecture for pneumonia detection in chest X-rays. *Pattern Recognition Letters, 143*, 67–74. doi:10.1016/j.patrec.2020.12.010

Ding, H., Pan, Z., Cen, Q., Li, Y., & Chen, S. (2020). Multi-scale fully convolutional network for gland segmentation using three-class classification. *Neurocomputing, 380*, 150–161. doi:10.1016/j.neucom.2019.10.097

Ding, L., Fan, L., Xu, X., Fu, J., & Xue, Y. (2019). Identification of core genes and pathways in type 2 diabetes mellitus by bioinformatics analysis. *Molecular Medicine Reports*. doi:10.3892/mmr.2019.10522 PMID:31524257

Dixit, A., Garg, P., Sethi, P., & Singh, Y. (2020, April). TVCCCS: Television Viewer's Channel Cost Calculation System On Per Second Usage. [). IOP Publishing.]. *IOP Conference Series. Materials Science and Engineering, 804*(1), 012046.

Dol, J., Richardson, B., Murphy, G. T., Aston, M., McMillan, D., & Campbell-Yeo, M. (2020). Impact of mobile health interventions during the perinatal period on maternal psychosocial outcomes: A systematic review. *JBI Evidence Synthesis, 18*(1), 30–55. doi:10.11124/JBISRIR-D-19-00191 PMID:31972680

Dong, K., Zhou, C., Ruan, Y., & Li, Y. (2020). MobileNetV2 Model for Image Classification. *2020 2nd International Conference on Information Technology and Computer Application (ITCA)*. 10.1109/ITCA52113.2020.00106

Dörr, M., Nohturfft, V., Brasier, N., Bosshard, E., Djurdjevic, A., Gross, S., Raichle, C. J., Rhinisperger, M., Stöckli, R., & Eckstein, J. (2019). The WATCH AF trial: SmartWATCHes for detection of atrial fibrillation. *JACC Clinical Electrophysiology, 5*(2), 199–208. doi:10.1016/j.jacep.2018.10.006 PMID:30784691

Dror, A. A., Eisenbach, N., Taiber, S., Morozov, N. G., Mizrachi, M., Zigron, A., Srouji, S., & Sela, E. (2020). Vaccine hesitancy: The next challenge in the fight against COVID-19. *European Journal of Epidemiology, 35*(8), 775–779. doi:10.100710654-020-00671-y PMID:32785815

Duggal, P. (2020). Prediction of thyroid disorders using advanced machine learning techniques. *In 2020 10th International Conference on Cloud Computing, Data Science & Engineering (Confluence)* (pp. 670-675). IEEE.

Durairaj, M. (2015). Prediction Of Diabetes Using Back Propagation Algorithm.

Ebiele, J., Ansah-Narh, T., Djiokap, S., Proven-Adzri, E., & Atemkeng, M. (2020, September). Conventional machine learning based on feature engineering for detecting pneumonia from chest X-rays. In Conference of the South African Institute of Computer Scientists and Information Technologists 2020 (pp. 149-155). doi:10.1145/3410886.3410898

Ehde, D. M., Roberts, M. K., Herring, T. E., & Alschuler, K. N. (2021). Willingness to obtain COVID-19 vaccination in adults with multiple sclerosis in the United States. *Multiple Sclerosis and Related Disorders*, *49*, 102788. doi:10.1016/j.msard.2021.102788 PMID:33508570

Elhaj, F. A., Salim, N., Harris, A. R., Swee, T. T., & Ahmed, T. (2016). Arrhythmia recognition and classification using combined linear and nonlinear features of ECG signals. Computer methods and programs in biomedicine, 127, 52-63. https:// doi:10.1016/j.cmpb.2015.12.024

Elliott Range, D. D., Dov, D., Kovalsky, S. Z., Henao, R., Carin, L., & Cohen, J. (2020). Application of a machine learning algorithm to predict malignancy in thyroid cytopathology. *Cancer Cytopathology*, *128*(4), 287–295. doi:10.1002/cncy.22238 PMID:32012493

Elshennawy, N. M., & Ibrahim, D. M. (2020). Deep-pneumonia framework using deep learning models based on chest x-ray images. *Diagnostics (Basel)*, *10*(9), 649. doi:10.3390/diagnostics10090649 PMID:32872384

Ephzibah, E. P. (2011). Cost Effective Approach on Feature Selection Using Genetic Algorithms and Fuzzy logic for Diabetes Diagnosis. *International Journal on Soft Computing*, *2*(1), 1–10. https://doi.org/10.5121/ijsc.2011.2101

Erickson, B. J., Korfiatis, P., Akkus, Z., & Kline, T. L. (2017). Machine Learning for Medical Imaging. *Radiographics*, *37*(2), 505–515. https://doi.org/10.1148/rg.2017160130

Eswaraiah, R., & Sreenivasa Reddy, E. (2014). Medical image watermarking technique for accurate tamper detection in ROI and exact recovery of ROI. *International Journal of Telemedicine and Applications*, *2014*, 2014. doi:10.1155/2014/984646 PMID:25328515

Etzioni-Friedman, T., & Etzioni, A. (2020). Adherence to Immunization: Rebuttal of Vaccine Hesitancy. *Acta Haematologica*, *1–5*. doi:10.1159/000511760 PMID:33202404

EUCDC. (2021). *COVID-19 Vaccine Tracker.* European Centre for Disease Prevention and Control. https://qap.ecdc.europa.eu/public/extensions/COVID-19/vaccine-tracker.html#distribution-tab.

European Centre for Disease Prevention and Control (EUCDC). (2023). *Ebola outbreak in Uganda, as of 3 January 2023.* Europa.

Fabbrocini, G., Triassi, M., Mauriello, M. C., Torre, G., Annunziata, M. C., Vita, V. D., & Monfrecola, G. (2010). Epidemiology of skin cancer: Role of some environmental factors. *Cancers (Basel), 2*(4), 1980–1989. doi:10.3390/cancers2041980 PMID:24281212

Fan, L., Huang, T., Lou, D., Peng, Z., He, Y., Zhang, X., Gu, N., & Zhang, Y. (2021). Artificial Intelligence-Aided Multiple Tumor Detection Method Based on Immunohistochemistry-Enhanced Dark-Field Imaging. *Analytical Chemistry, 94*(2), 1037–1045. doi:10.1021/acs.analchem.1c04000 PMID:34927419

Faris, H., Habib, M., Faris, M., Elayan, H., & Alomari, A. (2021). An intelligent multimodal medical diagnosis system based on patients' tole medical questions and structured symptoms for telemedicine. *Science Direct*. https://doi.org/10.1016/j.imu.2021.100513

Farokhian, F., Yang, C., Demirel, H., Wu, S., & Beheshti, I. (2017). Automatic parameters selection of Gabor filters with the imperialism competitive algorithm with application to retinal vessel segmentation. *Biocybernetics and Biomedical Engineering, 37*(1), 246–254. doi:10.1016/j.bbe.2016.12.007

Fauci, A. S. (2014). Ebola–underscoring the global disparities in health care resources. *The New England Journal of Medicine, 371*(12), 1084–1086. doi:10.1056/NEJMp1409494 PMID:25119491

Fedha, T. (2014). Impact of Mobile Telephone on Maternal Health Service Care: A Case of Njoro Division. *Open Journal of Preventive Medicine, 4*(5), 365–376. doi:10.4236/ojpm.2014.45044

Feroz, A., Rizvi, N., Sayani, S., & Saleem, S. (2017). Feasibility of mHealth intervention to improve uptake of antenatal and postnatal care services in peri-urban areas of Karachi: A qualitative exploratory study. *Journal of Hospital Management and Health Policy, 1*(4), 4. https://jhmhp.amegroups.com/article/view/3945. doi:10.21037/jhmhp.2017.10.02

Ferreira, J. R., Cardenas, D. A. C., Moreno, R. A., de Sá Rebelo, M. D. F., Krieger, J. E., & Gutierrez, M. A. (2020, July). Multi-view ensemble convolutional neural network to improve classification of pneumonia in low contrast chest x-ray images. In *2020 42nd Annual International Conference of the IEEE Engineering in Medicine & Biology Society (EMBC)* (pp. 1238-1241). IEEE. 10.1109/EMBC44109.2020.9176517

Filali, Y., Ennouni, A., Sabri, M. A., & Aarab, A. (2017, May). Multiscale approach for skin lesion analysis and classification. In *2017 International Conference on Advanced Technologies for Signal and Image Processing (ATSIP)* (pp. 1-6). IEEE. 10.1109/ATSIP.2017.8075545

Filali, Y., Ennouni, A., Sabri, M. A., & Aarab, A. (2018, April). A study of lesion skin segmentation, features selection and classification approaches. In *2018 International Conference on Intelligent Systems and Computer Vision (ISCV)* (pp. 1-7). IEEE. 10.1109/ISACV.2018.8354069

Filteau, J., Lee, S. J., & Jung, A. (2018, December). Real-time streaming application for IoT using Raspberry Pi and handheld devices. In *2018 IEEE Global Conference on Internet of Things (GCIoT)* (pp. 1-5). IEEE.10.1109/GCIoT.2018.8620141

Fink, S. (2015). Ebola spreads in sex prompt a CDC warning. *New York Times*.

Finnegan, E., Villarroel, M., Velardo, C., & Tarassenko, L. (2019). Automated method for detecting and reading seven-segment digits from images of blood glucose metres and blood pressure monitors. *Journal of Medical Engineering & Technology*, *43*(6), 341–355. doi:10.1080/03091902.2019.1673844 PMID:31679409

Fisher-Hoch, S. P., Khan, J. A., Rehman, S., Mirza, S., Khurshid, M., & McCormick, J. B. (1995). Crimean Congo-haemorrhagic fever treated with oral ribavirin. *Lancet*, *346*(8973), 472–474. doi:10.1016/S0140-6736(95)91323-8 PMID:7637481

Fleming, M., Ravula, S., Tatishchev, S. F., & Wang, H. L. (2012). Colorectal carcinoma: Pathologic aspects. *Journal of Gastrointestinal Oncology*, *3*(3), 153–173. doi:10.3978/j.issn.2078-6891.2012.030 PMID:22943008

Flutter Beautiful native apps in record time. (2021). Flutter. https://flutter.dev/

Flutter_mobile_vision (2021), Flutter. https://pub.dev/packages/flutter_mobile_vision

Flutter_tts (2021). Flutter. https://pub.dev/packages/flutter_tts

Fowler, R., Fletcher, T., Fischer, W. II, Lamontagne, F., Jacob, S., Brett-Major, D., Lawler, J. V., Jacquerioz, F. A., Houlihan, C., O'Dempsey, T., Ferri, M., Adachi, T., Lamah, M.-C., Bah, E. I., Mayet, T., Schieffelin, J., McLellan, S. L., Senga, M., Kato, Y., & Bausch, D. (2014). Caring for critically Ill patients with Ebola virus disease. Perspectives from West Africa. *American Journal of Respiratory and Critical Care Medicine*, *190*(7), 733–737. doi:10.1164/rccm.201408-1514CP PMID:25166884

Franco, J. S.-A. (2013). Thyroid disease and autoimmune diseases. In *Autoimmunity: From Bench to Bedside*. El Rosario University Press.

Fraz, M. M., Remagnino, P., Hoppe, A., Uyyanonvara, B., Rudnicka, A. R., Owen, C. G., & Barman, S. A. (2012). An Ensemble Classification-Based Approach Applied to Retinal Blood Vessel Segmentation. *IEEE Transactions on Biomedical Engineering*, *59*(9), 2538–2548. doi:10.1109/TBME.2012.2205687 PMID:22736688

Freeman, D., Loe, B. S., Chadwick, A., Vaccari, C., Waite, F., Rosebrock, L., Jenner, L., Petit, A., Lewandowsky, S., Vanderslott, S., Innocenti, S., Larkin, M., Giubilini, A., Yu, L.-M., McShane, H., Pollard, A. J., & Lambe, S. (2020). COVID-19 vaccine hesitancy in the UK: The Oxford coronavirus explanations, attitudes, and narratives survey (Oceans) II. *Psychological Medicine*, 1–15. doi:10.1017/S0033291720005188 PMID:33305716

Frid-Adar, M., Diamant, I., Klang, E., Amitai, M., Goldberger, J., & Greenspan, H. (2018). GAN-based synthetic medical image augmentation for increased CNN performance in liver lesion classification. *Neurocomputing*, *321*, 321–331. doi:10.1016/j.neucom.2018.09.013

Gabruseva, T., Poplavskiy, D., & Kalinin, A. (2020). Deep learning for automatic pneumonia detection. In *Proceedings of the IEEE/CVF conference on computer vision and pattern recognition workshops* (pp. 350-351). IEEE.

Gahalod, L., & Gupta, S. K. (2018). A Review on Digital Image Watermarking using 3-Level Discrete Wavelet Transform. *IJSRSET, 4099 Themed Section. Engineering and Technology*, *4*(1), 2395–1990.

Gang, L., Chutatape, O., & Krishnan, S. M. (2002). Detection and measurement of retinal vessels in fundus images using amplitude modified second-order Gaussian filter. *IEEE Transactions on Biomedical Engineering*, *49*(2), 168–172. doi:10.1109/10.979356 PMID:12066884

Gan, L., Chen, Y., Hu, P., Wu, D., Zhu, Y., Tan, J., Li, Y., & Zhang, D. (2021). Willingness to Receive SARS-CoV-2 Vaccination and Associated Factors among Chinese Adults: A Cross Sectional Survey. *International Journal of Environmental Research and Public Health*, *18*(4), 1993. doi:10.3390/ijerph18041993 PMID:33670821

Gao, Q., Wang, Y., Xu, W., & Jin, H. (2022). Predicting diagnostic gene biomarkers in patients with diabetic kidney disease based on weighted gene co-expression network analysis and machine-learning algorithms. *Research Square*. https://doi.org/10.21203/rs.3.rs-1696152/v1

Garg, P., Dixit, A., Sethi, P., & Pinheiro, P. R. (2020). Impact of node density on the qos parameters of routing protocols in opportunistic networks for smart spaces. *Mobile Information Systems*.

Garg, P., Dixit, A., & Sethi, P. (2019). Wireless sensor networks: An insight review. *International Journal of Advanced Science and Technology*, *28*(15), 612–627.

Garg, P., Dixit, A., & Sethi, P. (2022). Ml-fresh: Novel routing protocol in opportunistic networks using machine learning. *Computer Systems Science and Engineering*, *40*(2), 703–717.

Gayathri, S., Suchetha, M., & Latha, V. (2012). ECG Arrhythmia Detection and Classification Using Relevance Vector Machine. *Procedia Engineering*, *38*, 1333–1339. doi:10.1016/j.proeng.2012.06.164

Gelband, H., & Sloan, F. A. (Eds.). (2007). *Cancer control opportunities in low-and middle-income countries*. Academic Press.

geo. (2019). *Home*. GEO - NCBI. Nih.gov. https://www.ncbi.nlm.nih.gov/geo/

Gerke, S., Minssen, T., & Cohen, G. (2020). Ethical and legal challenges of artificial intelligence-driven healthcare. In *Artificial intelligence in healthcare* (pp. 295–336). Academic Press. doi:10.1016/B978-0-12-818438-7.00012-5

Gerussi, V., Peghin, M., Palese, A., Bressan, V., Visintini, E., Bontempo, G., Graziano, E., De Martino, M., Isola, M., & Tascini, C. (2021). Vaccine Hesitancy among Italian Patients Recovered from COVID-19 Infection towards Influenza and Sars-Cov-2 Vaccination. *Vaccines*, *9*(2), 172. doi:10.3390/vaccines9020172 PMID:33670661

Ghana Health Service. (2016). *The health sector in Ghana facts and figures 2015*. Ghana Health Service. https://www.ghanahealthservice.org/ghs-item-details.php?cid=5&scid=55&iid=134

Ghosh, P., Azam, S., Jonkman, M., Karim, A., Shamrat, F. M. J. M., Ignatious, E., Shultana, S., Beeravolu, A. R., & De Boer, F. (2021). Efficient Prediction of Cardiovascular Disease Using Machine Learning Algorithms With Relief and LASSO Feature Selection Techniques. *IEEE Access: Practical Innovations, Open Solutions*, *9*, 19304–19326. doi:10.1109/ACCESS.2021.3053759

Ghoushchi, S. J., Ranjbarzadeh, R., Dadkhah, A. H., Pourasad, Y., & Bendechache, M. (2021). An Extended Approach to Predict Retinopathy in Diabetic Patients Using the Genetic Algorithm and Fuzzy C-Means. *BioMed Research International,* 5597222. doi:10.1155/2021/5597222

Giger, M. L. (2018). Machine Learning in Medical Imaging. *Journal of the American College of Radiology*, *15*(3), 512–520. doi:10.1016/j.jacr.2017.12.028 PMID:29398494

GM, H., Gourisaria, M. K., Rautaray, S. S., & Pandey, M. (2021). Pneumonia detection using CNN through chest X-ray. [JESTEC]. *Journal of Engineering Science and Technology*, *16*(1), 861–876.

Goldberger, A. L. (2006). *Clinical Electrocardiography: A Simplified Approach* (7th ed.). Elsevier.

Goled, S. (2020, October 25). *Top 5 Neural Network Models For Deep Learning & Their Applications*. Analytics India Magazine. https://analyticsindiamag.com/top-5-neural-network-models-for-deep-learning-their-applications/

Gong, L., Thota, M., Yu, M., Duan, W., Swainson, M., Ye, X., & Kollias, S. (2021). A novel unified deep neural networks methodology for use by date recognition in retail food package image. *Signal, Image and Video Processing*, *15*(3), 449–457. https://doi.org/10.1007/s11760-020-01764-7

Gosavi, C. S., & Mali, S. N. (2017). Watermarking for Video using single channel block based schur decomposition. *Global Journal of Pure and Applied Mathematics*, *12*(2), 1575–1585.

Grzybowski, A., Brona, P., Lim, G., Ruamviboonsuk, P., Tan, G. S., Abramoff, M., & Ting, D. S. (2020). Artificial intelligence for diabetic retinopathy screening: A review. *Eye (London, England)*, *34*(3), 451–460. doi:10.103841433-019-0566-0 PMID:31488886

Guail, A. A. A., Jinsong, G., Oloulade, B. M., & Al-Sabri, R. (2022). A principal neighborhood aggregation-based graph convolutional network for pneumonia detection. *Sensors (Basel)*, *22*(8), 3049. doi:10.339022083049 PMID:35459035

Gu, J. Z., Zhu, J., Qiu, Q., Wang, Y., Bai, T., & Yin, Y. (2019). Prediction of immunohistochemistry of suspected thyroid nodules by use of machine learning–based radiomics. *AJR. American Journal of Roentgenology*, *213*(6), 1348–1357. doi:10.2214/AJR.19.21626 PMID:31461321

Gulati, S., & Bhogal, R. K. (2020). Classification of melanoma from dermoscopic images using machine learning. In *Smart Intelligent Computing and Applications: Proceedings of the Third International Conference on Smart Computing and Informatics*, Volume 1 (pp. 345-354). Springer. 10.1007/978-981-13-9282-5_32

Gurusamy, P. S. R., & Janagaraj, P. D. (2018). A Success Story: The Burden of Maternal, Neonatal and Childhood Mortality in Rwanda - Critical Appraisal of Interventions and Recommendations for the Future. *African Journal of Reproductive Health*, *22*(2), 9–16. doi:10.29063/ajrh2018/v22i2.1 PMID:30052329

Gu, X., Pan, L., Liang, H., & Yang, R. (2018, March). Classification of bacterial and viral childhood pneumonia using deep learning in chest radiography. In *Proceedings of the 3rd International Conference on Multimedia and Image Processing* (pp. 88-93). 10.1145/3195588.3195597

Habibi, S., Ahmadi, M., & Alizadeh, S. (2015). Type 2 Diabetes Mellitus Screening and Risk Factors Using Decision Tree: Results of Data Mining. *Global Journal of Health Science*, *7*(5). https://doi.org/10.5539/gjhs.v7n5p304

Habib, N., Hasan, M. M., & Rahman, M. M. (2020). Fusion of deep convolutional neural network with PCA and logistic regression for diagnosis of pediatric pneumonia on chest X-rays. *The New Biologist*, *10*(3), 62–76.

Hacking, C. (n.d.). Pneumonia: Radiology Reference Article. *Radiopaedia.org*. https://radiopaedia.org/articles/pneumonia

Haldar, N. A. H., Khan, F. A., Ali, A., & Abbas, H. (2017). Arrhythmia classification using Mahalan obis distance based improved Fuzzy C Means clustering for mobile health monitoring systems. *Neurocomputing*, *220*, 221–235. doi:10.1016/j.neucom.2016.08.042

Hamdi, T., Ali, J. B., Fnaiech, N., Di Costanzo, V., Fnaiech, F., Moreau, E., & Ginoux, J. M. (2017, February). Artificial neural network for blood glucose level prediction. In *2017 International Conference on Smart, Monitored and Controlled Cities (SM2C)* (pp. 91-95). IEEE. 10.1109/SM2C.2017.8071825

Harapan, H., Wagner, A. L., Yufika, A., Winardi, W., Anwar, S., Gan, A. K., Setiawan, A. M., Rajamoorthy, Y., Sofyan, H., & Mudatsir, M. (2020). Acceptance of a COVID-19 Vaccine in Southeast Asia: A Cross-Sectional Study in Indonesia. *Frontiers in Public Health*, *8*, 381. doi:10.3389/fpubh.2020.00381 PMID:32760691

Hasanzad, M., Aghaei Meybodi, H. R., Sarhangi, N., & Larijani, B. (2022). Artificial intelligence perspective in the future of endocrine diseases. *Journal of Diabetes and Metabolic Disorders*, *21*(1), 1–8. doi:10.100740200-021-00949-2 PMID:35673469

Hashmi, M. F., Katiyar, S., Keskar, A. G., Bokde, N. D., & Geem, Z. W. (2020). Efficient pneumonia detection in chest xray images using deep transfer learning. *Diagnostics (Basel)*, *10*(6), 417. doi:10.3390/diagnostics10060417 PMID:32575475

Heider, D., Pyka, M., & Barnekow, A. (2009). DNA watermarks in non-coding regulatory sequences. *BMC Research Notes*, *2*(1), 1–6. doi:10.1186/1756-0500-2-125 PMID:19583865

He, K., Zhang, X., Ren, S., & Sun, J. (2016). Deep Residual Learning for Image Recognition. *2016 IEEE Conference on Computer Vision and Pattern Recognition (CVPR)*, (pp. 770–778). IEEE. 10.1109/CVPR.2016.90

Heneghan, C. (2002). Characterization of changes in blood vessel width and tortuosity in retinopathy of prematurity using image analysis. *Medical Image Analysis*, *6*(4), 407–429. doi:10.1016/S1361-8415(02)00058-0 PMID:12426111

Hernandez, J. R., Amado, M., & Perez-Gonzalez, F. (2000). DCT-domain watermarking techniques for still images: Detector performance analysis and a new structure. *IEEE Transactions on Image Processing*, *9*(1), 55–68. doi:10.1109/83.817598 PMID:18255372

Ho, A. T., Zhu, X., & Guan, Y. L. (2004). Image content authentication using pinned sine transform. *EURASIP Journal on Advances in Signal Processing*, *2004*(14), 1–11. doi:10.1155/S111086570440506X

Horgan, R. P., & Kenny, L. C. (2011). "Omic" technologies: genomics, transcriptomics, proteomics and metabolomics. *The Obstetrician & Gynaecologist, 13*(3), 189–195. doi:10.1576/toag.13.3.189.27672

Hosseini, M. S., Chan, L., Tse, G., Tang, M., Deng, J., Norouzi, S., Rowsell, C., Plataniotis, K. N., & Damaskinos, S. (2019). *Atlas of Digital Pathology: A Generalized Hierarchical Histological Tissue Type-Annotated Database for Deep Learning*. Openaccess.thecvf.com. https://openaccess.thecvf.com/content_CVPR_2019/html/Hosseini_Atlas_of_Digital_Pathology_A_Generalized_Hierarchical_Histological_Tissue_Type-Annotated_CVPR_2019_paper.html

Houweling, T. A. J., Ronsmans, C., Campbell, O. M. R., & Kunst, A. E. (2007). Huge poor-rich inequalities in maternity care: An international comparative study of maternity and child care in developing countries. *Bulletin of the World Health Organization*, *85*(10), 745–754. doi:10.2471/BLT.06.038588 PMID:18038055

Hsieh, C. T., & Sou, P. Y. (2002, July). Blind cepstrum domain audio watermarking based on time energy features. In *2002 14th International Conference on Digital Signal Processing Proceedings. DSP 2002 (Cat. No. 02TH8628)* (*Vol. 2,* pp. 705-708). IEEE.

Hu, M. A. (2022). Development and preliminary validation of a machine learning system for thyroid dysfunction diagnosis based on routine laboratory tests. *Communication & Medicine*, 1–8. PMID:35603277

Ibrahim, I. M., & Abdulazeez, A. M. (2021). The Role of Machine Learning Algorithms for Diagnosing Diseases. *JASTT.* doi:10.38094/jastt20179

Ieracitano, C., Mammone, N., Versaci, M., Varone, G., Ali, A. R., Armentano, A., Calabrese, G., Ferrarelli, A., Turano, L., Tebala, C., Hussain, Z., Sheikh, Z., Sheikh, A., Sceni, G., Hussain, A., & Morabito, F. C. (2022). A fuzzy-enhanced deep learning approach for early detection of Covid-19 pneumonia from portable chest X-ray images. *Neurocomputing*, *481*, 202–215. doi:10.1016/j.neucom.2022.01.055 PMID:35079203

Iizuka, O., Kanavati, F., Kato, K., Rambeau, M., Arihiro, K., & Tsuneki, M. (2020). Deep Learning Models for Histopathological Classification of Gastric and Colonic Epithelial Tumours. *Scientific Reports*, *10*(1), 1504. doi:10.103841598-020-58467-9 PMID:32001752

Imaduddin, M. D., & Pullarao, G. (2014). Real Time Simulation Based on Image Protection Using Digital Watermarking Techniques. *International Journal of New Trends in Electronics and Communication (Vol. 2).*

Institute of Medicine (US) Committee on Quality of Health Care in America. (2000). *To Err is Human: Building a Safer Health System* (L. T. Kohn, J. M. Corrigan, & M. S. Donaldson, Eds.). National Academies Press. https://www.ncbi.nlm.nih.gov/books/NBK225182/

Invernizzi, A., Torre, A., Parrulli, S., Zicarelli, F., Schiuma, M., Colombo, V., Giacomelli, A., Cigada, M., Milazzo, L., Ridolfo, A., Faggion, I., Cordier, L., Oldani, M., Marini, S., Villa, P., Rizzardini, G., Galli, M., Antinori, S., Staurenghi, G., & Meroni, L. (2020). Retinal findings in patients with COVID-19: Results from the SERPICO-19 study. *EClinicalMedicine*, *27*, 100550. doi:10.1016/j.eclinm.2020.100550 PMID:32984785

Ioniţă, I. (2016). Prediction of thyroid disease using data mining techniques. *Broad Research in Artificial Intelligence and Neuroscience*, 115–124.

Irfan, A., Adivishnu, A. L., Sze-To, A., Dehkharghanian, T., Rahnamayan, S., & Tizhoosh, H. R. (2020, July). Classifying pneumonia among chest x-rays using transfer learning. In *2020 42nd Annual International Conference of the IEEE Engineering in Medicine & Biology Society (EMBC)* (pp. 2186-2189). IEEE. 10.1109/EMBC44109.2020.9175594

Islam, S. S., Haque, M. S., Miah, M. S. U., Sarwar, T. B., & Nugraha, R. (2022). Application of machine learning algorithms to predict the thyroid disease risk: An experimental comparative study. *PeerJ. Computer Science*, *8*, 898. doi:10.7717/peerj-cs.898 PMID:35494828

Jackins, V., Vimal, S., Kaliappan, M., & Lee, M. Y. (2020). AI-based smart prediction of clinical disease using random forest classifier and Naive Bayes. *The Journal of Supercomputing*. . doi:10.100711227-020-03481-x

Jain, R., Nagrath, P., Kataria, G., Kaushik, V. S., & Hemanth, D. J. (2020). Pneumonia detection in chest X-ray images using convolutional neural networks and transfer learning. *Measurement*, *165*, 108046. doi:10.1016/j.measurement.2020.108046

Jain, S., & Pise, N. (2015). Computer aided melanoma skin cancer detection using image processing. *Procedia Computer Science*, *48*, 735–740. doi:10.1016/j.procs.2015.04.209

Jaiswal, V., Negi, A., & Pal, T. (2021). A review on current advances in machine learning based diabetes prediction. *Primary Care Diabetes*, *15*(3), 435–443. https://doi.org/10.1016/j.pcd.2021.02.005

Jakkula, V. (n.d.). *Tutorial on Support Vector Machine (SVM)*. CCS. https://course.ccs.neu.edu/cs5100f11/resources/jakkula.pdf

Jatav S., & Sharma, V. (2018). An algorithm for predictive data mining approach in medical diagnosis. *IJCSIT, 10*(1). doi:10.5121/ijcsit.2018.10102

Javed Mehedi Shamrat, F. M., Ghosh, P., Sadek, M. H., & Kazi, Md. A., & Shultana, S. (2020). Implementation of Machine Learning Algorithms to Detect the Prognosis Rate of Kidney Disease. *2020 IEEE International Conference for Innovation in Technology (INOCON)*. IEEE. 10.1109/INOCON50539.2020.9298026

Jaworek-Korjakowska, J., & Tadeusiewicz, R. (2015, August). Determination of border irregularity in dermoscopic color images of pigmented skin lesions. In *Annual International Conference of the IEEE Engineering in Medicine and Biology Society*, (Vol. 2015, pp. 2665-2668). IEEE.

Jenkins, R. A., Torugsa, K., & Markowitz, L. E. (2000). Willingness to participate in HIV-1 vaccine trials among young Thai men. *Sexually Transmitted Infections*, *76*(5), 386–392. doi:10.1136ti.76.5.386 PMID:11141858

Jha, D., Smedsrud, P. H., Riegler, M. A., Halvorsen, P., de Lange, T., Johansen, D., & Johansen, H. D. (2019). Kvasir-SEG: A Segmented Polyp Dataset. *ArXiv:1911.07069* https://arxiv.org/abs/1911.07069

Jha, R. B., Bhattacharjee, V., & Mustafi, A. (2022). Increasing the Prediction Accuracy for Thyroid Disease: A Step Towards Better Health for Society. *Wireless Personal Communications*, *122*(2), 1921–1938. doi:10.100711277-021-08974-3

Jiang, B., Dong, N., Shou, J., Cao, L., Hu, K., Liu, W., & Qi, X. (2021). Effectiveness of artificial intelligent cardiac remote monitoring system for evaluating asymptomatic myocardial ischemia in patients with coronary heart disease. *American Journal of Translational Research*, *13*(10), 11653. PMID:34786091

Jiang, X., & Mojon, D. (2003). Adaptive local thresholding by verification-based multithreshold probing with application to vessel detection in retinal images. *IEEE Transactions on Pattern Analysis and Machine Intelligence*, *25*(1), 131–137. doi:10.1109/TPAMI.2003.1159954

Jin, P., Ji, X., Kang, W., Li, Y., Liu, H., Ma, F., Ma, S., Hu, H., Li, W., & Tian, Y. (2020). Artificial intelligence in gastric cancer: A systematic review. *Journal of Cancer Research and Clinical Oncology*, *146*(9), 2339–2350. doi:10.100700432-020-03304-9 PMID:32613386

Joby, A. (2021, July 19). *What Is K-Nearest Neighbor? An ML Algorithm to Classify Data*. Learn.g2. https://learn.g2.com/k-nearest-neighbor

Joffe, S. (2014). Evaluating novel therapies during the Ebola epidemic. *Journal of the American Medical Association*, *312*(13), 1299–1300. doi:10.1001/jama.2014.12867 PMID:25211645

Johnson, M. O. (2000). Personality correlates of HIV vaccine trial participation. *Personality and Individual Differences*, *29*(3), 459–467. doi:10.1016/S0191-8869(99)00206-8

Joshi, R. D., & Dhakal, C. K. (2021). Predicting Type 2 Diabetes Using Logistic Regression and Machine Learning Approaches. *International Journal of Environmental Research and Public Health*, *18*(14), 7346. https://doi.org/10.3390/ijerph18147346

Jung, W. H., & Lee, S. G. (2017). An arrhythmia classification method in utilizing the weighted KNN and the fitness rule. *IRBM*, *38*(3), 138–148. doi:10.1016/j.irbm.2017.04.002

Kahn, S. E., Hull, R. L., & Utzschneider, K. M. (2006). Mechanisms linking obesity to insulin resistance and type 2 diabetes. *Nature*, *444*(7121), 840–846. https://doi.org/10.1038/nature05482

Kamble, M. V. A Review of Different Techniques on Digital Image Watermarking Scheme. *International Journal of Innovative Science, Engineering & Technology, 3*(2).

Kanagarathinam, K., & Sekar, K. (2019). Text detection and recognition in raw image dataset of seven segment digital energy meter display. *Energy Reports, 5*, 842–852.

Kandhasamy, J. Pradeep., & Balamurali, S. (2015, May). Performance Analysis of Classifier Models to Predict Diabetes Mellitus [Review of Performance Analysis of Classifier Models to Predict Diabetes Mellitus]. *Procedia Computer Science, 47.* doi:10.1016/j.procs.2015.03.182

Karageorgos, G., Andreadis, I., Psychas, K., Mourkousis, G., Kiourti, A., Lazzi, G., & Nikita, K. S. (2018). The promise of mobile technologies for the health care system in the developing world: A systematic review. *IEEE Reviews in Biomedical Engineering, 12*, 100–122. doi:10.1109/RBME.2018.2868896 PMID:30188840

Karahalil, B. (2016). Overview of Systems Biology and Omics Technologies. *Current Medicinal Chemistry, 23*(37), 4221–4230. https://doi.org/10.2174/0929867323666160926150617

Karthik, S. Sudha, M. (2018). A Survey on Machine Learning Approaches in Gene Expression Classification in Modelling Computational Diagnostic System for Complex Diseases. *8*(2).

Karuppaiah, G., Velayutham, J., Hansda, S., Narayana, N., Bhansali, S., & Manickam, P. (2022). Towards the development of reagent-free and reusable electrochemical aptamer-based cortisol sensor. *Bioelectrochemistry (Amsterdam, Netherlands), 145*, 108098. doi:10.1016/j.bioelechem.2022.108098 PMID:35325786

Kashani, A. H., Asanad, S., Chan, J. W., Singer, M. B., Zhang, J., Sharifi, M., Khansari, M. M., Abdolahi, F., Shi, Y., Biffi, A., Chui, H., & Ringman, J. M. (2021). Past, present and future role of retinal imaging in neurodegenerative disease. *Progress in Retinal and Eye Research, 83*, 100938. doi:10.1016/j.preteyeres.2020.100938 PMID:33460813

Kather, J. N., Krisam, J., Charoentong, P., Luedde, T., Herpel, E., Weis, C.-A., Gaiser, T., Marx, A., Valous, N. A., Ferber, D., Jansen, L., Reyes-Aldasoro, C. C., Zörnig, I., Jäger, D., Brenner, H., Chang-Claude, J., Hoffmeister, M., & Halama, N. (2019). Predicting survival from colorectal cancer histology slides using deep learning: A retrospective multicenter study. *PLoS Medicine, 16*(1), e1002730. doi:10.1371/journal.pmed.1002730 PMID:30677016

Kather, J. N., Pearson, A. T., Halama, N., Jäger, D., Krause, J., Loosen, S. H., Marx, A., Boor, P., Tacke, F., Neumann, U. P., Grabsch, H. I., Yoshikawa, T., Brenner, H., Chang-Claude, J., Hoffmeister, M., Trautwein, C., & Luedde, T. (2019). Deep learning can predict microsatellite instability directly from histology in gastrointestinal cancer. *Nature Medicine, 25*(7), 1054–1056. doi:10.103841591-019-0462-y PMID:31160815

Kaul, K., Tarr, J. M., Ahmad, S. I., Kohner, E. M., & Chibber, R. (2012). Introduction to Diabetes Mellitus. *Advances in Experimental Medicine and Biology, 771*, 1–11. doi:10.1007/978-1-4614-5441-0_1 PMID:23393665

Kavitha, K. K., Koshti, A., & Dunghav, P. (2012). Steganography using least significant bit algorithm. *International Journal of Engineering Research and Applications (IJERA).*

Kermany, D., Zhang, K., & Goldbaum, M. (2018). Labeled optical coherence tomography (OCT) and chest x-ray images for classification. Mendeley Data. doi:10.17632/rscbjbr9sj.2

Khalea, A. F., Owis, M. I., & Yassine, I. A. (2015). A novel technique for cardiac arrhythmia classification using spectral correlation and support vector machines. *Expert Systems with Applications*, *42*(21), 8361–8368. doi:10.1016/j.eswa.2015.06.046

Khanam, J. J., & Foo, S. Y. (2021). A comparison of machine learning algorithms for diabetes prediction. *ICT Express*, *7*(4), 432–439. doi:10.1016/j.icte.2021.02.004

Khandare, S., & Shrawankar, U. (2016). Image bit depth plane digital watermarking for secured classified image data transmission. *Procedia Computer Science*, *78*, 698–705. doi:10.1016/j.procs.2016.02.119

Khan, K. B., Khaliq, A. A., Jalil, A., Iftikhar, M. A., Ullah, N., Aziz, M. W., Ullah, K., & Shahid, M. (2019). A review of retinal blood vessels extraction techniques: Challenges, taxonomy, and future trends. *Pattern Analysis & Applications*, *22*(3), 767–802. doi:10.100710044-018-0754-8

Khanna, A., Rani, P., Garg, P., Singh, P. K., & Khamparia, A. (2021). An Enhanced Crow Search Inspired Feature Selection Technique for Intrusion Detection Based Wireless Network System. *Wireless Personal Communications*, 1–18.

Kharazmi, P., AlJasser, M. I., Lui, H., Wang, Z. J., & Lee, T. K. (2016). Automated detection and segmentation of vascular structures of skin lesions seen in Dermoscopy, with an application to basal cell carcinoma classification. *IEEE Journal of Biomedical and Health Informatics*, *21*(6), 1675–1684. doi:10.1109/JBHI.2016.2637342 PMID:27959832

Kharghanian, R., & Ahmadyfard, A. (2012). Retinal Blood Vessel Segmentation Using Gabor Wavelet and Line Operator. *International Journal of Machine Learning and Computing*, *2*(5), 593–597. doi:10.7763/IJMLC.2012.V2.196

Khorshid, S. F., & Abdulazeez, A. M. (2021). Breast Cancer Diagnosis Based On K-Nearest Neighbors: A Review. *PalArch's Journal of Archaeology of Egypt / Egyptology*, *18*(4), 1927–1951. https://archives.palarch.nl/index.php/jae/article/view/6601

Kim, J. H., Marks, F., & Clemens, J. D. (2021). Looking beyond COVID-19 vaccine phase 3 trials. *Nature Medicine*, *27*(2), 205–211. doi:10.103841591-021-01230-y PMID:33469205

Kn, A. (2015). Can she make it? Transportation barriers to accessing maternal and child health care services in rural Ghana. *BMC Health Services Research*, *15*(1), 333–333. doi:10.118612913-015-1005-y PMID:26290436

Kochner, B. (1998). Course tracking and contour extraction of retinal vessels from color fundus photographs: most efficient use of steerable filters for model-based image analysis. In K. M. Hanson (Ed.), *Medical Imaging 1998: Image Processing* (pp. 755–761)., doi:10.1117/12.310955

Kohavi, R. (1995, August). A study of cross-validation and bootstrap for accuracy estimation and model selection [Review of A study of cross-validation and bootstrap for accuracy estimation and model selection]. *IJCAI'95: Proceedings of the 14th international joint conference on Artificial intelligence* – (Volume 2). IEEE.

Ko, L. T., Chen, J. E., Shieh, Y. S., Hsin, H. C., & Sung, T. Y. (2012). Nested quantization index modulation for reversible watermarking and its application to healthcare information management systems. *Computational and Mathematical Methods in Medicine*, *2012*, 2012. doi:10.1155/2012/839161 PMID:22194776

Ko, L. T., Chen, J. E., Shieh, Y. S., & Sung, T. Y. (2012, June). A novel fractional discrete cosine transform based reversible watermarking for biomedical image applications. In *2012 International Symposium on Computer, Consumer and Control* (pp. 36-39). IEEE. 10.1109/IS3C.2012.19

Korkmaz, H., Canayaz, E., Birtane Akar, S., & Altikardes, Z. A. (2019). Fuzzy logic based risk assessment system giving individualized advice for metabolic syndrome and fatal cardiovascular diseases. *Technology and Health Care*, *27*, 59–66. https://doi.org/10.3233/thc-199007

Krissian, K., Malandain, G., Ayache, N., Vaillant, R., & Trousset, Y. (2000). Model-Based Detection of Tubular Structures in 3D Images. *Computer Vision and Image Understanding*, *80*(2), 130–171. doi:10.1006/cviu.2000.0866

Krizhevsky, A., Sutskever, I., & Hinton, G. E. (2012). ImageNet Classification with Deep Convolutional Neural Networks. *Advances in Neural Information Processing Systems, 25*, 1097–1105. https://papers.nips.cc/paper/2012/hash/c399862d3b9d6b76c8436e924a68c45b-Abstract.html

Krosin, M. T., Klitzman, R., Levin, B., Cheng, J., & Ranney, M. L. (2006). Problems in comprehension of informed consent in rural and peri-urban Mali, West Africa. *Clinical Trials*, *3*(3), 306–313. doi:10.1191/1740774506cn150oa PMID:16895047

Kudina, O., & de Boer, B. (2021). Co-designing diagnosis: Towards a responsible integration of Machine Learning decision-support systems in medical diagnostics. *Journal of Evaluation in Clinical Practice.* Wiley. doi:10.1111/jep.13535

Kumar Jaiswal, R., & Ravi, S. (2018). Robust Imperceptible Digital Image Watermarking based on Discrete Wavelet & Cosine Transforms. *International Journal of Advanced Research in Computer Engineering & Technology (IJARCET), 7*(2).

Kumar, I., Bhatt, C., Vimal, V., & Qamar, S. (2022). Automated white corpuscles nucleus segmentation using deep neural network from microscopic blood smear. *Journal of Intelligent & Fuzzy Systems*, (Preprint), 1-14.

Kumari, S., Kumar, D., & Mittal, M. (2021, May). An ensemble approach for classification and prediction of diabetes mellitus using soft voting classifier [Review of An ensemble approach for classification and prediction of diabetes mellitus using soft voting classifier]. *International Journal of Cognitive Computing in Engineering, 2,* 40-46. doi:10.1016/j.ijcce.2021.01.001

Kumari, V. A., & Chitra, R. (2013). Classification of Diabetes Disease Using Support Vector Machine. [IJERA]. *International Journal of Engineering Research and Applications*, *3*, 1797–1801.

Kumar, L., & Singh, K. U. (2020). An analysis of different watermarking schemes for medical image authentication. *European Journal of Molecular & Clinical Medicine*, *7*(4), 2250–2259.

Kumar, S., Nilsen, W. J., Abernethy, A., Atienza, A., Patrick, K., Pavel, M., Riley, W. T., Shar, A., Spring, B., Spruijt-Metz, D., Hedeker, D., Honavar, V., Kravitz, R., Lefebvre, R. C., Mohr, D. C., Murphy, S. A., Quinn, C., Shusterman, V., & Swendeman, D. (2013). Mobile health technology evaluation: The mHealth evidence workshop. *American Journal of Preventive Medicine*, *45*(2), 228–236. doi:10.1016/j.amepre.2013.03.017 PMID:23867031

Kundu, R., Das, R., Geem, Z. W., Han, G. T., & Sarkar, R. (2021). Pneumonia detection in chest X-ray images using an ensemble of deep learning models. *PLoS One*, *16*(9), e0256630.

Kuppusamy, K., & Thamodaran, K. (2012). Optimized image watermarking scheme based on PSO. *Procedia Engineering*, *38*, 493–503. doi:10.1016/j.proeng.2012.06.061

Kutlu, Y., & Kuntalp, D. (2011). A multi-stage automatic arrhythmia recognition and classification system. *Computers in Biology and Medicine*, *41*(1), 37–45. doi:10.1016/j.compbiomed.2010.11.003 PMID:21183163

Lai, Z., & Deng, H. (2018). Medical Image Classification Based on Deep Features Extracted by Deep Model and Statistic Feature Fusion with Multilayer Perceptron□. *Computational Intelligence and Neuroscience*, *2018*, 1–13. doi:10.1155/2018/2061516 PMID:30298088

Laouamer, L., AlShaikh, M., Nana, L., & Pascu, A. C. (2015). Robust watermarking scheme and tamper detection based on threshold versus intensity. *Journal of Innovation in Digital Ecosystems*, *2*(1-2), 1–12. doi:10.1016/j.jides.2015.10.001

Lattoofi, N. F., Al-Sharuee, I. F., Kamil, M. Y., Obaid, A. H., Mahidi, A. A., & Omar, A. A. (2019, December). Melanoma skin cancer detection based on ABCD rule. In *2019 First International Conference of Computer and Applied Sciences (CAS)* (pp. 154-157). IEEE. 10.1109/CAS47993.2019.9075465

Lazarus, J. V., Ratzan, S. C., Palayew, A., Gostin, L. O., Larson, H. J., Rabin, K., Kimball, S., & El-Mohandes, A. (2021a). A global survey of potential acceptance of a COVID-19 vaccine. *Nature Medicine*, *27*(2), 225–228. doi:10.103841591-020-1124-9 PMID:33082575

Lee, C.-S., & Wang, M.-H. (2011). A Fuzzy Expert System for Diabetes Decision Support Application. *IEEE Transactions on Systems, Man, and Cybernetics. Part B, Cybernetics*, *41*(1), 139–153. https://doi.org/10.1109/tsmcb.2010.2048899

Lee, S. H., Nurmatov, U. B., Nwaru, B. I., Mukherjee, M., Grant, L., & Pagliari, C. (2016). Effectiveness of mHealth interventions for maternal, newborn and child health in low- and middle-income countries: Systematic review and meta-analysis. *Journal of Global Health*, *6*(1), 010401. doi:10.7189/jogh.06.010401 PMID:26649177

Lee, S., Cho, Y., & Kim, S.-Y. (2017). Mapping mHealth (mobile health) and mobile penetrations in sub-Saharan Africa for strategic regional collaboration in mHealth scale-up: An application of exploratory spatial data analysis. *Globalization and Health, 13*(1), 63. doi:10.118612992-017-0286-9 PMID:28830540

Li, J. Q., Dukes, P. V., Lee, W., Sarkis, M., & Vo-Dinh, T. (2022). Machine learning using convolutional neural networks for SERS analysis of biomarkers in medical diagnostics. *Journal of Raman Spectroscopy*. Wiley. doi:10.1002/jrs.6447

Liang, G., & Zheng, L. (2020). A transfer learning method with deep residual network for pediatric pneumonia diagnosis. *Computer Methods and Programs in Biomedicine, 187*, 104964. doi:10.1016/j.cmpb.2019.06.023 PMID:31262537

Liaw, A., & Wiener, M. (2002). Classification and Regression by randomForest. *R News, 2*(3). https://cogns.northwestern.edu/cbmg/LiawAndWiener2002.pdf. doi:10.1057/9780230509993

Li, J., Pan, C., Zhang, S., Spin, J. M., Deng, A., Leung, L. L., Dalman, R. L., Tsao, P. S., & Snyder, M. (2018). Decoding the genomics of abdominal aortic aneurysm. *Cell, 174*(6), 1361–1372. doi:10.1016/j.cell.2018.07.021 PMID:30193110

Li, K., Fathan, M. I., Patel, K., Zhang, T., Zhong, C., Bansal, A., Rastogi, A., Wang, J. S., & Wang, G. (2021). Colonoscopy polyp detection and classification: Dataset creation and comparative evaluations. *PLoS One, 16*(8), e0255809. doi:10.1371/journal.pone.0255809 PMID:34403452

Linhares, R. R. (2016). Arrhythmia detection from heart rate variability by SDFA method. *International Journal of Cardiology, 224*, 27–32. doi:10.1016/j.ijcard.2016.08.286 PMID:27611914

Linsangan, N. B., Adtoon, J. J., & Torres, J. L. (2018, November). Geometric analysis of skin lesion for skin cancer using image processing. In *2018 IEEE 10th International Conference on Humanoid, Nanotechnology, Information Technology, Communication and Control, Environment and Management (HNICEM)* (pp. 1-5). IEEE. 10.1109/HNICEM.2018.8666296

Liu, G., Liu, H., & Kadir, A. (2012). Wavelet-based color pathological image watermark through dynamically adjusting the embedding intensity. *Computational and Mathematical Methods in Medicine, 2012*, 2012. doi:10.1155/2012/406349 PMID:23243463

Liu, Y., Geng, H., Duan, B., Yang, X., Ma, A., & Ding, X. (2021). Identification of Diagnostic CpG Signatures in Patients with Gestational Diabetes Mellitus via Epigenome-Wide Association Study Integrated with Machine Learning. *BioMed Research International, 2021*, 1–10. https://doi.org/10.1155/2021/1984690

Liu, Z., Li, L., Li, T., Luo, D., Wang, X., & Luo, D. (2020). Does a Deep Learning–Based Computer-Assisted Diagnosis System Outperform Conventional Double Reading by Radiologists in Distinguishing Benign and Malignant Lung Nodules? *Frontiers in Oncology, 10*, 545862. doi:10.3389/fonc.2020.545862 PMID:33163395

Lock, K. (2000). Health impact assessment. *BMJ (Clinical Research Ed.), 320*(7246), 1395–1398. doi:10.1136/bmj.320.7246.1395 PMID:10818037

Lukmanto, R. B. Suharjito, N. A., & Akbar, H. (2019). Early Detection of Diabetes Mellitus using Feature Selection and Fuzzy Support Vector Machine. *Procedia Computer Science, 157*, 46–54. doi:10.1016/j.procs.2019.08.140

Luz, E. J. D. S., Nunes, T. M., De Albuquerque, V. H. C., Papa, J. P., & Menotti, D. (2013). ECG arrhythmia classification based on optimum-path forest. *Expert Systems with Applications*, *40*(9), 3561–3573. doi:10.1016/j.eswa.2012.12.063

Lv, B., & Jiang, Y. (2021). Prediction of Short-Term Stock Price Trend Based on Multiview RBF Neural Network. *Computational Intelligence and Neuroscience*, *2021*, 1–13. doi:10.1155/2021/8495288 PMID:34876898

Ma, Y., Chen, X., Cheng, K., Li, Y., & Sun, B. (2021). LDPolypVideo Benchmark: A Large-Scale Colonoscopy Video Dataset of Diverse Polyps. Medical Image Computing and Computer Assisted Intervention – MICCAI 2021, (pp. 387–396). Springer. doi:10.1007/978-3-030-87240-3_37

Maggo, C., & Garg, P. (2022). From linguistic features to their extractions: Understanding the semantics of a concept. *2022 Fifth International Conference on Computational Intelligence and Communication Technologies (CCICT)*, (pp. 427-431). Research Gate. doi:10.1109/CCiCT56684.2022.00082

Mahajan, P. H., & Bhalerao, P. B. (2014). A Review of Digital Watermarking Strategies. *International Journal of Advanced Research in Computer Science And Management Studies, 7.*

Mahase, E. (2020). Covid-19: Oxford researchers halt vaccine trial while adverse reaction is investigated. *BMJ (Clinical Research Ed.)*, *370*, m3525. doi:10.1136/bmj.m3525 PMID:32907856

Malakar, S., Roy, S. D., Das, S., Sen, S., Velasquez, J. D., & Sarkar, R. (2022).*nComputer Based Diagnosis of Some Chronic Diseases: A Medical Journey of the Last Two Decades*. Springer. https://doi.org/10.1007/s11831-022-09776-x

Manickam, P., Kanagavel, V., Sonawane, A., Thipperudraswamy, S. P., & Bhansali, S. (2019). Electrochemical systems for healthcare applications. *Bioelectrochemical Interface Engineering*, 385-409.

Manickam, P., Mariappan, S. A., Murugesan, S. M., Hansda, S., Kaushik, A., Shinde, R., & Thipperudraswamy, S. P. (2022). Artificial intelligence (AI) and internet of medical things (IoMT) assisted biomedical systems for intelligent healthcare. *Biosensors (Basel)*, *12*(8), 562. doi:10.3390/bios12080562 PMID:35892459

Manogaran, G., Chilamkurti, N., & Hsu, C. H. (2018). Emerging trends, issues, and challenges in Internet of Medical Things and wireless networks. *Personal and Ubiquitous Computing*, *22*(5), 879–882. doi:10.100700779-018-1178-6

Marie-Sainte, L., Almohaini, A. & Saba. (2019). Current Techniques for Diabetes Prediction: Review and Case Study. *Applied Sciences, 9*(21), 4604. doi:10.3390/app9214604

Marinho, P. M., Marcos, A. A. A., Romano, A. C., Nascimento, H., & Belfort, R. Jr. (2020). Retinal findings in patients with COVID-19. *Lancet*, *395*(10237), 1610. doi:10.1016/S0140-6736(20)31014-X PMID:32405105

Marselli, L., Thorne, J., Dahiya, S., Sgroi, D. C., Sharma, A., Bonner-Weir, S., Marchetti, P., & Weir, G. C. (2010). Gene Expression Profiles of Beta-Cell Enriched Tissue Obtained by Laser Capture Microdissection from Subjects with Type 2 Diabetes. *PLoS One*, *5*(7), e11499. https://doi.org/10.1371/journal.pone.0011499

Martinez-Perez, M. E., Hughes, A. D., Thom, S. A., Bharath, A. A., & Parker, K. H. (2007). Segmentation of blood vessels from red-free and fluorescein retinal images. *Medical Image Analysis*, *11*(1), 47–61. doi:10.1016/j.media.2006.11.004 PMID:17204445

Martis, R. J., Acharya, U. R., Prasad, H., Chua, C. K., Lim, C. M., & Suri, J. S. (2013). Application of higher order statistics for atrial arrhythmia classification. *Biomedical Signal Processing and Control*, *8*(6), 888–900. doi:10.1016/j.bspc.2013.08.008

Maulana, Y. I. R., Badriyah, T., & Syarif, I. (2018). Influence of Logistic Regression Models For Prediction and Analysis of Diabetes Risk Factors. *EMITTER International Journal of Engineering Technology*, *6*(1), 151–167. doi:10.24003/emitter.v6i1.258

Mayo clinic staff. (June 2022), *Pneumonia*. May Clinic. https://www.mayoclinic.org/diseases-conditions/pneumonia/sym ptoms-causes/syc-20354204

McNabb, M., Chukwu, E., Ojo, O., Shekhar, N., Gill, C. J., Salami, H., & Jega, F. (2015). Assessment of the Quality of Antenatal Care Services Provided by Health Workers Using a Mobile Phone Decision Support Application in Northern Nigeria: A Pre/Post-Intervention Study. *PLoS One*, *10*(5), e0123940. doi:10.1371/journal.pone.0123940 PMID:25942018

Mehta, B., & Rani, S. (2014). Segmentation of broken characters of handwritten Gurmukhi script. *International Journal of Engineering Science*, *3*, 95–105.

Melin, P., Amezcua, J., Valdez, F., & Castillo, O. (2014). A new neural network model based on the LVQ algorithm for multi-class classification of arrhythmias. *Information Sciences*, *279*, 483–497. doi:10.1016/j.ins.2014.04.003

Memari, N., Ramli, A. R., Saripan, M. I. B., Mashohor, S., & Moghbel, M. (2019). Retinal Blood Vessel Segmentation by Using Matched Filtering and Fuzzy C-means Clustering with Integrated Level Set Method for Diabetic Retinopathy Assessment. *Journal of Medical and Biological Engineering*, *39*(5), 713–731. doi:10.100740846-018-0454-2

Mendonca, A. M., & Campilho, A. (2006). Segmentation of retinal blood vessels by combining the detection of centerlines and morphological reconstruction. *IEEE Transactions on Medical Imaging*, *25*(9), 1200–1213. doi:10.1109/TMI.2006.879955 PMID:16967805

Mercan, Ö. B., Kılıç, V., & Şen, M. (2021). Machine learning-based colorimetric determination of glucose in artificial saliva with different reagents using a smartphone coupled μPAD. *Sensors and Actuators. B, Chemical*, *329*, 129037. doi:10.1016/j.snb.2020.129037

Miller, R. A. (1994). Medical Diagnostic Decision Support Systems -Past, Present, and Future. *Journal of the American Medical Informatics Association*, *1*(1), 8–27. https://doi.org/10.1136/jamia.1994.95236141

Mirshahvalad, R., & Zanjani, N. A. (2017). Diabetes prediction using ensemble perceptron algorithm. In *2017 9th International Conference on Computational Intelligence and Communication Networks (CICN),* pp. 190–194. IEEE.

Mirza, S., Mittal, S., & Zaman, M. (2018). Decision Support Predictive model for prognosis of diabetes using SMOTE and Decision tree. *International Journal of Applied Engineering Research: IJAER*, *13*, 9277–9282. http://www.ripublication.com/ijaer18/ijaerv13n11_73.pdf

Misawa, M., Kudo, S., Mori, Y., Hotta, K., Ohtsuka, K., Matsuda, T., Saito, S., Kudo, T., Baba, T., Ishida, F., Itoh, H., Oda, M., & Mori, K. (2020). Development of a computer-aided detection system for colonoscopy and a publicly accessible large colonoscopy video database (with video). *Gastrointestinal Endoscopy*. doi:10.1016/j.gie.2020.07.060 PMID:32745531

Mishra, A. K., & Raghav, S. (2010). Local fractal dimension based ECG arrhythmia classification. *Biomedical Signal Processing and Control*, *5*(2), 114–123. doi:10.1016/j.bspc.2010.01.002

Mittal, P., & Gill, N. (2016, May). A computational hybrid model with two level classification using SVM and neural network for predicting the diabetes disease [Review of A computational hybrid model with two level classification using SVM and neural network for predicting the diabetes disease]. *Journal of Theoretical and Applied Information Technology*.

Miyazaki, A. (2005). An improved correlation-based watermarking method for images using a nonlinear programming algorithm. NSIP 2005. Abstracts. IEEE- Nonlinear Signal and Image Processing. IEEE.

Miyazaki, A. (2005, May). An improved correlation-based watermarking method for images using a nonlinear programming algorithm. In NSIP 2005. Abstracts. IEEE-Eurasip Nonlinear Signal and Image Processing, 2005. (p. 5). IEEE. doi:10.1109/NSIP.2005.1502212

Mj, H., R, O., G, R., Jc, N., & O, J. (1992). Enhancement after feline immunodeficiency virus vaccination. *Veterinary Immunology and Immunopathology*, *35*(1–2), 191–197. doi:10.1016/0165-2427(92)90131-9 PMID:1337397

Moderna. (2020). *Moderna Announces Primary Efficacy Analysis in Phase 3 COVE Study for Its COVID-19 Vaccine Candidate and Filing Today with U.S. FDA for Emergency Use Authorization.* Moderna, Inc. https://investors.modernatx.com/news-releases/news-release-details/moderna-announces-primary-efficacy-analysis-phase-3-cove-study/

Mohammedhasan, M., & Uğuz, H. (2020). A New Early Stage Diabetic Retinopathy Diagnosis Model Using Deep Convolutional Neural Networks and Principal Component Analysis. *Traitement Du Signal, 37*(5), 711–722. doi:10.18280/ts.370503

Mohite, J. (2020). OCR Using Flutter. Optical character recognition is a Flutter World. *The Medium.* https://medium.com/flutterworld/ocr-using-flutter-6f5765af49a6#:~:text=Optical%20character%20recognition%20is%20a%20process%20of%20conversion%20of%20typed,images%20that%20contains%20the%20text

Mokhnache, S., Bekkouche, T., & Chikouche, D. (2018). A Robust Watermarking Scheme Based on DWT and DCT Using Image Gradient. *International Journal of Applied Engineering Research, 13*(4). Research India Publications.

Moor, J. (2019). The Dartmouth College Artificial Intelligence Conference: The Next Fifty Years. *AI Magazine, 27*(4), 87–87. doi:10.1609/aimag.v27i4.1911

Mosavi, A. Faizollahzadeh ardabili, S., & R. Várkonyi-Kóczy, A. (2019). *List of Deep Learning Models.* Preprints. doi:10.20944/preprints201908.0152.v1

Moussa, R., Gerges, F., Salem, C., Akiki, R., Falou, O., & Azar, D. (2016, October). Computer-aided detection of Melanoma using geometric features. In *2016 3rd Middle East Conference on Biomedical Engineering (MECBME)* (pp. 125-128). IEEE. 10.1109/MECBME.2016.7745423

Moyer, C. A., Dako-Gyeke, P., & Adanu, R. A. (2013). Facility-based delivery and maternal and early neonatal mortality in sub-Saharan Africa: A regional review of the literature. *African Journal of Reproductive Health, 17*, 30–43. PMID:24069765

Muhammad, L. J., & Algehyne, E. A. (2021). Fuzzy based expert system for diagnosis of coronary artery disease in nigeria. *Health and Technology, 11*(2), 319–329. https://doi.org/10.1007/s12553-021-00531-z

Mujahid, M., Rustam, F., Álvarez, R., Luis Vidal Mazón, J., Díez, I. D. L. T., & Ashraf, I. (2022). Pneumonia Classification from X-ray images with inception-v3 and convolutional neural network. *Diagnostics (Basel), 12*(5), 1280. doi:10.3390/diagnostics12051280 PMID:35626436

Mupapa, K., Massamba, M., Kibadi, K., Kuvula, K., Bwaka, A., Kipasa, M., Colebunders, R., & Muyembe-Tamfum, J. J. (1999). Treatment of Ebola hemorrhagic fever with blood transfusions from convalescent patient. *The Journal of Infectious Diseases, 179*(s1), S18–S23. doi:10.1086/514298 PMID:9988160

Murat Kirisci, M. Ubeydullah, S., & Yilmaz, H. (2019). An ANFIS perspective for the diagnosis of type II diabetes. *ANNALS of FUZZY MATHEMATICS and INFORMATICS, 17*(2), 101–113. doi:10.30948/afmi.2019.17.2.101

Murugeswari, S., & Sukanesh, R. (2017). Investigations of severity level measurements for diabetic macular oedema using machine learning algorithms. *Irish Journal of Medical Science (1971 -), 186*(4), 929–938. doi:10.1007/s11845-017-1598-8

Musabyimana, A., Ruton, H., Gaju, E., Berhe, A., Grépin, K. A., Ngenzi, J., Nzabonimana, E., Hategeka, C., & Law, M. R. (2018). Assessing the perspectives of users and beneficiaries of a community health worker mHealth tracking system for mothers and children in Rwanda. *PLoS One*, *13*(6), e0198725. doi:10.1371/journal.pone.0198725 PMID:29879186

Musale, S., & Ghiye, V. (2018, January). Smart reader for visually impaired. In *2018 2nd International Conference on Inventive Systems and Control (ICISC)* (pp. 339-342). IEEE. doi:10.1109/ICISC.2018.8399091

N., R. (2020). Arrhythmia Detection Based on Hybrid Features of T-Wave in Electrocardiogram. In J. Thomas, P. Karagoz, B. Ahamed, & P. Vasant (Eds.), *Deep Learning Techniques and Optimization Strategies in Big Data Analytics* (pp. 1-20). IGI Global. . doi:10.4018/978-1-7998-1192-3.ch001

Nachega, J. B., Skinner, D., Jennings, L., Magidson, J. F., Altice, F. L., Burke, J. G., Lester, R. T., Uthman, O. A., Knowlton, A. R., Cotton, M. F., Anderson, J. R., & Theron, G. B. (2016). Acceptability and feasibility of mHealth and community-based directly observed antiretroviral therapy to prevent mother-to-child HIV transmission in South African pregnant women under Option B+: An exploratory study. *Patient Preference and Adherence*, *10*, 683–690. doi:10.2147/PPA.S100002 PMID:27175068

Nakhleh, M. K., Baram, S., Jeries, R., Salim, R., Haick, H., & Hakim, M. (2016). Artificially intelligent nanoarray for the detection of preeclampsia under real-world clinical conditions. *Advanced Materials Technologies*, *1*(9), 1600132. doi:10.1002/admt.201600132

Nanjundegowda, R., & Meshram, V. (2018). Arrhythmia recognition and classification using kernel ICA and higher order spectra. *Int J Eng Technol*, *7*(2), 256–262. doi:10.14419/ijet.v7i2.9535

Nanonets: Intelligent document processing with. (2022). Nanonets. https://nanonets.com/

National Institute of Diabetes and Digestive and Kidney Diseases. (2016, December). *What is Diabetes?* National Institute of Diabetes and Digestive and Kidney Diseases. https://www.niddk.nih.gov/health-information/diabetes/overview/what-is-diabetes

Navarro, F., Escudero-Vinolo, M., & Bescós, J. (2018). Accurate segmentation and registration of skin lesion images to evaluate lesion change. *IEEE Journal of Biomedical and Health Informatics*, *23*(2), 501–508. doi:10.1109/JBHI.2018.2825251 PMID:29993849

Naveen, P., & Diwan, B. (2021, March). Pre-trained VGG-16 with CNN Architecture to classify X-Rays images into Normal or Pneumonia. In *2021 International Conference on Emerging Smart Computing and Informatics (ESCI)* (pp. 102-105). IEEE 10.1109/ESCI50559.2021.9396997

Negi, A., & Jaiswal, V. (2016, December 1). A first attempt to develop a diabetes prediction method based on different global datasets. *IEEE Xplore*. doi:10.1109/PDGC.2016.7913152

Neumann-Böhme, S., Varghese, N. E., Sabat, I., Barros, P. P., Brouwer, W., van Exel, J., Schreyögg, J., & Stargardt, T. (2020a). Once we have it, will we use it? A European survey on willingness to be vaccinated against COVID-19. *The European Journal of Health Economics*, *21*(7), 977–982. doi:10.100710198-020-01208-6 PMID:32591957

Nganga, K. (2022). *Building A Multiclass Image Classifier Using MobilenetV2 and TensorFlow*. Engineering Education (EngEd) Program. https://www.section.io/engineering-education/building-a-multiclass-image-classifier-using-mobilenet-v2-and-tensorflow/

Nie, D. (2011, March). Classification of melanoma and clark nevus skin lesions based on Medical Image Processing Techniques. In *2011 3rd International Conference on Computer Research and Development* (*Vol. 3,* pp. 31-34). IEEE.

Nilashi, M., Bin Ibrahim, O., Mardani, A., Ahani, A., & Jusoh, A. (2016). A soft computing approach for diabetes disease classification. *Health Informatics Journal*, *24*(4), 379–393. https://doi.org/10.1177/1460458216675500

Nirmaladevi, M., Appavu, S., & Swathi, U. V. (2013). An amalgam KNN to predict diabetes mellitus. *2013 IEEE International Conference ON Emerging Trends in Computing, Communication and Nanotechnology (ICECCN),* (pp. 691-695). IEEE.

Niswati, Z., Mustika, F. A., & Paramita, A. (2018). Fuzzy logic implementation for diagnosis ofDiabetes Mellitusdisease at Puskesmas in East Jakarta. *Journal of Physics: Conference Series*, *1114*, 012107. https://doi.org/10.1088/1742-6596/1114/1/012107

Nkuma-Udah, K. I., Chukwudebe, G. A., & Ekwonwune, E. N. (2018). Medical Diagnosis Expert System for Malaria and Related Diseases for Developing Countries. *Scientific Research.* https://doi.org/10.4236/etsn.2018.72002

Nnam, N. M. (2015). Improving maternal nutrition for better pregnancy outcomes. *The Proceedings of the Nutrition Society*, *74*(4), 454–459. doi:10.1017/S0029665115002396 PMID:26264457

Nogueira-Rodríguez, A., Domínguez-Carbajales, R., López-Fernández, H., Iglesias, Á., Cubiella, J., Fdez-Riverola, F., Reboiro-Jato, M., & Glez-Peña, D. (2021). Deep Neural Networks approaches for detecting and classifying colorectal polyps. *Neurocomputing*, *423*, 721–734. doi:10.1016/j.neucom.2020.02.123

Nogueira-Rodríguez, A., Reboiro-Jato, M., Glez-Peña, D., & López-Fernández, H. (2022). Performance of Convolutional Neural Networks for Polyp Localization on Public Colonoscopy Image Datasets. *Diagnostics (Basel)*, *12*(4), 898. doi:10.3390/diagnostics12040898 PMID:35453946

Okokpujie, K., Orimogunje, A., Noma-Osaghae, E., Olaitan, A. (2017). An Intelligent Online Diagnostic System with Epidemic Alert. *2*(9).

Omoregbe, N. A. I., Ndaman, I. O., Misra, S., Abayomi-alli, O. O., & Damasevitius, R. (2020), Text Messaging-Based Medical Diagnosis Using Natural Language Processing and Fuzzy Logic. *Hindawi.* https://doi.org/10.1155/2020/8839524

Osareh, A., & Shadgar, B. (2008) Retinal Vessel Extraction Using Gabor Filters and Support Vector Machines. in Communications in Computer and Information Science, (pp. 356–363). Springer. doi:10.1007/978-3-540-89985-3_44

Osowski, S., Markiewicz, T., & Hoai, L. T. (2008). Recognition and classification system of arrhythmia using ensemble of neural networks. *Measurement*, *41*(6), 610–617. doi:10.1016/j.measurement.2007.07.006

Ouyang, F. S., Guo, B., Ouyang, L., Liu, Z., Lin, S., Meng, W., Huang, X., Chen, H., Qiu-gen, H., & Yang, S. (2019). Comparison between linear and nonlinear machine-learning algorithms for the classification of thyroid nodules. *European Journal of Radiology*, *113*, 251–25. doi:10.1016/j.ejrad.2019.02.029 PMID:30927956

Özbay, Y., & Tezel, G. (2010). A new method for classification of ECG arrhythmias using neural network with adaptive activation function. *Digital Signal Processing*, *20*(4), 1040–1049. doi:10.1016/j.dsp.2009.10.016

Pandey, D., & Pandey, K. (2021, September). An Assistive Technology-based Approach towards Helping Visually Impaired People. In *2021 9th International Conference on Reliability, Infocom Technologies and Optimization (Trends and Future Directions)(ICRITO)* (pp. 1-5). IEEE.

Pandey, K., Yadav, V., Pandey, D., & Vikhram, S. (2021). MAGIC-I as an Assistance for the Visually Impaired People. *Recent Advances in Computer Science and Communications (Formerly: Recent Patents on Computer Science), 14*(9), 3012-3024.

Pandiaraj, M., Benjamin, A. R., Madasamy, T., Vairamani, K., Arya, A., Sethy, N. K., Bhargava, K., & Karunakaran, C. (2014). A cost-effective volume miniaturized and microcontroller based cytochrome c assay. *Sensors and Actuators. A, Physical*, *220*, 290–297. doi:10.1016/j.sna.2014.10.018

Pandya, J. B., & Gupta, R. V. (2018). A Study of ROI based Image Watermarking Techniques. *International Journal of Scientific Research in Computer Science. Engineering and Information Technology*, *3*(1), 1213–1217.

Pant, B., Bordoloi, D., & Gangodkar, D. (2021). A neural network classifier for payload-based online worms detection. *Webology*, *18*(5), 3235–3240.

Pan, W. W., Gardner, T. W., & Harder, J. L. (2021). Integrative Biology of Diabetic Retinal Disease: Lessons from Diabetic Kidney Disease. *Journal of Clinical Medicine*, *10*(6), 1254. https://doi.org/10.3390/jcm10061254

Parida, P., Dash, J., & Bhoi, N. (2020). Retinal Blood Vessel Extraction from Fundus Images Using Enhancement Filtering and Clustering. *ELCVIA. Electronic Letters on Computer Vision and Image Analysis*, *19*(1), 38. doi:10.5565/rev/elcvia.1239

Park, S., & Han, K. (2018). Methodologic Guide for Evaluating Clinical Performance and Effect of Artificial Intelligence Technology for Medical Diagnosis and Prediction, 286(3).

Park, J., Lee, W., & Huh, K. Y. (2022). Model order reduction by radial basis function network for sparse reconstruction of an industrial natural gas boiler. *Case Studies in Thermal Engineering*, *37*, 102288. doi:10.1016/j.csite.2022.102288

Parmar, A. K. (2018). A review on random forest: An ensemble classifier. *In International Conference on Intelligent Data Communication Technologies and Internet of Things* (pp. 758-763). Springer.

Parry, J., & Stevens, A. (2001). Prospective health impact assessment: Pitfalls, problems, and possible ways forward. *BMJ (Clinical Research Ed.)*, *323*(7322), 1177–1182. doi:10.1136/bmj.323.7322.1177 PMID:11711414

Patel, A. B., Kuhite, P. N., Alam, A., Pusdekar, Y., Puranik, A., Khan, S. S., Kelly, P., Muthayya, S., Laba, T.-L., Almeida, M. D., & Dibley, M. J. (2019). M-SAKHI-Mobile health solutions to help community providers promote maternal and infant nutrition and health using a community-based cluster randomized controlled trial in rural India: A study protocol. *Maternal and Child Nutrition*, *15*(4), e12850. doi:10.1111/mcn.12850 PMID:31177631

Paul, E., Steptoe, A., & Fancourt, D. (2021). Attitudes towards vaccines and intention to vaccinate against COVID-19: Implications for public health communications. *The Lancet Regional Health - Europe*, *1*, 100012. doi:10.1016/j.lanepe.2020.100012

Pei, D., Yang, T., & Zhang, C. (2020). Estimation of Diabetes in a High-Risk Adult Chinese Population Using J48 Decision Tree Model. *Diabetes, Metabolic Syndrome and Obesity*, *13*, 4621–4630. https://doi.org/10.2147/dmso.s279329

Peng, E., Peursum, P., & Li, L. (2012, December). Product barcode and expiry date detection for the visually impaired using a smartphone. In *2012 International Conference on Digital Image Computing Techniques and Applications (DICTA)* (pp. 1-7). IEEE. doi:10.1109/DICTA.2012.6411673

Perez, L., & Wang, J. (2017). The Effectiveness of Data Augmentation in Image Classification using Deep Learning. *ArXiv:1712.04621*. https://arxiv.org/abs/1712.04621

Permana, B. A. C., Ahmad, R., Bahtiar, H., Sudianto, A., & Gunawan, I. (2021). Classification of diabetes disease using decision tree algorithm (C4.5). *Journal of Physics: Conference Series*, *1869*(1), 012082. doi:10.1088/1742-6596/1869/1/012082

Perona, P., & Malik, J. (1990). Scale-space and edge detection using anisotropic diffusion. *IEEE Transactions on Pattern Analysis and Machine Intelligence*, *12*(7), 629–639. doi:10.1109/34.56205

Petrellis, N. (2018, July). The Effect of the Training Set Size in a Skin Disorder Classification Application. In *2018 41st International Conference on Telecommunications and Signal Processing (TSP)* (pp. 1-5). IEEE. 10.1109/TSP.2018.8441474

Petticrew, M., Whitehead, M., Macintyre, S. J., Graham, H., & Egan, M. (2004). Evidence for public health policy on inequalities: 1: the reality according to policymakers. *Journal of Epidemiology and Community Health*, *58*(10), 811–816. doi:10.1136/jech.2003.015289 PMID:15365104

Pfizer Inc. (n.d.). *Pfizer and BioNTech Conclude Phase 3 Study of COVID-19 Vaccine Candidate, Meeting All Primary Efficacy Endpoints.* Pfizer. https://www.pfizer.com/news/press-release/press-release-deta il/pfizer-and-biontech-conclude-phase-3-study-covid-19-vacci ne

Pham, T. T., Talukder, A. M., Walsh, N. J., Lawson, A. G., Jones, A. J., Bishop, J. L., & Kruse, E. J. (2018). Clinical and epidemiological factors associated with suicide in colorectal cancer. *Supportive Care in Cancer*, *27*(2), 617–621. doi:10.100700520-018-4354-3 PMID:30027329

Phasinam, K. M., Mondal, T., Novaliendry, D., Yang, C.-H., Dutta, C., & Shabaz, M. (2022). Analyzing the Performance of Machine Learning Techniques in Disease Prediction. *Journal of Food Quality*, *2022*, 1–9. doi:10.1155/2022/7529472

Pickholtz, R., Schilling, D., & Milstein, L. (1982). Theory of spread-spectrum communications-a tutorial. *IEEE Transactions on Communications*, *30*(5), 855–884. doi:10.1109/TCOM.1982.1095533

Pohjois-Suomen sosiaalialan osaamiskeskus [Northern Finland's Center of Expertise in the Social Sector]. (2018). *Monipuoliset tuen muodot kotona asumiseen Lapissa – Toimivan kotihoidon käsikirja. Toimiva kotihoito Lappiin – Monipuoliset tuen muodot kotona asumiseen -hanke [Versatile forms of support for living at home in Lapland- Manual for functional home care. Functional home care in Lapland- Multifaceted forms of support for living at home project].* Grano Oy, Helsinki.

Popayorm, S., Titijaroonroj, T., Phoka, T., & Massagram, W. (2019, July). Seven segment display detection and recognition using predefined HSV color slicing technique. In *2019 16th International Joint Conference on Computer Science and Software Engineering (JCSSE)* (pp. 224-229). IEEE. doi:10.1109/JCSSE.2019.8864189

Posonia, A. M., Vigneshwari, S., & Rani, D. J. (2020, December 1). Machine Learning based Diabetes Prediction using Decision Tree J48. *IEEE Xplore*. doi:10.1109/ICISS49785.2020.9316001

Prajapati H, Jain A, Pal SK (2017). An enhance expert system for diagnosis of diabetes using fuzzy rules over PIMA dataset. *4*(9), 225-230.

Prasad, V. R., Rao, T. S., & Babu, M. S. P. (2016). Thyroid disease diagnosis via hybrid architecture composing rough data sets theory and machine learning algorithms. *Soft Computing*, *20*(3), 1179–1189. doi:10.100700500-014-1581-5

Prerana, P. S. (2015). Predictive data mining for diagnosis of thyroid disease using neural network. *International Journal of Research in Management, Science & Technology*, 75-80.

Priyanka, B., Krishna, D. P., & Purushottam, E. (2014). Attestation Performance on Digital Watermarking. [IJCSNS]. *International Journal of Computer Science and Network Security*, *14*(1), 94.

Pustokhina, I. V., Pustokhin, D. A., Lydia, E. L., Garg, P., Kadian, A., & Shankar, K. (2021). Hyperparameter search based Convolutionneural network with Bi-LSTM model for intrusion detection system in multimedia big data environment. *Multimedia Tools and Applications*, 1–18.

Qiu X, Wong G, Audet J, Bello A, Fernando L, et al. (2014). Reversion of advanced Ebola virus disease in nonhuman primates with ZMapp. *Nature 514*(7520):47–53.

Quinlan, J. R. (1986). Induction of decision trees. *Machine Learning*, *1*(1), 81–106. https://doi.org/10.1007/bf00116251

R., P., & P., A. (2013). Diagnosis of diabetic retinopathy using machine learning techniques. Ictact *Journal on Soft Computing, 03*(04), 563–575. doi:10.21917/ijsc.2013.0083

Raabe, M. L., Issel, C. J., & Montelaro, R. C. (1999). In vitro antibody-dependent enhancement assays are insensitive indicators of in vivo vaccine enhancement of equine infectious anemia virus. *Virology*, *259*(2), 416–427. doi:10.1006/viro.1999.9772 PMID:10388665

Rader, C., & Brenner, N. (1976). A new principle for fast Fourier transformation. *IEEE Transactions on Acoustics, Speech, and Signal Processing*, *24*(3), 264–266. doi:10.1109/TASSP.1976.1162805

Raghu, N. (2020). Arrhythmia detection based on hybrid features of T-wave in electrocardiogram. In *Deep Learning Techniques and Optimization Strategies in Big Data Analytics* (pp. 1–20). IGI Global.

Rahman, F., & Mandaogade, N. N. (2014). Digital audio watermarking techniques with musical audio feature classification. *Int. J. Curr. Eng. Technol*, *4*(5).

Rahman, R. M., & Afroz, F. (2013). Comparison of Various Classification Techniques Using Different Data Mining Tools for Diabetes Diagnosis. *Journal of Software Engineering and Applications*, *06*(03), 85–97. https://doi.org/10.4236/jsea.2013.63013

Rahman, T., Chowdhury, M. E., Khandakar, A., Islam, K. R., Islam, K. F., Mahbub, Z. B., Kadir, M. A., & Kashem, S. (2020). Transfer learning with deep convolutional neural network (CNN) for pneumonia detection using chest X-ray. *Applied Sciences (Basel, Switzerland)*, *10*(9), 3233. doi:10.3390/app10093233

Raisinghani, S. S. (2019). In International Conference on Advances in Computing and Data Sciences. *Thyroid prediction using machine learning techniques*, 140-150.

Rajaraman, S., Candemir, S., Kim, I., Thoma, G., & Antani, S. (2018). Visualization and interpretation of convolutional neural network predictions in detecting pneumonia in pediatric chest radiographs. *Applied Sciences (Basel, Switzerland)*, *8*(10), 1715. doi:10.3390/app8101715 PMID:32457819

Rajasenbagam, T., Jeyanthi, S., & Pandian, J. A. (2021). Detection of pneumonia infection in lungs from chest X-ray images using deep Convolutionalal neural network and content-based image retrieval techniques. *Journal of Ambient Intelligence and Humanized Computing*, 1–8.

Rajendra, P., & Latifi, S. (2021). Prediction of diabetes using logistic regression and ensemble techniques. *Computer Methods and Programs in Biomedicine Update, 1,* 100032. doi:10.1016/j.cmpbup.2021.100032

Rajesh, K. (2012, September). Application of Data Mining Methods and Techniques for Diabetes Diagnosis (V. Sangeetha, Ed.) [Review of Application of Data Mining Methods and Techniques for Diabetes Diagnosis]. International Journal of Engineering and Innovative Technology (IJEIT), 2,(3).

Rajeswari, K., & Vaithiyanathan, V. (2011). Fuzzy based modeling for diabetic diagnostic decision support using Artificial Neural Network. *IJCSNS International Journal of Computer Science and Network Security, 11*(4), 126. http://paper.ijcsns.org/07_book/201104/20110419.pdf

Rajpurkar, P., Irvin, J., Zhu, K., Yang, B., Mehta, H., Duan, T., & Ng, A. Y. (2017). *Chexnet: Radiologist-level pneumonia detection on chest x-rays with deep learning.* arXiv:1711.05225.

Rajput, R., & Borse, R. (2017, August). Alternative product label reading and speech conversion: an aid for blind person. In *2017 International Conference on Computing, Communication, Control and Automation (ICCUBEA)* (pp. 1-6). IEEE. doi:10.1109/ICCUBEA.2017.8463923

Rakshit, S., Manna, S., & Biswas, S. (2017). *Prediction of Diabetes Type-II Using a Two-Class Neural Network* [Review of Prediction of Diabetes Type-II Using a Two-Class Neural Network]. Computational Intelligence, Communications, and Business Analytics, Springer Singapore.

Ramya, M. (2020). Prediction And Providing Medication For Thyroid Disease Using Machine Learning Technique (SVM). *Turkish Journal of Computer and Mathematics Education (TURCOMAT)*, 1099-1107.

Rangayyan, R. M. (2008). Detection of blood vessels in the retina with multiscale Gabor filters. *Journal of Electronic Imaging, 17*(2), 023018. doi:10.1117/1.2907209

Rangayyan, R. M.. (2007) Detection of Blood Vessels in the Retina Using Gabor Filters. in *2007 Canadian Conference on Electrical and Computer Engineering*, (pp. 717–720). IEEE. 10.1109/CCECE.2007.184

Rao, A. R. (2020). A machine learning approach to predict thyroid disease at early stages of diagnosis. *In 2020 IEEE International Conference for Innovation in Technology (INOCON)* (pp. 1-4). IEEE. 10.1109/INOCON50539.2020.9298252

Rashid, A. (2016). Digital watermarking applications and techniques: A brief review. *International Journal of Computer Applications Technology and Research, 5*(3), 147–150. doi:10.7753/IJCATR0503.1006

Ratawal, K. & Zade, A. (2021). Medical Diagnostic Systems Using Artificial Intelligence (AI) Algorithms. *08*(8).

Raval, D., & Bhatt, D. (2016). *Malaram K Kumhar, Vishal Parikh, Daiwat Vyas*. Medical Diagnosis System Using Machine Learning. doi:10.090592/IICSC.2016.026

Rawat, J., Singh, A., Bhadauria, H. S., Virmani, J., & Devgun, J. S. (2017). Classification of acute lymphoblastic leukaemia using hybrid hierarchical classifiers. *Multimedia Tools and Applications*, *76*(18), 19057–19085. doi:10.100711042-017-4478-3

Rawat, J., Singh, A., Bhadauria, H. S., Virmani, J., & Devgun, J. S. (2018). Leukocyte classification using adaptive neuro-fuzzy inference system in microscopic blood images. *Arabian Journal for Science and Engineering*, *43*(12), 7041–7058. doi:10.100713369-017-2959-3

Rawat, J., Virmani, J., Singh, A., Bhadauria, H. S., Kumar, I., & Devgan, J. S. (2022). FAB classification of acute leukemia using an ensemble of neural networks. *Evolutionary Intelligence*, *15*(1), 99–117. doi:10.100712065-020-00491-9

Ray, A., & Chaudhuri, A. K. (2020). Smart healthcare disease diagnosis and patient management: Innovation, improvement and skill development. *Machine Learning with Applications.* https://doi.org/10.1016/j.mlwa.2020.100011

Razak, N. A. (2018). Digital Image watermarking base on DWT and SVD techniques. [JNCET]. *J Netw Commun Emerging Technol*, *8*(02).

Razazzadeh, N., & Khalili, M. (2015, May). A high performance algorithm to diagnosis of skin lesions deterioration in dermatoscopic images using new feature extraction. In *2015 IEEE 28th Canadian Conference on Electrical and Computer Engineering (CCECE)* (pp. 1207-1212). IEEE. 10.1109/CCECE.2015.7129449

Razia, S. S. (2020). Machine learning techniques for thyroid disease diagnosis: a systematic review. *Modern Approaches in Machine Learning and Cognitive Science: A Walkthrough*, 203-212.

Razia, S., & Narasinga Rao, M. R. (2016). Machine learning techniques for thyroid disease diagnosis-a review. *Indian Journal of Science and Technology*, *9*(28), 1–9. doi:10.17485/ijst/2016/v9i28/93705

Ren, S., He, K., Girshick, R., & Sun, J. (2017). Faster R-CNN: Towards Real-Time Object Detection with Region Proposal Networks. *IEEE Transactions on Pattern Analysis and Machine Intelligence*, *39*(6), 1137–1149. doi:10.1109/TPAMI.2016.2577031 PMID:27295650

Riahi-Madvar, H., Dehghani, M., Seifi, A., Salwana, E., Shamshirband, S., Mosavi, A., & Chau, K. (2019). Comparative analysis of soft computing techniques RBF, MLP, and ANFIS with MLR and MNLR for predicting grade-control scour hole geometry. *Engineering Applications of Computational Fluid Mechanics*, *13*(1), 529–550. doi:10.1080/19942060.2019.1618396

Riahi-Madvar, H., & Seifi, A. (2018). Uncertainty analysis in bed load transport prediction of gravel bed rivers by ANN and ANFIS. *Arabian Journal of Geosciences*, *11*(21), 688. doi:10.100712517-018-3968-6

Riaz, S., & Lee, S. W. (2013, January). Image authentication and restoration by multiple watermarking techniques with advance encryption standard in digital photography. In *2013 15th International Conference on Advanced Communications Technology (ICACT)* (pp. 24-28). IEEE.

Rigla, M., Martínez-Sarriegui, I., García-Sáez, G., Pons, B., & Hernando, M. E. (2018). Gestational diabetes management using smart mobile telemedicine. *Journal of Diabetes Science and Technology*, *12*(2), 260–264. doi:10.1177/1932296817704442 PMID:28420257

Robert, L., & Shanmugapriya, T. (2009). A study on digital watermarking techniques. *International journal of Recent trends in Engineering*, *1*(2), 223.

Robertson, G., Lehmann, E. D., Sandham, W., & Hamilton, D. (2011). Blood Glucose Prediction Using Artificial Neural Networks Trained with the AIDA Diabetes Simulator: A Proof-of-Concept Pilot Study. *Journal of Electrical and Computer Engineering*, *2011*, 1–11. doi:10.1155/2011/681786

Roček, A., Slavíček, K., Dostál, O., & Javorník, M. (2016). A new approach to fully-reversible watermarking in medical imaging with breakthrough visibility parameters. *Biomedical Signal Processing and Control*, *29*, 44–52. doi:10.1016/j.bspc.2016.05.005

Rogerson, B., Lindberg, R., Baum, F., Dora, C., Haigh, F., Simoncelli, A. M., Parry Williams, L., Peralta, G., Pollack Porter, K. M., & Solar, O. (2020). Recent Advances in Health Impact Assessment and Health in All Policies Implementation: Lessons from an International Convening in Barcelona. *International Journal of Environmental Research and Public Health*, *17*(21), 7714. doi:10.3390/ijerph17217714 PMID:33105669

Roman, I., Santana, R., Mendiburu, A., & Lozano, J. A. (2020). In-depth analysis of SVM kernel learning and its components. *Neural Computing & Applications*, *33*(12), 6575–6594. doi:10.100700521-020-05419-z

Ronneberger, O., Fischer, P., & Brox, T. (2015). U-Net: Convolutional Networks for Biomedical Image Segmentation. *Lecture Notes in Computer Science*, *9351*, 234–241. doi:10.1007/978-3-319-24574-4_28

Ruela, M., Barata, C., & Marques, J. S. (2013). What is the role of color symmetry in the detection of melanomas? In Advances in Visual Computing: 9th International Symposium, ISVC 2013, Proceedings, *9*(Part I), 1–10. IEEE.

Ryu, S. (2012). Book Review: MHealth: New Horizons for Health through Mobile Technologies: Based on the Findings of the Second Global Survey on eHealth (Global Observatory for eHealth Series, Volume 3). *Healthcare Informatics Research*, *18*(3), 231–233. doi:10.4258/hir.2012.18.3.231

Sabri, M. A., Filali, Y., El Khoukhi, H., & Aarab, A. (2020, June). Skin cancer diagnosis using an improved ensemble machine learning model. In *2020 International Conference on Intelligent Systems and Computer Vision (ISCV)* (pp. 1-5). IEEE. 10.1109/ISCV49265.2020.9204324

Sadasivam, M., Sakthivel, A., Nagesh, N., Hansda, S., Veerapandian, M., Alwarappan, S., & Manickam, P. (2020). Magnetic bead-amplified voltammetric detection for carbohydrate antigen 125 with enzyme labels using aptamer-antigen-antibody sandwiched assay. *Sensors and Actuators. B, Chemical*, *312*, 127985. doi:10.1016/j.snb.2020.127985

Sahebi, H. R., & Ebrahimi, S. (2015). A Fuzzy Classifier Based on Modified Particle Swarm Optimization for Diabetes Disease Diagnosis. *Advances in Computer Science: An International Journal, 4*(3), 11–17. http://www.acsij.org/acsij/article/view/90/86

Sakthivel, A., Chandrasekaran, A., Sadasivam, M., Manickam, P., & Alwarappan, S. (2021). Sulphur doped graphitic carbon nitride as a dual biosensing platform for the detection of cancer biomarker CA15–3. *Journal of the Electrochemical Society, 168*(1), 017507. doi:10.1149/1945-7111/abd927

Sanakal, R., & Jayakumari, Smt. T. (2014). Prognosis of Diabetes Using Data mining Approach-Fuzzy C Means Clustering and Support Vector Machine. *International Journal of Computer Trends and Technology, 11*(2), 94–98. doi:10.14445/22312803/ijctt-v11p120

Sánchez-Peralta, L. F., Pagador, J. B., Picón, A., Calderón, Á. J., Polo, F., Andraka, N., Bilbao, R., Glover, B., Saratxaga, C. L., & Sánchez-Margallo, F. M. (2020). PICCOLO White-Light and Narrow-Band Imaging Colonoscopic Dataset: A Performance Comparative of Models and Datasets. *Applied Sciences (Basel, Switzerland), 10*(23), 8501. doi:10.3390/app10238501

Sandler, M., Howard, A., Zhu, M., Zhmoginov, A., & Chen, L. C. (2018). Mobilenetv2: Inverted residuals and linear bottlenecks. In *Proceedings of the IEEE Conference on Computer Vision and Pattern Recognition* (pp. 4510-4520).

Saraswat, L., Mohanty, L., Garg, P., & Lamba, S. (2022). Plant Disease Identification Using Plant Images. *2022 Fifth International Conference on Computational Intelligence and Communication Technologies (CCICT)*, (pp. 79-82). Research Gate. doi:10.1109/CCiCT56684.2022.00026

Sarker, I. H. (2021). Machine learning: Algorithms, real-world applications, and research directions. *SN Computer Science*, 1-21.

Satpathy, S., Mohan, P., Das, S., & Debbarma, S. (2019). *A new healthcare diagnosis system using an loT-based fuzzy classifier with FPGA*. Springerhttps://doi.org/10.1007/s11227-019-03013-2 doi:.

Sauramäki, J. M., Adusei-Mensah, F., Hakalehto, J., Armon, R., & Hakalehto, E. (2022). 7 Pandemic situation and safe transportation, storage, and distribution for food catering and deliveries. In E. Hakalehto (Ed.), Microbiology of Food Quality: Challenges in Food Production and Distribution During and After the Pandemics (pp. 149–172). De Gruyter. .

Saxena, A., Singh Tomar, S., Jain, G., & Gupta, R. (2021). Deep learning based Diagnosis of diseases using Image Classification. *2021 11th International Conference on Cloud Computing, Data Science & Engineering (Confluence)*. IEEE. 10.1109/Confluence51648.2021.9377154

Saxena, R., Sharma, S. K., & Gupta, M. (2021, April). Role of K-nearest neighbour in detection of Diabetes Mellitus [Review of Role of K-nearest neighbour in detection of Diabetes Mellitus]. *Turkish Journal of Computer and Mathematics Education, 12*(10).

Saxena, R. (2021). Role of K-nearest neighbour in detection of Diabetes Mellitus. [TURCOMAT]. *Turkish Journal of Computer and Mathematics Education, 12*(10), 373–376. https://doi.org/10.17762/turcomat.v12i10.4182

Seetha, C., Goollawattanaporn, S., & Tanprasert, C. (2013). Transparent digital watermark on Drug's images. *Procedia Computer Science*, *21*, 302–309. doi:10.1016/j.procs.2013.09.040

Sempionatto, J. R., Montiel, V. R. V., Vargas, E., Teymourian, H., & Wang, J. (2021). Wearable and mobile sensors for personalized nutrition. *ACS Sensors*, *6*(5), 1745–1760. doi:10.1021/acssensors.1c00553 PMID:34008960

Sethi, P., Garg, P., Dixit, A., & Singh, Y. (2020, April). Smart number cruncher–a voice based calculator. *IOP Conference Series. Materials Science and Engineering*, *804*(1), 012041.

Sey, A. (2011). 'We use it different, different': Making sense of trends in mobile phone use in Ghana. *New Media & Society*, *13*(3), 375–390. doi:10.1177/1461444810393907

Shalu, K., A. (2018, December). A color-based approach for melanoma skin cancer detection. In *2018 First International Conference on Secure Cyber Computing and Communication (ICSCCC)* (pp. 508-513). IEEE. 10.1109/ICSCCC.2018.8703309

Shankar, K. L., Lakshmanaprabu, S. K., Gupta, D., Maseleno, A., & de Albuquerque, V. H. C. (2020). Optimal feature-based multi-kernel SVM approach for thyroid disease classification. *The Journal of Supercomputing*, *76*(2), 1128–1143. doi:10.100711227-018-2469-4

Shapcott, M., Hewitt, K. J., & Rajpoot, N. (2019). Deep Learning With Sampling in Colon Cancer Histology. *Frontiers in Bioengineering and Biotechnology*, *7*, 52. doi:10.3389/fbioe.2019.00052 PMID:30972333

Sharma, H., Jain, J. S., Bansal, P., & Gupta, S. (2020, January). Feature extraction and classification of chest x-ray images using CNN to detect pneumonia. In *2020 10th International Conference on Cloud Computing, Data Science & Engineering (Confluence)* (pp. 227-231). IEEE. 10.1109/Confluence47617.2020.9057809

Sharma, R., Gupta, S., & Garg, P. (2022). Model for Predicting Cardiac Health using Deep Learning Classifier. *2022 Fifth International Conference on Computational Intelligence and Communication Technologies (CCICT)*, (pp. 25-30). Research Gate. doi:10.1109/CCiCT56684.2022.00017

Sharma, T., & Shah, M. (2021). A comprehensive review of machine learning techniques on diabetes detection. *Visual Computing for Industry, Biomedicine, and Art, 4*(1). doi:10.1186/s42492-021-00097-7

Sharma, A., Singh, A. K., & Ghrera, S. P. (2015). Secure hybrid robust watermarking technique for medical images. *Procedia Computer Science*, *70*, 778–784. doi:10.1016/j.procs.2015.10.117

Sharma, N., & Garg, P. (2022). Ant colony based optimization model for QoS-Based task scheduling in cloud computing environment. Measurement. *Sensors (Basel)*, 100531.

Sheik Abdullah, A., & Selvakumar, S. (2018). Assessment of the risk factors for type II diabetes using an improved combination of particle swarm optimization and decision trees by evaluation with Fisher's linear discriminant analysis. *Soft Computing*, *23*(20), 9995–10017. https://doi.org/10.1007/s00500-018-3555-5

Shelhamer, E., Long, J., & Darrell, T. (2017). Fully Convolutional Networks for Semantic Segmentation. *IEEE Transactions on Pattern Analysis and Machine Intelligence*, *39*(4), 640–651. doi:10.1109/TPAMI.2016.2572683 PMID:27244717

Shenoy, V. N., & Aalami, O. O. (2017). Utilizing smartphone-based machine learning in medical monitor data collection: Seven segment digit recognition. *AMIA ... Annual Symposium Proceedings - AMIA Symposium. AMIA Symposium*, *2017*, 1564.

Siegel, R. L., Miller, K. D., Wagle, N. S., & Jemal, A. (2023). Cancer statistics, 2023. *CA: a Cancer Journal for Clinicians*, *73*(1), 17–48. doi:10.3322/caac.21763 PMID:36633525

Siettos, C., Anastassopoulou, C., Russo, L., Grigoras, C., & Mylonakis, E. (2015). Modeling the 2014 Ebola Virus Epidemic – Agent-Based Simulations, Temporal Analysis and Future Predictions for Liberia and Sierra Leone. *PLoS Currents*, *7*. doi:10.1371/currents.outbreaks.8d5984114855fc425e699e1a18cdc6c9 PMID:26064785

Silva, J., Histace, A., Romain, O., Dray, X., & Granado, B. (2013). Toward embedded detection of polyps in WCE images for early diagnosis of colorectal cancer. *International Journal of Computer Assisted Radiology and Surgery*, *9*(2), 283–293. doi:10.100711548-013-0926-3 PMID:24037504

Simarjeet, K., Singla, J., Nkenyereye, L., Jha, S., Parashar, D., El-Sappagh, G. P., Islam, S., & Islam, S. M. (2020). *Medical Diagnostic Systems Using Artificial Intelligence (AI) Algorithms: Principles and Perspectives.* IEEE. doi:10.1109/ACCESS.2020.3042273

Simon, A. E., Wu, A. W., Lavori, P. W., & Sugarman, J. (2007). Preventive misconception: Its nature, presence, and ethical implications of research. *American Journal of Preventive Medicine*, *32*(5), 370–374. doi:10.1016/j.amepre.2007.01.007 PMID:17478261

Simonyan, K., & Zisserman, A. (2014). Very deep convolutional networks for large-scale image recognition. *arXiv preprint arXiv:1409.1556.*

Simonyan, K., & Zisserman, A. (2014). *Very Deep Convolutional Networks for Large-Scale Image Recognition.* ArXiv.org. https://arxiv.org/abs/1409.1556

Simplilearn. (2022, September 1). *What Are Restricted Boltzmann Machines? A Beginner's Guide to RBMs.* Simplilearn. https://www.simplilearn.com/restricted-boltzmann-machines-rbms-article

Singh Gill, H., Ibrahim Khalaf, O., Alotaibi, Y., Alghamdi, S., & Alassery, F. (2022). Multi-Model CNN-RNN-LSTM Based Fruit Recognition and Classification. *Intelligent Automation & Soft Computing*, *33*(1), 637–650. doi:10.32604/iasc.2022.022589

Singh Gill, H., & Singh Khehra, B. (2020). Efficient image classification technique for weather degraded fruit images. *IET Image Processing*, *14*(14), 3463–3470. doi:10.1049/iet-ipr.2018.5310

Singh, A. K., Kumar, B., Singh, G., & Mohan, A. (2017). BMedical image watermarking: techniques and applications. *Book series on Multimedia Systems and Applications.*

Singh, D. P., Bordoloi, D., & Shukla, S. (2021). Utilizing Steganography and Cryptography to Conceal Information Within BMP Images. *Webology*, *18*(5), 3005–3009.

Singh, Y. S., Devi, B. P., & Singh, K. M. (2013). A review of different techniques on digital image watermarking scheme. *International Journal of Engine Research*, *2*(3), 194–200.

Sinha, M. K., Rai, R., & Kumar, G. (2014). Literature survey on digital watermarking. *International Journal of Computer Science and Information Technologies*, *5*(5), 6538–6542.

Sirish Kaushik, V., Nayyar, A., Kataria, G., & Jain, R. (2020). Pneumonia detection using Convolutionalal neural networks (CNNs). In *Proceedings of First International Conference on Computing, Communications, and Cyber-Security (IC4S 2019)* (pp. 471-483). Springer, Singapore.

Sisodia, D., & Sisodia, D. S. (2018). Prediction of Diabetes using Classification Algorithms. *Procedia Computer Science*, *132*, 1578–1585. https://doi.org/10.1016/j.procs.2018.05.122

Soares, J. V. B., Leandro, J. J. G., Cesar, R. M., Jelinek, H. F., & Cree, M. J. (2006). Retinal vessel segmentation using the 2-D Gabor wavelet and supervised classification. *IEEE Transactions on Medical Imaging*, *25*(9), 1214–1222. doi:10.1109/TMI.2006.879967 PMID:16967806

Sofka, M., & Stewart, C. V. (2006). Retinal Vessel Centerline Extraction Using Multiscale Matched Filters, Confidence and Edge Measures. *IEEE Transactions on Medical Imaging*, *25*(12), 1531–1546. doi:10.1109/TMI.2006.884190 PMID:17167990

Solanki, A. C., & Bakaraniya, P. V. (2018). Different video watermarking techniques-a review. *International Journal of Scientific Research in Computer Science. Engineering and Information Technology*, *3*(1), 1890–1894.

Soliman, O. S., & AboElhamd, E. (2014). *Classification of Diabetes Mellitus using Modified Particle Swarm Optimization and Least Squares Support Vector Machine*. ArXiv:1405.0549 https://arxiv.org/abs/1405.0549

Sonawane, A., Nasim, S., Shah, P., Ramaswamy, S., Urizar, G., Manickam, P., Mujawar, M., & Bhansali, S. (2020). Communication—Detection of Salivary Cortisol Using Zinc Oxide and Copper Porphyrin Composite Using Electrodeposition and Plasma-Assisted Deposition. *ECS Journal of Solid State Science and Technology: JSS*, *9*(6), 061022. doi:10.1149/2162-8777/aba856

Sondaal, S. F. V., Browne, J. L., Amoakoh-Coleman, M., Borgstein, A., Miltenburg, A. S., Verwijs, M., & Klipstein-Grobusch, K. (2016). Assessing the Effect of mHealth Interventions in Improving Maternal and Neonatal Care in Low- and Middle-Income Countries: A Systematic Review. *PLoS One*, *11*(5), e0154664. doi:10.1371/journal.pone.0154664 PMID:27144393

Soni, E., Nagpal, A., Garg, P., & Pinheiro, P. R. (2022). Assessment of Compressed and Decompressed ECG Databases for Telecardiology Applying a ConvolutionNeural Network. *Electronics (Basel)*, *11*(17), 2708.

Sonuç, E. (2021). Thyroid Disease Classification Using Machine Learning Algorithms. In Journal of Physics: Conference Series IOP Publishing., 012140.

Sood, S. (2014). Digital Watermarking Using Hybridization of Optimization Techniques: A Review. *International Journal of Computer Science and Information Technologies*, *5*(4), 5249–5251.

Soomro, T. A., Afifi, A. J., Zheng, L., Soomro, S., Gao, J., Hellwich, O., & Paul, M. (2019). Deep Learning Models for Retinal Blood Vessels Segmentation: A Review. *IEEE Access: Practical Innovations, Open Solutions*, *7*, 71696–71717. doi:10.1109/ACCESS.2019.2920616

Sousa, A. S., Ferrito, C., & Paiva, J. A. (2018). Intubation-associated pneumonia: An integrative review. *Intensive & Critical Care Nursing*, *44*, 45–52. doi:10.1016/j.iccn.2017.08.003 PMID:28869146

Sousa, G. G. B., Fernandes, V. R. M., & Paiva, A. C. D. (2019, August). Optimized deep learning architecture for the diagnosis of pneumonia through chest X-rays. In *International Conference on Image Analysis and Recognition* (pp. 353-361). Springer. 10.1007/978-3-030-27272-2_31

Sreejini, K. S., & Govindan, V. K. (2015). Improved multiscale matched filter for retina vessel segmentation using PSO algorithm. *Egyptian Informatics Journal*, *16*(3), 253–260. doi:10.1016/j.eij.2015.06.004

Sridar, K., & Shanthi, D. (2014, October). Medical diagnosis system for the diabetes mellitus by using back propagation-apriori algorithms [Review of Medical diagnosis system for the diabetes mellitus by using back propagation-apriori algorithms]. *Journal of Theoretical and Applied Information Technology*, *68*(1), 36–43.

Staal, J., Abramoff, M. D., Niemeijer, M., Viergever, M. A., & van Ginneken, B. (2004). Ridge-Based Vessel Segmentation in Color Images of the Retina. *IEEE Transactions on Medical Imaging*, *23*(4), 501–509. doi:10.1109/TMI.2004.825627 PMID:15084075

Stafford, I. S., Kellermann, M., Mossotto, E., Beattie, R. M., MacArthur, B. D., & Ennis, S. (2020). A systematic review of the applications of artificial intelligence and machine learning in autoimmune diseases. *NPJ Digital Medicine*, *3*(1), 1–11. doi:10.103841746-020-0229-3 PMID:32195365

Staprans, S. I., Hamilton, B. L., Follansbee, S. E., Elbeik, T., Barbosa, P., Grant, R. M., & Feinberg, M. B. (1995). Activation of virus replication after vaccination of HIV-1-infected individuals. *The Journal of Experimental Medicine*, *182*(6), 1727–1737. doi:10.1084/jem.182.6.1727 PMID:7500017

Stephen, O., Sain, M., Maduh, U. J., & Jeong, D. U. (2019). An efficient deep learning approach to pneumonia classification in healthcare. *Journal of Healthcare Engineering*, *2019*, 1–7. doi:10.1155/2019/4180949 PMID:31049186

Strisciuglio, N. (2015) Multiscale blood vessel delineation using B-COSFIRE filters. In Lecture Notes in Computer Science (including subseries Lecture Notes in Artificial Intelligence and Lecture Notes in Bioinformatics), pp. 300–312. Springer. doi:10.1007/978-3-319-23117-4_26

Subudhi, A., Pattnaik, S., & Sabut, S. (2016). Blood vessel extraction of diabetic retinopathy using optimized enhanced images and matched filter. *Journal of Medical Imaging (Bellingham, Wash.)*, *3*(4), 044003. doi:10.1117/1.JMI.3.4.044003 PMID:27981066

Suganya, R. (2016, April). An automated computer aided diagnosis of skin lesions detection and classification for dermoscopy images. In *2016 International Conference on Recent Trends in Information Technology (ICRTIT)* (pp. 1-5). IEEE. 10.1109/ICRTIT.2016.7569538

Sumankuuro, J., Wulifan, J. K., Angko, W., Crockett, J., Derbile, E. K., & Ganle, J. K. (2020). Predictors of maternal mortality in Ghana: Evidence from the 2017 GMHS Verbal Autopsy data. *The International Journal of Health Planning and Management*, *35*(6), 1512–1531. doi:10.1002/hpm.3054 PMID:32901986

Sun, Y., & Zhang, D. (2019, June). Machine Learning Techniques for Screening and Diagnosis of Diabetes: a Survey [Review of Machine Learning Techniques for Screening and Diagnosis of Diabetes: a Survey]. *Tehnicki vjesnik - Technical Gazette, 26*(3). https://hrcak.srce.hr/221017

Sundar, R. S., & Vadivel, M. (2016, March). Performance analysis of melanoma early detection using skin lession classification system. In *2016 International Conference on Circuit, Power and Computing Technologies (ICCPCT)* (pp. 1-5). IEEE. 10.1109/ICCPCT.2016.7530182

Swiderska-Chadaj, Z., Pinckaers, H., van Rijthoven, M., Balkenhol, M., Melnikova, M., Geessink, O., Manson, Q., Sherman, M., Polonia, A., Parry, J., Abubakar, M., Litjens, G., van der Laak, J., & Ciompi, F. (2019). Learning to detect lymphocytes in immunohistochemistry with deep learning. *Medical Image Analysis*, *58*, 101547. doi:10.1016/j.media.2019.101547 PMID:31476576

Szegedy, C., Liu, W., Jia, Y., Sermanet, P., Reed, S., Anguelov, D., Erhan, D., & Vanhoucke, V. (2015). Going deeper with convolutions. *2015 IEEE Conference on Computer Vision and Pattern Recognition (CVPR)*. IEEE. 10.1109/CVPR.2015.7298594

Szepesi, P., & Szilágyi, L. (2022). Detection of pneumonia using Convolutionalal neural networks and deep learning. *Biocybernetics and Biomedical Engineering*, *42*(3), 1012–1022. doi:10.1016/j.bbe.2022.08.001

Tajbakhsh, N., Gurudu, S. R., & Liang, J. (2016). Automated Polyp Detection in Colonoscopy Videos Using Shape and Context Information. *IEEE Transactions on Medical Imaging*, *35*(2), 630–644. doi:10.1109/TMI.2015.2487997 PMID:26462083

Takore, T. T., Kumar, P. R., & Devi, G. L. (2016, March). A modified blind image watermarking scheme based on DWT, DCT and SVD domain using GA to optimize robustness. In 2016 international conference on electrical, electronics, and optimization techniques (ICEEOT) (pp. 2725-2729). IEEE.

Tan, J. H., Acharya, U. R., Chua, K. C., Cheng, C., & Laude, A. (2016). Automated extraction of retinal vasculature. *Medical Physics*, *43*(5), 2311–2322. doi:10.1118/1.4945413 PMID:27147343

Taser, P. Y. (2021). Application of Bagging and Boosting Approaches Using Decision Tree-Based Algorithms in Diabetes Risk Prediction. *Proceedings*, *74*(1), 6. https://doi.org/10.3390/proceedings2021074006

Tasnim, Z., Chakraborty, S., Shamrat, F. M. J. M., Chowdhury, A. N., Nuha, H. A., Karim, A., Zahir, S. B., & Billah, M. (2021). Deep Learning Predictive Model for Colon Cancer Patient using CNN-based Classification. *International Journal of Advanced Computer Science and Applications*, *12*(8). doi:10.14569/IJACSA.2021.0120880

Temurtas, F. (2009). A comparative study on thyroid disease diagnosis using neural networks. *Expert Systems with Applications*, *36*(1), 944–949. doi:10.1016/j.eswa.2007.10.010

Thakkar, H., Shah, V., Yagnik, H., & Shah, M. (2021). Comparative anatomization of data mining and fuzzy logic techniques used in diabetes prognosis. *Clinical EHealth*, *4*, 12–23. doi:10.1016/j.ceh.2020.11.001

The Moderna COVID-19 (mRNA-1273) vaccine: What you need to know. (n.d.). WHO. https://www.who.int/news-room/feature-stories/detail/the-moderna-covid-19-mrna-1273-vaccine-what-you-need-to-know

Thomas M, Das MK & Ari S (2015). Automatic ECG arrhythmia classification using dual tree complex wavelet based features. *262 International Journal of Engineering & Technology AEU-International Journal of Electronics and Communications, 69*)(4), 715-721. . doi:10.1016/j.aeue.2014.12.013

Titus, L. J., Clough-Gorr, K., Mackenzie, T. A., Perry, A., Spencer, S. K., Weiss, J., Abrahams-Gessel, S., & Ernstoff, M. S. (2013). Recent skin self-examination and doctor visits in relation to melanoma risk and tumour depth. *British Journal of Dermatology*, *168*(3), 571–576. doi:10.1111/bjd.12003 PMID:22897437

Toğaçar, M., Ergen, B., Cömert, Z., & Özyurt, F. (2020). A deep feature learning model for pneumonia detection applying a combination of mRMR feature selection and machine learning models. *IRBM*, *41*(4), 212–222. doi:10.1016/j.irbm.2019.10.006

Top 10 Deep Learning Algorithms in Machine Learning [2022]. (n.d.). ProjectPro. https://www.projectpro.io/article/deep-learning-algorithms/443

Tseng, K. K., He, X., Kung, W. M., Chen, S. T., Liao, M., & Huang, H. N. (2014). Wavelet-based watermarking and compression for ECG signals with verification evaluation. *Sensors (Basel)*, *14*(2), 3721–3736. doi:10.3390140203721 PMID:24566636

Tseng, P. Y., Chen, Y. T., Wang, C. H., Chiu, K. M., Peng, Y. S., Hsu, S. P., Chen, K.-L., Yang, C.-Y., & Lee, O. K. S. (2020). Prediction of the development of acute kidney injury following cardiac surgery by machine learning. *Critical Care (London, England)*, *24*(1), 1–13. doi:10.118613054-020-03179-9 PMID:32736589

Tyagi, A. M. (2018). Interactive thyroid disease prediction system using machine learning technique. *In 2018 Fifth international conference on parallel, distributed and grid computing (PDGC)* (pp. 689-693). IEEE.

UNICEF. (2021). *Pneumonia*. UNICEF. https://data.unicef.org/topic/child-health/pneumonia/

Usman, A. G., Ghali, U. M., Degm, M. A. A., Muhammad, S. M., Hincal, E., Kurya, A. U., Işik, S., Hoti, Q., & Abba, S. I. (2022). Simulation of liver function enzymes as determinants of thyroidism: A novel ensemble machine learning approach. *Bulletin of the National Research Center*, *46*(1), 1–10. doi:10.118642269-022-00756-6

Utzinger, J. (2004). Health impact assessment: Concepts, theory, techniques, and applications. *Bulletin of the World Health Organization*, *82*(12), 954–954.

Uvaliyeva, I., Belginova, S., & Ismukhamedova, A. (2018). Development and implementation of the algorithm of differential diagnostics. *IEEE 12th International Conference on Application of Information and Communication Technologies (AICT)*. IEEE. doi:10.1109/ICAICT.2018.8747116

Vadapalli, P. (2020, May 29). [*Deep Learning Techniques You Should Know About*. UpGrad Blog. https://www.upgrad.com/blog/top-deep-learning-techniques-you-should-know-about/]. *Top (Madrid)*, *10*.

Varshney, S. L., & Garg, P. (2022). A Comprehensive Survey on Event Analysis Using Deep Learning. *2022 Fifth International Conference on Computational Intelligence and Communication Technologies (CCICT)*, (pp. 146-150). Research Gate. doi:10.1109/CCiCT56684.2022.00037

Varshni, D., Thakral, K., Agarwal, L., Nijhawan, R., & Mittal, A. (2019, February). Pneumonia detection using CNN based feature extraction. In *2019 IEEE international conference on electrical, computer and communication technologies (ICECCT)* (pp. 1-7). IEEE.

Varshni, D., Thakral, K., Agarwal, L., Nijhawan, R., & Mittal, A. (2019, February). Pneumonia detection using CNN based feature extraction. In *2019 IEEE International Conference on Electrical, Computer and Communication Technologies (ICECCT)* (pp. 1-7). IEEE. 10.1109/ICECCT.2019.8869364

Vecchia, C. L., Negri, E., Alicandro, G., & Scarpino, V. (2020). Attitudes towards influenza vaccine and a potential COVID-19 vaccine in Italy and differences across occupational groups, September 2020. *Environmental Health*, *111*(6), 445–448. doi:10.23749/mdl.v111i6.10813 PMID:33311419

Vidya, M., & Karki, M. V. (2020, July). Skin cancer detection using machine learning techniques. In *2020 IEEE international conference on electronics, computing and communication technologies (CONECCT)* (pp. 1-5). IEEE.

Viknesh, C. K., Kumar, P. N., & Seetharaman, R. (2019, January). Computer aided diagnostic system for the classification of skin cancer using dermoscopic images. In *2019 Third International Conference on Inventive Systems and Control (ICISC)* (pp. 342-345). IEEE. 10.1109/ICISC44355.2019.9036327

Viscaino, M., Torres Bustos, J., Muñoz, P., Auat Cheein, C., & Cheein, F. A. (2021). Artificial intelligence for the early detection of colorectal cancer: A comprehensive review of its advantages and misconceptions. *World Journal of Gastroenterology*, *27*(38), 6399–6414. doi:10.3748/wjg.v27.i38.6399 PMID:34720530

Voysey, M., Costa Clemens, S. A., Madhi, S. A., Weckx, L. Y., Folegatti, P. M., Aley, P. K., Angus, B., Baillie, V. L., Barnabas, S. L., Bhorat, Q. E., Bibi, S., Briner, C., Cicconi, P., Clutterbuck, E. A., Collins, A. M., Cutland, C. L., Darton, T. C., Dheda, K., & Dold, C. (2021).Single-dose administration and the influence of the timing of the booster dose on immunogenicity and efficacy of ChAdOx1 nCoV-19 (AZD1222) vaccine: A pooled analysis of four randomised trials. *Lancet*. doi:10.1016/S0140-6736(21)00432-3 PMID:33617777

Waljee, A. K., Weinheimer-Haus, E. M., Abubakar, A., Ngugi, A. K., Siwo, G. H., Kwakye, G., Singal, A. G., Rao, A., Saini, S. D., Read, A. J., Baker, J. A., Balis, U., Opio, C. K., Zhu, J., & Saleh, M. N. (2022). Artificial intelligence and machine learning for early detection and diagnosis of colorectal cancer in sub-Saharan Africa. *Gut*, *71*(7), 1259–1265. doi:10.1136/gutjnl-2022-327211 PMID:35418482

Wang, J. S., Chiang, W. C., Hsu, Y. L., & Yang, Y. T. C. (2013). ECG arrhythmia classification using a probabilistic neural network with a feature reduction method. *Neurocomputing*, *116*, 38–45. doi:10.1016/j.neucom.2011.10.045

Wang, X., Zhai, M., Ren, Z., Ren, H., Li, M., Quan, D., Chen, L., & Qiu, L. (2021). Exploratory study on classification of diabetes mellitus through a combined Random Forest Classifier. *BMC Medical Informatics and Decision Making*, *21*(1), 105. Advance online publication. doi:10.118612911-021-01471-4 PMID:33743696

Wang, Z. J., Turko, R., Shaikh, O., Park, H., Das, N., Hohman, F., Kahng, M., & Polo Chau, D. H. (2021). CNN Explainer: Learning Convolutional Neural Networks with Interactive Visualization. *IEEE Transactions on Visualization and Computer Graphics*, *27*(2), 1396–1406. doi:10.1109/TVCG.2020.3030418 PMID:33048723

Wang, Z., Wang, Z., Zhou, Z., & Ren, Y. (2016). Crucial genes associated with diabetic nephropathy explored by microarray analysis. *BMC Nephrology*, *17*(1), 128. doi:10.118612882-016-0343-2 PMID:27613243

Whipple, A., Bridges, M., Hanson, A., Maddipatla, D., & Atashbar, M. (2022, July). A Fully Flexible Handheld Wireless Estrogen Sensing Device. In *2022 IEEE International Conference on Flexible and Printable Sensors and Systems (FLEPS)* (pp. 1-4). IEEE. 10.1109/FLEPS53764.2022.9781499

WHO & World Bank. (2014). *Trends in Maternal Mortality: 1990 to 2013*. World Health Organization. http://VH7QX3XE2P.search.serialssolutions.com/?V=1.0&L=VH7QX3XE2P&S=AC_T_B&C=Trends%20in%20Maternal%20Mortality%20:%201990%20to%202013&T=marc&tab=BOOKS

WHO (2014). *Ground zero in Guinea: The Ebola outbreak smoulders - undetected - for more than 3 months. A retrospective on the first cases of the outbreak*. WHO.

WHO. (2006). *WHO Constitution, Basic Documents, Forty-fifth edition, Supplement, October 2006.* WHO. https://www.who.int/about/who-we-are/constitution

WHO. (2021). *Coronavirus disease (COVID-19): Vaccines*. WHO. https://www.who.int/news-room/q-a-detail/coronavirus-disease-(covid-19)-vaccines

WHO. (2021). *Pneumonia* WHO. https://www.who.int/news-room/fact-sheets/detail/pneumonia

WHO. (2021a). *Health impact assessment*. WHO. https://www.who.int/westernpacific/health-topics/health-impa
ct-assessment

WHO. (2021b). *Maternal and reproductive health*. WHO. https://www.who.int/data/maternal-newborn-child-adolescent-ageing/advisory-groups/gama/activities-of-gama

WHO. (n.d.). Vaccines and immunization: What is vaccination? Retrieved March 9, 2021, from https://www.who.int/news-room/q-a-detail/vaccines-and-immuni zation-what-is-vaccination

WHO. UNICEF, UNFPA, The World Bank, & United Nations Population Division. (2014). Trends in maternal mortality: 1990 to 2013: Estimates by WHO, UNICEF, UNFPA, The World Bank and the United Nations Population Division. WHO.

Willcox, J. C., van der Pligt, P., Ball, K., Wilkinson, S. A., Lappas, M., McCarthy, E. A., & Campbell, K. J. (2015). Views of Women and Health Professionals on mHealth Lifestyle Interventions in Pregnancy: A Qualitative Investigation. *JMIR mHealth and uHealth, 3*(4). https://doi.org/10.2196/mhealth.4869

Witter, S., & Adjei, S. (2007). Start-stop funding, its causes and consequences: A case study of the delivery exemptions policy in Ghana. *The International Journal of Health Planning and Management, 22*(2), 133–143. https://doi.org/10.1002/hpm.867

Wolfgang, R. B., Podilchuk, C. I., & Delp, E. J. (1999). Perceptual watermarks for digital images and video. *Proceedings of the IEEE, 87*(7), 1108–1126. doi:10.1109/5.771067

World Health Organization. (2022). *Diabetes*. World Health Organization. https://www.who.int/health-topics/diabetes#tab=tab_1

World Health Organization. *(2022). Visual impairment and blindness.* WHO. https://www.who.int/news-room/fact-sheets/detail/blindness-a nd-visual-im payment

World health organization. (n.d.). *Cancer*. WHO. https://www.who.int/health-topics/cancer#tab=tab_1 (Accessed July, 06, 2020)

Wu, C. F., & Hsieh, W. S. (2000). Digital watermarking using zerotree of DCT. *IEEE Transactions on Consumer Electronics, 46*(1), 87–94. doi:10.1109/30.826385

Wu, G., Imhoff-Kunsch, B., & Girard, A. W. (2012). Biological mechanisms for nutritional regulation of maternal health and fetal development. *Paediatric and Perinatal Epidemiology*, *26*, 4–26.

Wu, H., Xie, P., Zhang, H., Li, D., & Cheng, M. (2020). Predict pneumonia with chest X-ray images based on convolutional deep neural learning networks. *Journal of Intelligent & Fuzzy Systems*, *39*(3), 2893–2907. doi:10.3233/JIFS-191438

Wu, P., Duan, F., Luo, C., Liu, Q., Qu, X., Liang, L., & Wu, K. (2020). Characteristics of Ocular Findings of Patients with Coronavirus Disease 2019 (COVID-19) in Hubei Province, China. *JAMA Ophthalmology*, *138*(5), 575–578. doi:10.1001/jamaophthalmol.2020.1291 PMID:32232433

Wu, Y., Zhao, P., Li, W., Cao, M.-Q., Du, L., & Chen, J.-C. (2019). The effect of remote health intervention based on internet or mobile communication network on hypertension patients: Protocol for a systematic review and meta-analysis of randomized controlled trials. *Medicine*, *98*(9), e14707. https://doi.org/10.1097/MD.0000000000014707

Xiao, Y., Li, J., Zhong, J., Chen, D., Shi, J., & Jin, H. (2022). Diagnostic Performance of Diffusion-Weighted Imaging for Colorectal Cancer Detection: An Updated Systematic Review and Meta-Analysis. *Frontiers in Oncology*, *12*, 656095. doi:10.3389/fonc.2022.656095 PMID:35814462

Xu, Z., Shi, D., & Tu, Z. ((2021). Research on Diagnostic Information of Smart Medical Care Based on Big Data. *Hindawi*. doi:10.1155/2021/9977358

Xu, A., Tian, M.-W., Firouzi, B., Alattas, K. A., Mohammadzadeh, A., & Ghaderpour, E. (2022). A New Deep Learning Restricted Boltzmann Machine for Energy Consumption Forecasting. *Sustainability*, *14*(16), 10081. doi:10.3390u141610081

Yadav, D. C. (2020). Prediction of thyroid disease using decision tree ensemble method. *Human-Intelligent Systems Integration*, 89-95.

Yadav, D. C., & Pal, S. (2019). To generate an ensemble model for women thyroid prediction using data mining techniques. *Asian Pacific Journal of Cancer Prevention*, *20*(4), 1275–1281. doi:10.31557/APJCP.2019.20.4.1275 PMID:31031212

Yadav, P. S., Khan, S., Singh, Y. V., Garg, P., & Singh, R. S. (2022). A Lightweight Deep Learning-Based Approach for Jazz Music Generation in MIDI Format. *Computational Intelligence and Neuroscience*, 2022.

Yadav, V., & Verma, N. (2016). Secure Multimedia Data using Digital Watermarking: A Review. *International Journal of Engineering Research and General Science*, *4*(1), 181–187.

Yamada, M., Saito, Y., Imaoka, H., Saiko, M., Yamada, S., Kondo, H., Takamaru, H., Sakamoto, T., Sese, J., Kuchiba, A., Shibata, T., & Hamamoto, R. (2019). Development of a real-time endoscopic image diagnosis support system using deep learning technology in colonoscopy. *Scientific Reports*, *9*(1), 14465. Advance online publication. doi:10.103841598-019-50567-5 PMID:31594962

Yamashita, R., Nishio, M., Do, R. K. G., & Togashi, K. (2018). Convolutional neural networks: An overview and application in radiology. *Insights Into Imaging*, *9*(4), 611–629. doi:10.100713244-018-0639-9 PMID:29934920

Yang, C. Q., Gardiner, L., Wang, H., Hueman, M. T., & Chen, D. (2019). Creating prognostic systems for well-differentiated thyroid cancer using machine learning. *Frontiers in Endocrinology*, *10*, 288. doi:10.3389/fendo.2019.00288 PMID:31139148

Yang, F. Z. (2022). Machine learning applications in drug repurposing. *Interdisciplinary Sciences, Computational Life Sciences*, 1–7. PMID:35066811

Ye, Y., Xiong, Y., Zhou, Q., Wu, J., Li, X., & Xiao, X. (2020). Comparison of Machine Learning Methods and Conventional Logistic Regressions for Predicting Gestational Diabetes Using Routine Clinical Data: A Retrospective Cohort Study. *Journal of Diabetes Research*, *2020*, 1–10. https://doi.org/10.1155/2020/4168340

Yip, M. S., Leung, H. L., Li, P. H., Cheung, C. Y., Dutry, I., Li, D., Daëron, M., Bruzzone, R., Peiris, J. S., & Jaume, M. (2016). Antibody-dependent enhancement of SARS coronavirus infection and its role in the pathogenesis of SARS. *Hong Kong Medical Journal, Xianggang Yi Xue Za Zhi*, *22*(3 Suppl 4), 25–31.

Yip, M. S., Leung, N. H. L., Cheung, C. Y., Li, P. H., Lee, H. H. Y., Daëron, M., Peiris, J. S. M., Bruzzone, R., & Jaume, M. (2014). Antibody-dependent infection of human macrophages by severe acute respiratory syndrome coronavirus. *Virology Journal*, *11*(1), 82. doi:10.1186/1743-422X-11-82 PMID:24885320

Ylenia, C., Chiara, D. L., Giovanni, I., Lucia, R., Donatella, V., Tiziana, S., Vincenzo, G., Ciro, V., & Stefania, S. (2021). A Clinical Decision Support System based on fuzzy rules and classification algorithms for monitoring the physiological parameters of type-2 diabetic patients. *Mathematical Biosciences and Engineering*, *18*(3), 2654–2674. https://doi.org/10.3934/mbe.2021135

Yue, Z., Ma, L., & Zhang, R. (2020). Comparison and validation of deep learning models for the diagnosis of pneumonia. *Computational Intelligence and Neuroscience*, *2020*, 1–8. doi:10.1155/2020/8876798 PMID:33014032

Yu, K.-H., Beam, A. L., & Kohane, I. S. (2018). Artificial intelligence in healthcare. *Nature Biomedical Engineering*, *2*(10), 719–731. doi:10.103841551-018-0305-z PMID:31015651

Yu, M. K., Ma, J., Fisher, J., Kreisberg, J. F., Raphael, B. J., & Ideker, T. (2018). Visible Machine Learning for Biomedicine. *Cell*, *173*(7), 1562–1565. doi:10.1016/j.cell.2018.05.056 PMID:29906441

Yu, X., Wang, S. H., & Zhang, Y. D. (2021). CGNet: A graph-knowledge embedded Convolutionalal neural network for detection of pneumonia. *Information Processing & Management*, *58*(1), 102411.

Zadeh, A. E., Khazaee, A., & Ranaee, V. (2010). Classification of the electrocardiogram signals using supervised classifiers and efficient features. Computer methods and programs in biomedicine, 99(2), 179-194. doi:10.1016/j.cmpb.2010.04.013

Zadeh, L. A. (1969) Biological Applications of the Theory of Fuzzy Set and Systems, In: Proctor, L.D., Ed., *The Proceedings of an International Symposium on Biocybernetics of the Central Nervous System, Little,* 199-206. Brown and Company.

Zadeh, L. A. (1965). Fuzzy sets. *Information and Control, 8*(3), 338–353. https://doi.org/10.1016/s0019-9958(65)90241-x

Zaidi, M. R., Fisher, D. E., & Rizos, H. (2020). Biology of melanocytes and primary melanoma. *Cutaneous Melanoma*, 3-40.

Zana, F., & Klein, J.-C. (2001). Segmentation of vessel-like patterns using mathematical morphology and curvature evaluation. *IEEE Transactions on Image Processing, 10*(7), 1010–1019. doi:10.1109/83.931095 PMID:18249674

Zhang, Y., Weng, Y., & Lund, J. (2022). *Applications of Explainable Artificial Intelligence in Diagnosis and Surgery.* MDPI. https://doi.org/10.3390/diagnostics12020237

Zhang, J., Xu, J., Hu, X., Chen, Q., Tu, L., Huang, J., & Cui, J. (2017). Diagnostic Method of Diabetes Based on Support Vector Machine and Tongue Images. *BioMed Research International, 2017*, 1–9. https://doi.org/10.1155/2017/7961494

Zhang, M., Luo, H., Xi, Z., & Rogaeva, E. (2015). Drug Repositioning for Diabetes Based on "Omics" Data Mining. *PLoS One, 10*(5), e0126082. https://doi.org/10.1371/journal.pone.0126082

Zhang, X. L., Lee, V. C. S., Rong, J., Liu, F., & Kong, H. (2022). Multi-channel convolutional neural network architectures for thyroid cancer detection. *PLoS One, 17*(1), 0262128. doi:10.1371/journal.pone.0262128 PMID:35061759

Zhou, H. (2021). Design of Medical Diagnostic System Based on Artificial Intelligence. *Journal of Physics: Conference Series, 2037*, 012081. doi:10.1088/1742-6596/2037/1/012081

Zhu, W., Xie, L., Han, J., & Guo, X. (2020). The Application of Deep Learning in Cancer Prognosis Prediction. *Cancers (Basel), 12*(3), 603. doi:10.3390/cancers12030603 PMID:32150991

Zou, Q., Qu, K., Luo, Y., Yin, D., Ju, Y., & Tang, H. (2018). Predicting Diabetes Mellitus With Machine Learning Techniques. *Frontiers in Genetics, 9*. doi:10.3389/fgene.2018.00515

Żurawski, C., & Skłodowski, P. (2013). Standard Deviation-Based Image Fidelity Measure for Digital Watermarking. In XIV International Conference-System Modelling and Control. Łódź.

About the Contributors

Rijwan Khan received his B. Tech Degree in Computer Science & Engineering from BIT, M. Tech in Computer Science & Engineering from IETE, and Ph.D.in Computer Engineering from Jamia Millia Islamia, New Delhi. He has 16 years of Academic & Research Experience in various areas of Computer Science. He is currently working as Professor and Head of Department Computer Science and Engineering at ABES Institute of Technology, Ghaziabad U.P. He is author of three subject books. He published more than 30 research papers in different journals and conferences. He has been nominated in the board of reviewers of various peer-reviewed and refereed Journals. He is Editor of five research books. He is Editor of seven special issues of SCI and Scopus indexed journals. He was session chaired in three International conferences & Keynote speakers in some the national and International conferences.

Indrajeet Kumar received his B Tech in Computer Science & Engineering from Sant Longowal Institute of Engineering and Technology, Punjab in 2009 and M Tech in Computer Engineering with specialization in Computer Networks from J.C. Bose University of Science and Technology, YMCA, formerly YMCA University of Science and Technology, Faridabad in 2013. He received his PhD on Analysis and Classification of Breast density Classification using Mammographic Images from G.B Pant Institute of Engineering & Technology, Pauri garhwal, Veer Madho Singh Bhandari Uttarakhand Technical University, Dehradun, Uttarakhand, India in 2019. During his PhD he worked on enhancing the potential of most commonly available mammographic images for differential diagnosis between atypical cases of breast density pattern classification. He served in academia in various reputed organizations like Galgotias Institutions, Greater Noida, India and Graphic era Hill University, Dehradun, Uttarakhand, India for more than 6 years. His research interests include application of machine learning, Deep learning and soft computing techniques for analysis of medical images.

***

Kriti received her B.Tech in Electronics and Communication Engineering from Maharishi Markandeshwar University, Ambala, Haryana in the year 2013 and M.Tech in Electronics and Communication Engineering from JUIT, Waknaghat, Himachal Pradesh in the year 2015. She has completed her PhD in the field of Biomedical Image Processing from Thapar Institute of Engineering and Technology, Patiala, Punjab in the year 2020. She is working as an assistant professor at DIT University, Dehradun, Uttarakhand, India. Her research interests include application of digital image processing, machine learning and soft computing techniques for analysis of biomedical images.

Frank Adusei-Mensah has a research interest in Infectious disease epidemiology and safe applications of natural products for disease control. Dr Adusei-Mensah is also experienced in several extraction techniques and chemical analytical work (NMR, HPLC, and GC -mass spectrometry). He has broad experimental research experience in pharmacy and in public health. He has also carried some work on social media.

Avinav Agarwal is pursuing a B Tech.

Kiran B received a B.E in Instrumentation Technology and an M.Tech in Digital Electronics and Communication from Visvesvaraya Technological University, Belgaum, Karnataka. Currently pursuing a PhD in Electronics Engineering JAIN (Deemed-to-be University). Bengaluru. He has 8 years of teaching experience in UG and PG and Industry experience of 2 years. He has presented paper at National and International conference and Journals. His current research interests include design of CMOS Data Converters and Application Specific ICs.

Hritik Bhandari graduated from DIT university in the filed of Information Technology.(IT)

Sonali Dash has principal research interests in the field of Image Processing, Speech Processing, Pattern Recognition, Texture analysis, and Biomedical Image Processing. Texture analysis and classification is the research area for PhD. Currently working on Fundus Imaging on Diabetic Retinopathy and Glaucoma detection and Smart Transport Network System. Future research plans are on Biomedical Image Processing, Intelligent Transportation System for vehicle detection and Speech Processing. Dash has particular expertise and interest in Image, Speech, and Signal Processing.

Puneet Garg has completed PhD from YMCA. He is working as Assistant Professor in Department of Computer Science & Engineering Deptt.

Ivy Inkum is a statistician and practical nurse.

Chakresh Jain received his Ph.D. specialization in Bioinformatics (biotechnology) from Jiwaji University, Gwalior, India, focusing on computational designing of non-coding RNAs using machine learning methods. He is an Assistant Professor, Department of Biotechnology, Jaypee Institute of Information Technology, Noida, India. He is CSIR-UGC-NET [LS] qualified and member of International Association of Engineers (IAENG) and life member of IETE, New Delhi, India. His research interests include development of computational algorithms for quantification of biological features to understand the complex biological phenomenon and diseases such as cancer and neurodegenerative diseases apart from drug target identification and mutational analysis for revealing the antibiotic resistance across the microbes through computer based docking, molecular modelling and dynamics, non-coding RNAs identification, machine learning, data analytics, and systems biology based approaches.

Manjunatha K. N. received B.E in Instrumentation Technology and M.Tech in VLSI and Embedded Systems from Visvesvaraya Technological University, Belgaum, India in 2009 and 2011 respectively. Completed PhD in JAIN Deemed-to-be-University on power optimization in LTE networks in 2020. Currently working as Assistant Professor in Department of Robotics and Automation, School of Electrical Engineering, JAIN Deemed-to-be-University. He has 10 years of teaching experience in UG and PG. His research interests include design of very large scale integration (VLSI) architectures for low power application, Application Specific Integrated Circuits (ASIC) in Communication and Artificial intelligence. He has attended a number of workshops across India and presented papers in National and International Conferences. He has published more than 20 research articles in journals of National and International repute. He has also worked on funded projects by ISRO and State Council for Science and Technology.

Inderpreet Kaur has a B-Tech, MTech in CSE .She has completed her PhD From Mewar University.Currentely working as aProfessor in the department of CSE,Galgotia's College of Engineering and Technology, Greater noida INDIA. She has more than 17 Years of Teaching and Research Experience. Her areas of interest and research includes Computer Networks Security, Blockchain Technology, Cyber security.She has published various papers in peer reviewed international/national journals and conferences. She has also published number of book chapters in reputed publications like Springer.

Prashant Kaushik is pursuing a B Tech.

Aishani Kulshreshtha is pursuing a B Tech.

Chirag Mishra is currently pursuing a Bachelor's in Technology from ABES Engineering College Ghaziabad Uttar Pradesh.

Renu Mishra has completed her Ph.D (Information Technology) from School of IT, Rajiv Gandhi Proudyogiki Vishwavidyalaya (RGPV), Bhopal, INDIA in 2022. She has M-Tech. (Honors, Information Technology Branch) with 77.23%, from Technocrats Institute of Technology (TIT)-Bhopal (M.P.) / Rajiv Gandhi Proudyogiki Vishwavidyalaya (RGPV), Bhopal (M.P.) in year 2008 and B-Tech. (Information Technology Branch) with 66.29%, from Institute of Integral technology -Lucknow (U.P.) / Uttar Pradesh Technical University (UPTU), Lucknow (U.P.) in year 2005 She has 17 years of Teaching Experience,her area of research is Blockchain Technology, Mobile Ad-hoc Networks, Computer Networks, Wireless sensor network, Cryptography & Network Security etc.Renu also published various Book and book chapters.

Raghu N has ten years of experience in Academic and Research. He received the Ph.D. (2020) in Electronics Engineering from Jain University, and B.E. in Electronics and Telecommunications Engineering from VTU University, Karnataka. His research interests were in RF Communication and Image Processing. He has published his research findings in various Scopus indexed Journals and International conferences. He is a member of various professional bodies.

Mamta Narwaria is currently an Assistant Professor of computer science at the Galgotia's college of Engineering. She received a Bachelor's and Master's degree in Computer Science and Engineering from R.G.P.V University, Bhopal. She served for 15 years in the field of education and pursuing her Ph.D. degree in computer science & engineering. She supervised undergraduate and post- graduate students (Bachelor's and Master's) by research and training. Her research interests include data science, machine learning, computer vision for medical imaging, and big data problems in Healthcare."

Jeff Oduro is a medical doctor.

Dorcas Ofosu-Budu is a clinical and social psychologist.

Dhiraj Pandey received his Ph.D. in Computer Science and Engineering from Manipal University Jaipur in August 2018. He received his B.Tech degree in Information Technology from CCS University Meerut in the year 2003 and his M.Tech degree from the University School of Information Technology, GGSIPU, New Delhi in the year 2007. He has more than 19 years of academic experience. He joined the Department of Computer Science and Engineering at JSS Academy of Technical Education Noida in January 2011 and currently working as Associate Professor there. His recent research interests include assistive technologies, image processing, and information security allied areas.He is a senior member of IEEE.

Kavita Pandey is currently working as an Assistant Professor (Senior Grade) in Jaypee Institute of Information Technology (JIIT), Noida. She has more than 18 years of academic experience. She received her B.Tech. in Computer Science and Engineering from M.D. University in 2002 and M.Tech. (CS) from Banasthali Vidyapeeth University in year 2003. She has obtained her Ph.D. (CS) from JIIT, Noida, India in January, 2017. She is an editor of a book named as "Artificial Intelligence, Machine Learning and Mental Health in Pandemics: A Computational Approach", Elsevier. Her research interests include Soft Computing, Machine Learning, Vehicular Ad hoc Networks, Internet of Things and Optimization Techniques. She has published 50+ articles in International journals and conferences including Wiley, IEEE, Springer, Inderscience, etc. She worked as a guest editor of special issue, "Advances in Computational Intelligence and Applications" in International Journal of Information Retrieval Research (IJIRR), IGI Global, ESCI, Web of Science. She worked as a reviewer in many international journals of renowned publishers including Elsevier, Inderscience, IEEE Access, etc.

Jyoti Rawat received her diploma (Hons.) in 2007 with Information Technology from Govt. Polytechnic Srinagar, Uttarakhand; B.Tech (Hons.) in Information Technology from Rajasthan Technical University, Kota, in 2010 and M.Tech in Computer Science and Engineering from Graphic Era University, Dehradun, Uttarakhand, India. She has completed her PhD in Computer Science and Engineering from G B Pant Engineering College, Pauri, Uttarakhand and During her PhD, she worked on enhancing the potential of pathological analysis on microscopic blood imaging for differential diagnosis between different types of leukaemia. She is working as an assistant professor at DIT University, Dehradun, Uttarakhand, India. Her research interests include application of digital image processing, machine learning and soft computing techniques for analysis of medical images.

Gupteswar Sahu received the M.Tech and Ph.D. degrees in Electronics and communication Engineering from IIT Guwahati and NIT Jamshedpur, India, in 2008 and 2018 respectively. He is currently working as an Associate Professor in the Department of Electronics and Communication Engineering, Raghu Engineering College, Andhra Pradesh,Visakhapatnam, 531162, India. His current research interests include signal processing, image processing and applications of soft computing in electrical and electronics engineering.

Harshita Saxena is pursuing a B Tech.

Sandeep Saxena has received his Ph.D. degree in CSE from NIT Durgapur, West Bengal. He has received his MS degree in Information Security from the Indian Institute of Information Technology, Prayagraj. He has received his B. Tech degree in CSE from U.P.T.U. Lucknow. He has more than 15 Years of Teaching and Research Experience. His areas of interest and research include Security and Privacy in Blockchain Technology and Cloud Computing, Architecture Design for Cloud Computing, and Access control techniques in Cloud Computing and Blockchain Technology. He has performed the role of a key member in more than 10 International Conferences as a Keynote Speaker/Organizing Secretary/ Organizing Chair/ Session Chair. He has written 3 technical books for UP Technical University, Lucknow, and published multiple research papers in reputed international journals and conferences. He haspublished more than 30 research papers in reputed peer-reviewed journals/conferences indexed by (Scopus, SCIE, Google Scholars, DBLP) with high impact factors, more than 10 Patents published, and 2 Patents are granted. He is participating in multiple professional societies like IEEE (Senior Member), IAASSE (Senior Member), Life Time Member in CSI, and Life Time Member in CRSI. He has been working on various research & development Activities, University Syllabus Design, and mentoring innovation and incubation-related developments to students. He has served as a reviewer and member of editorial boards of several prestigious Conferences/Journals /Transactions like IEEE, SPRINGERS, and other Scopus Indexed International Journals. He was contributory to various prestigious Accreditation bodies like NAAC, NBA, and others.

Avinash Kumar Sharma is working as Associate Professor, Department of CSE, ABES Institute of Technology, Ghaziabad. Sharma's areas of interest are Cloud Computing, Data Structure, etc.

Sushant Sharma is a Sophomore pursuing a B.Tech. in CSE from ABESIT Ghaziabad, India. Sharma is a developer, programmer, and enthusiastic learner.

Sharma is learning Web Development, App Development, Machine Learning, and Web 3 Enthusiast.

Akhilesh Srivastava is the alumnus of KNIT and Delhi Technological University. Currently working as Assistant Professor in Department of Computer Science & Engineering Deptt in ABES EC, Ghaziabad.

Pankaj Tripathi is pursuing a PhD.

Pranav Tripathi is a student pursuing BTech with CSE branch with specialization in AI.

Mayank Upadhyay received his B Tech in Computer science and Engineering from Graphic Era Hill University, Bhimtal and M Tech in Computer science and Engineering from DIT University Dehradun, India. He is working as an engineer at ICP & Medical, Larson and Toubro services, Mysore, India. His research interests include application of machine learning and soft computing techniques.

Deepak Vishwakarma graduated from DIT University in the field of Information Technology.

Index

G

I

L

M

N

P

R

S

T

U

V

W

X